Donald School
EMBRYO
AS A PERSON AND AS A PATIENT

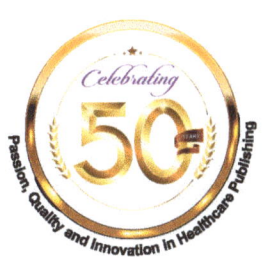

Donald School
EMBRYO
AS A PERSON AND AS A PATIENT

Editors

Asim Kurjak MD PhD
Professor
Department of Obstetrics and Gynecology
Medical School Universities of Zagreb and Sarajevo
Professor (Emeritus)
University Sarajevo School of Science and Technology
Ilidža, Bosnia and Herzegovina
President
International Academy of Perinatal Medicine
Founder and Director
Ian Donald Inter-University School of Medical Ultrasound
Zagreb, Croatia

Frank A Chervenak MD
Chair, Obstetrics and Gynecology
Lenox Hill Hospital
Zucker School of Medicine, Hofstra/Northwell
New York, USA

Foreword
Milan Stanojevic

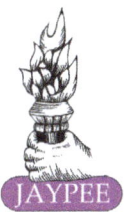

JAYPEE BROTHERS MEDICAL PUBLISHERS
The Health Sciences Publisher
New Delhi | London | Panama

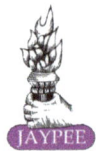

Jaypee Brothers Medical Publishers (P) Ltd

Headquarters
Jaypee Brothers Medical Publishers (P) Ltd.
4838/24, Ansari Road, Daryaganj
New Delhi 110 002, India
Phone: +91-11-43574357
Fax: +91-11-43574314
E-mail: jaypee@jaypeebrothers.com

Overseas Offices

JP Medical Ltd.
83, Victoria Street, London
SW1H 0HW (UK)
Phone: +44-20 3170 8910
Fax: +44(0)20 3008 6180
E-mail: info@jpmedpub.com

Jaypee-Highlights Medical Publishers Inc.
City of Knowledge, Bld. 235, 2nd Floor, Clayton
Panama City, Panama
Phone: +1 507-301-0496
Fax: +1 507-301-0499
E-mail: cservice@jphmedical.com

Jaypee Brothers Medical Publishers (P) Ltd.
Bhotahity, Kathmandu, Nepal
Phone: +977-9741283608
E-mail: kathmandu@jaypeebrothers.com

Website: www.jaypeebrothers.com
Website: www.jaypeedigital.com

© 2020, Jaypee Brothers Medical Publishers

The views and opinions expressed in this book are solely those of the original contributor(s)/author(s) and do not necessarily represent those of editor(s) of the book.

All rights reserved. No part of this publication may be reproduced, stored or transmitted in any form or by any means, electronic, mechanical, photocopying, recording or otherwise, without the prior permission in writing of the publishers.

All brand names and product names used in this book are trade names, service marks, trademarks or registered trademarks of their respective owners. The publisher is not associated with any product or vendor mentioned in this book.

Medical knowledge and practice change constantly. This book is designed to provide accurate, authoritative information about the subject matter in question. However, readers are advised to check the most current information available on procedures included and check information from the manufacturer of each product to be administered, to verify the recommended dose, formula, method and duration of administration, adverse effects and contraindications. It is the responsibility of the practitioner to take all appropriate safety precautions. Neither the publisher nor the author(s)/editor(s) assume any liability for any injury and/or damage to persons or property arising from or related to use of material in this book.

This book is sold on the understanding that the publisher is not engaged in providing professional medical services. If such advice or services are required, the services of a competent medical professional should be sought.

Every effort has been made where necessary to contact holders of copyright to obtain permission to reproduce copyright material. If any have been inadvertently overlooked, the publisher will be pleased to make the necessary arrangements at the first opportunity. The **CD/DVD-ROM** (if any) provided in the sealed envelope with this book is complimentary and free of cost. **Not meant for sale.**

Inquiries for bulk sales may be solicited at: jaypee@jaypeebrothers.com

Embryo as a Person and as a Patient

First Edition: **2020**

ISBN: 978-93-5270-912-0

Dedicated to

Our sons and grandchildren
—**Asim Kurjak**
My sons and hopefully to future grandchildren
—**Frank A Chervenak**

Contributors

Ambra Iuculano MD
Department of Prenatal and
Preimplantation Genetic Diagnosis and
Fetal Therapy
Microcitemico Pediatric Hospital
"A Cao"
Cagliari, Italy

Asim Kurjak MD PhD
Professor
Department of Obstetrics and
Gynecology
Medical School Universities of Zagreb
and Sarajevo
Professor (Emeritus)
University Sarajevo School of Science
and Technology
Ilidža, Bosnia and Herzegovina
President
International Academy of Perinatal
Medicine
Founder and Director
Ian Donald Inter-University School of
Medical Ultrasound
Zagreb, Croatia

Cristina Peddes MD
Department of Prenatal and
Preimplantation Genetic Diagnosis and
Fetal Therapy
Microcitemico Pediatric Hospital
"A Cao"
Cagliari, Italy

Eberhard Merz MD
Professor and Head
Center for Ultrasound and Prenatal
Medicine
Frankfurt/Main, Germany

Elitza Markova-Car PhD
Associate Professor
University of Rijeka
Department of Biotechnology
Rijeka, Croatia

Frank A Chervenak MD
Chair, Obstetrics and Gynecology
Lenox Hill Hospital
Zucker School of Medicine, Hofstra/
Northwell
New York, USA

Giovanni Monni MD PhD
Professor, Head and Chairman
Department of Prenatal and
Preimplantation Genetic Diagnosis and
Fetal Therapy
Microcitemico Pediatric Hospital
"A Cao"
Cagliari, Italy

Gwang Jun Kim MD PhD
Professor and Head
Department of Obstetrics and
Gynecology
Chung-Ang University Hospital
Seoul, Korea

Iris Žunić Išasegi MD
PhD Candidate
Croatian Institute for Brain Research
Center of Research Excellence for
Basic, Clinical and Translational
Neuroscience
University of Zagreb, School of
Medicine
Zagreb, Croatia

Ivica Kostović MD MSc DSc
Professor Emeritus of Neuroscience
and Anatomy
Honorary Director
Croatian Institute for Brain Research
Center of Research Excellence for
Basic, Clinical and Translational
Neuroscience
University of Zagreb, School of
Medicine
Department of Medical Sciences
Fellow
Croatian Academy of Sciences and Arts
Zagreb, Croatia

Joseph G Schenker MD FACOG FRCOG
Department of Obstetrics and
Gynecology
Hebrew University
Hadassah Medical Center
Jerusalem, Israel

Kenji Kanenishi MD PhD
Associate Professor
Department of Perinatology and
Gynecology
Kagawa University Graduate School of
Medicine
Kagawa, Japan

Kresimir Pavelic MD PhD
Professor
Department of Biotechnology
University of Rijeka
Rijeka, Croatia
and
Juraj Dobrila University of Pula
Pula, Croatia

Lara Spalldi Barišić MD MA
PhD Candidate, SSST University
Department of Obstetrics and
Gynecology
Private Clinic Veritas
Director of Croatian Branch of Ian
Donald Inter-University School of
Medical Ultrasound
Zagreb, Croatia

Laurence B McCullough PhD
Professor
Department of Obstetrics and
Gynecology
Lenox Hill Hospital
Zucker School of Medicine, Hofstra/
Northwell
New York, USA

Maria Carla Monni MD
Department of Prenatal and
Preimplantation Genetic Diagnosis and
Fetal Therapy
Microcitemico Pediatric Hospital
"A Cao"
Cagliari, Italy

Megumi Ito MD
Department of Perinatology and Gynecology
Kagawa University Graduate School of Medicine, Kagawa, Japan

Mohamed Ahmed Mostafa AboEllail MD PhD
Assistant Professor
Department of Perinatology and Gynecology
Kagawa University Graduate School of Medicine, Kagawa, Japan

Nobuhiro Mori MD PhD
Clinical Lecturer
Department of Perinatology and Gynecology
Kagawa University Graduate School of Medicine, Kagawa, Japan

Ritsuko K Pooh MD PhD
CRIFM Clinical Research Institute of Fetal Medicine PMC
Osaka, Japan

Sandra Kraljevic Pavelic PhD
Associate Professor
Department of Biotechnology
University of Rijeka
Center for High-throughput Technologies, Rijeka, Croatia

Sanja Kupesic Plavsic MD PhD
Professor
Department of Obstetrics and Gynecology
Associate Dean
Office of Faculty Development
Paul L Foster School of Medicine
Texas Tech University Health Sciences Center El Paso
El Paso, Texas, USA

Sonila Pashaj MD
Center for Ultrasound and Prenatal Medicine
Frankfurt/Main, Germany

Srećko Gajović MD PhD
Professor and Chairman
Department of Histology and Embryology
Croatian Institute for Brain Research
University of Zagreb School of Medicine
Zagreb, Croatia

Toshiyuki Hata MD PhD
Professor and Chairman
Department of Perinatology and Gynecology
Kagawa University Graduate School of Medicine
Kagawa, Japan

Uiko Hanaoka MD PhD
Lecturer
Department of Perinatology and Gynecology
Kagawa University Graduate School of Medicine
Kagawa, Japan

Valentina Corda MD
Department of Prenatal and Preimplantation Genetic Diagnosis and Fetal Therapy
Microcitemico Pediatric Hospital "A Cao"
Cagliari, Italy

Željka Krsnik MSc PhD
Assistant Professor of Neuroscience
Assistant Director
Center of Research Excellence for Basic, Clinical and Translational Neuroscience
Croatian Institute for Brain Research
Department of Neuroscience
School of Medicine
University of Zagreb
Zagreb, Croatia

Foreword

The issue of the beginning of life and in particular the beginning of human life is fascinating throughout the entire history. This question remains unanswered, which is the reason why it is of great interest for scientists and general public. The intrauterine development of the human was the mystery for many centuries, while in the past decades possibility to look inside the uterus developed, arising many dilemmas and unanswered questions. The discussion on some of the unanswered questions and dilemmas on development of human embryo will be found in the chapters of this unique monograph from different points of view. Prominent neuroscientists, embryologists, experts in three dimensional ultrasonography, experts studding behavior, medical ethicists, geneticists, sonoembryologists are looking at the human embryo from their point of view which is under the scope of their scientific interest. This makes the book a unique master art, giving the readers an opportunity to, together with the authors, go into the uniqueness of embryonic world. That is why this book is enthusiastically recommended not only to the advanced professionals from the medical field such as obstetricians, ultrasonographers and experts in ultrasonography, reproductive health specialists, but also to those who are interested in ethics, philosophy and neuroscience.

Milan Stanojevic MD PhD
Professor
Neonatal Unit, Department of Obstetrics and Gynecology
Medical School University of Zagreb
Zagreb, Croatia

Acknowledgments

We are thankful to painter Zlatan Vehabović (graduated from the Academy of Fine Arts in Zagreb, Croatia), who designed cover of the book with all his artistic elegance.

Lastly, we would like to thank Shri Jitendar P Vij (Group Chairman), Mr Ankit Vij (Managing Director), Ms Chetna Malhotra Vohra (Associate Director-Content Strategy), and Ms Kritika Dua (Senior Development Editor) of M/s Jaypee Brothers Medical Publishers (P) Ltd, New Delhi, India, for their untiring support.

Contents

1. **Neurogenetic Processes in the Lateral Telencephalon during Intrauterine Development of the Human Embryo**   1
   Ivica Kostović, Iris Žunić Išasegi, Željka Krsnik
   - Development between 22 days to 7 Postconceptual Weeks   3

2. **Morphogenetic and Differentiation Powers of the Human Embryo**   12
   Srećko Gajović
   - From the Fertilization to the Activation of the New Genome   12

3. **Sonoembryology**   19
   Ritsuko K Pooh
   - Modern Embryology   19
   - Abnormalities at Embryonal Stage   22

4. **Controversies on the Beginning of Human Life**   28
   Asim Kurjak, Lara Spalldi Barišić
   - Science and Religion: Models of the Interaction   29
   - The Scientific Study of the Science and Religion   29
   - Academia and Religious Beliefs   30
   - The Definition of "Life"   30
   - The Facts of Human Embryogenesis   32
   - Influence of the Genetics and Epigenetics   34
   - Personality   34
   - Embryo as a Patient   35
   - Legal Status of the Embryo   38
   - Arguments for Beginning of Human Life and Human Person at Fertilization   39
   - Arguments against the Beginning of Human Life at Fertilization   40
   - Different Religious Teachings and Historical Aspects   41
   - Clinical Controversies   42
   - Visualization of Early Human Development   43
   - New Possibilities for Studying Embryonic Movements and Behavior   45

5. **Embryonic and Early Fetal Abnormalities Diagnosed with Three-dimensional Ultrasound in the 1st Trimester**   51
   Eberhard Merz, Sonila Pashaj
   - Embryonic Period   51
   - Normal Sonographic Development of the Embryo   51
   - Fetal Period   52
   - Embryonic/Fetal Malformations   52
   - Yolk Sac Abnormality   52
   - Umbilical Cord Cyst   52
   - Acrania, Anencephaly and Exencephaly   52
   - Encephalocele   53
   - Holoprosencephaly   53

- Dandy–Walker Malformation 54
- Cleft Lip/Palate 54
- Retro-/Micrognathia 55
- Low Set Ears 55
- Enlarged Nuchal Translucency 55
- Cystic Hygroma 56
- Fetal Hydrops 56
- Spina Bifida 56
- Heart Defects 56
- Abdominal Wall Defects 57
- Urinary Tract Anomalies 59
- Limb Anomalies 60
- Conjoined Twins 60
- Single Umbilical Artery 60

6. Behavior of the Embryo   65
Toshiyuki Hata, Uiko Hanaoka, Mohamed Ahmed Mostafa AboEllail, Nobuhiro Mori, Kenji Kanenishi, Megumi Ito

- Neurological Development of the Embryo 65
- Two-dimensional Sonographic Study on Embryonic Behavior 65
- Four-dimensional Ultrasound Study on Embryonic Behavior 66

7. Pre-embryo: Medical, Moral and Legal Aspects   75
Joseph G Schenker

- Events of Fertilization 75
- Pre-embryo Development in vitro 75
- Pre-embryo Culture Conditions 75
- Composition of the Embryo Culture Medium 76
- Pre-embryo Cryopreservation 76
- Pre-embryo Assessment—Noninvasive Methods 77
- Genetic Testing of Pre-embryo 77
- Legal Status of the Preimplanted Pre-embryo 78
- Moral Status of Pre-embryo 79
- Human Genome Editing 79
- Mitochondria Manipulation: A Three-parent Babies 80

8. The Moral Status of the Embryo in Professional Obstetric Ethics   82
Frank A Chervenak, Laurence B McCullough

- Ethics 82

9. Invasive Diagnostic Procedures in Embryonic Period   89
Giovanni Monni, Ambra Iuculano, Cristina Peddes, Maria Carla Monni, Valentina Corda

- Genetic-obstetric Counseling 89
- Ultrasound and Prenatal Invasive Techniques 89
- Embryonic Invasive Diagnostic Procedures Chorionic Villus Sampling–Preimplantation Genetic Diagnosis 89

10. The First Four Weeks: Ultrasound and Doppler Assessment of Normal and Abnormal Implantation   96
Sanja Kupesic Plavsic

- Ultrasound and Doppler Studies of the Endometrium 96

11. Ultrasonographic Evaluation of Embryonic Cardiac Development — 105
Gwang Jun Kim

- Carnegie Stage 9 (19–21 Days of Conception, 5 Gestational Weeks), CRL 2 mm *106*
- Carnegie Stage 10 (22–23 Days of Conception, 5 Weeks 1–3 Days of Gestation), CRL 2.5 mm *106*
- Carnegie Stage 11–12 (23–26 Days of Conception, 5 Weeks 2–5 Days of Gestation), CRL 3–3.5 mm *106*
- Carnegie Stage 13 (28 Days of Conception, 6 Weeks of Gestation), (9.5 Days of Rat Embryo), CRL 4.5 mm *106*
- Carnegie Stage 14 (32 Days of Conception, 6 Weeks 4 Days of Gestation), 10 Days of Rat Embryo, CRL 6 mm *107*
- Carnegie Stage 15 (36 Days of Conception, 7 Weeks 1 Day of Gestation), 11.5 Days of Rat Embryo, CRL 8 mm *107*
- Carnegie Stage 16 (40 Days of Conception, 7 Weeks 6 Days of Gestation), CRL 10 mm *108*
- Carnegie Stage 17 (42 Days of Conception, 8 Weeks of Gestation) 12.5 Days in the Rat Embryo, CRL 11 mm *109*
- Carnegie Stage 18 (44 Days of Conception, 8 Weeks 2 Days of Gestation), 13 Days in the Rat Embryo, CRL 13 mm *110*
- Carnegie Stage 19–21 (48–52 Days of Conception, 8 Weeks 2–5 Days of Gestation) 13.5 Ed in the Rat Embryo, CRL 16–23 mm *110*
- Carnegie Stage 22 (54 Days of Conception, 9 Weeks 1 Day of Gestation), 14.5 Ed in the Rat Embryo, CRL 26 mm *113*

12. Preimplantation Genetic Diagnosis — 116
Elitza Markova-Car, Krešimir Pavelić

- Biopsy Techniques *116*
- Use of Polymerase Chain Reaction *116*
- Microarray Platforms *118*
- Next Generation Sequencing *118*

13. Vanishing Twin Syndrome — 121
Maria Carla Monni, Ambra Iuculano, Cristina Peddes, Valentina Corda, Giovanni Monni

- Vanishing Twin Syndrome in ART Pregnancies *121*
- Effects of Vanishing Twin Syndrome on Surviving Twin *123*
- Influence of Vanishing Twin Syndrome on Maternal Serum Markers *124*
- Influence of Vanishing Twin Syndrome on Nips *125*
- Influence of Vanishing Twin Syndrome on Invasive Prenatal Diagnosis *126*
- How Early can the Suspicion of Vanishing Twin Syndrome be Posed? *127*

14. Genomic Editing, Human Enhancement and Transhumanism: A Brief Overview — 131
Kresimir Pavelic, Sandra Kraljevic Pavelic

- Genomic Editing *131*
- Human Enhancement *134*
- Designing a Baby with GE *135*
- Transhumanism and "The Culture of Life" *137*
- Living Indefinitely Long *139*

Index — 145

CHAPTER 1

Neurogenetic Processes in the Lateral Telencephalon during Intrauterine Development of the Human Embryo

Ivica Kostović, Iris Žunić Išasegi, Željka Krsnik

INTRODUCTION

Almost all functions which are characteristic for humans or make us human are integrated in the cerebral cortex. At the present, it is difficult to state when cerebral functions begin in a prenatal human brain and, and even more difficult to mark a crucial developmental phase in which humans begin to develop as cortical beings. Based on the fact that in the adult cortex all cortical functions are performed throughout chemical synapses, it is reasonable to propose that beginning of synaptogenesis in the human cortex marks an essential phase in development of human beings. As early as 1973, Molliver et al.[1] presented evidence on synapses in a human telencephalon at 8.5 postconceptional weeks (PCW), at the beginning of fetal period. The rationale of this review is to discuss organization of the embryonic cortical anlage and embryonic precortical organization in human brain. In this review, we will discuss classical neuroembryological data, recent evidences on development of human embryological cortex, and our own data from previous papers, various textbook chapters,[2-5] and Zagreb Neuroembryological Collection.[6,7] Focus will be put on period from 6 to 7 postovulation weeks (POW) which roughly corresponds to 8–9 weeks of postmenstrual period. In our review, we will try to see whether there is something characteristic for human brain development in this late embryonic stage. Namely, organization of human embryonic brain is very similar to the monkey brain[8] and early embryonic stages are very similar to development in other mammals. Human developmental neuroanatomists and neuroembryologists should answer the question if there is something in the organization of embryonic telencephalon that is characteristic for humans. It was already shown that some of the features of the human embryonic cortex are characteristic for the primate brains, such as an early appearance of Cajal-Retzius cells and subventricular zone (SVZ). Evaluating literature for this review, we have found that there is a lack of studies on histogenetic processes and development of connections and communication between neuronal cells. On the contrary, several current studies are focused on volumetric and other types of measurements of the developing cerebral vesicles during transitional period between embryo and fetus.[9-11] In addition, contemporary researchers sometimes ignore classical developmental studies and present superficial interpretation of classical studies, e.g. seminal studies of His (1904)[12] and precise atlas and reconstruction of Hochstetter's (1919).[13]

One of the serious issue in comparing embryological studies and clinical data is the problem of staging and timing of human embryos. For embryonic period, it is recommended to use postfertilization (postconceptional) age and embryological staging.[8,14,15] Staging of embryonic development was systematically performed by Streeter[16-20] on the Carnegie Collection and systematically presented by O'Rahilly and his group.[14,15,21-24]

In our review, we will use postconceptual age for embryonic period, but we will also refer to standard clinical timing (menstrual age—8.6 weeks). O'Rahilly and Gardner[14] pointed out the fact that there is no menstruation age, because immediately after menstruation embryo does not exist.

In our Zagreb Neuroembryological Collection, we have used crown-rump length (CRL) measurements and careful histological analysis for evaluation of maturational phases, such as presence of embryonic zones, their development, and developmental status. Following the recommendation of O'Rahilly and Gardner,[14] we express prospective developmental age as "at 20 mm CRL" instead of 20 mm stage.

Finally, there is a problem of terminology. Frequently used term for the late embryonic human cortex is "primordial plexiform layer" introduced by Marin-Padilla,[25,26] based on the observation on developing cat, and not on developing human cortex. Term "plexiform" may be misleading because this layer situated between ventricular zone (VZ) or SVZ and pial surface is predominantly cellular, while only outer (toward pia) part is fibrillar or plexiform. This is properly described by His[12] and is called mantle layer or *Mantelschicht* or intermediate zone. Recently, this compartment is called the "preplate" and this term is predominantly used by the current literature.[5,27] For terminology, we recommend recent review by Bystron et al.[27] with upgraded terminology of The Boulder Committee (1970)[28] and Kostović and Judaš.[5] However, we suggest that neuroembryological researchers compare current terminology and descriptions with classical descriptions of embryonic zones and terminology presented by His,[12] The Boulder Committee,[28] Kostović[29] and O'Rahilly and Muller.[24]

In the present review, we will focus on the developmental period before formation of the cortical plate (CP), in order to discuss first cortical network in late embryonic human telencephalic wall with emphasis on status of histogenetic processes and intercellular communication though the intracellular junctions.[30-36] First, we will briefly describe histogenetic processes after appearance of telencephalic vesicles (4 PCW, stages 10-13), then we will discuss *in extenso* crucial phase of development at 20 mm CRL (7 PCW—corresponds to stage 20), and finally, we will describe the earliest appearance of the CP at 22–24 mm CRL (8 PCW), corresponding to stages 22 and 23.

Morphogenesis will be only briefly outlined and the focus will be on histogenetic status. Histogenetic events in the human embryonic and fetal cortex are following (Fig. 1.1)—neuronal proliferation and migration, glial proliferation, specification of morphological and molecular neuronal phenotypes (growth of dendrites, dendritic spines and axons), specification of glial morphological and molecular phenotypes (astroglia, oligodendroglia and microglia), aggregation of specific neuronal population, establishment of neuronal circuitry and connectivity (growth of axonal pathways and synaptogenesis), elimination of exuberant connectivity elements, and myelination.[5] From the graphical presentation (Fig. 1.1), it is obvious that the main cellular histogenetic processes during embryonic period are— proliferation, migration, and molecular specification. End of the embryonic period starts with the process of neuronal aggregation into cytoarchitectonic zones, initial ingrowth and outgrowth of axons, and initial neurochemical maturation. The fact that intensity of different histogenetic events varies or may be even limited to certain developmental period is important in analysis of environmental and intrinsic factors on development of embryonic cortical anlage. Developmental periods

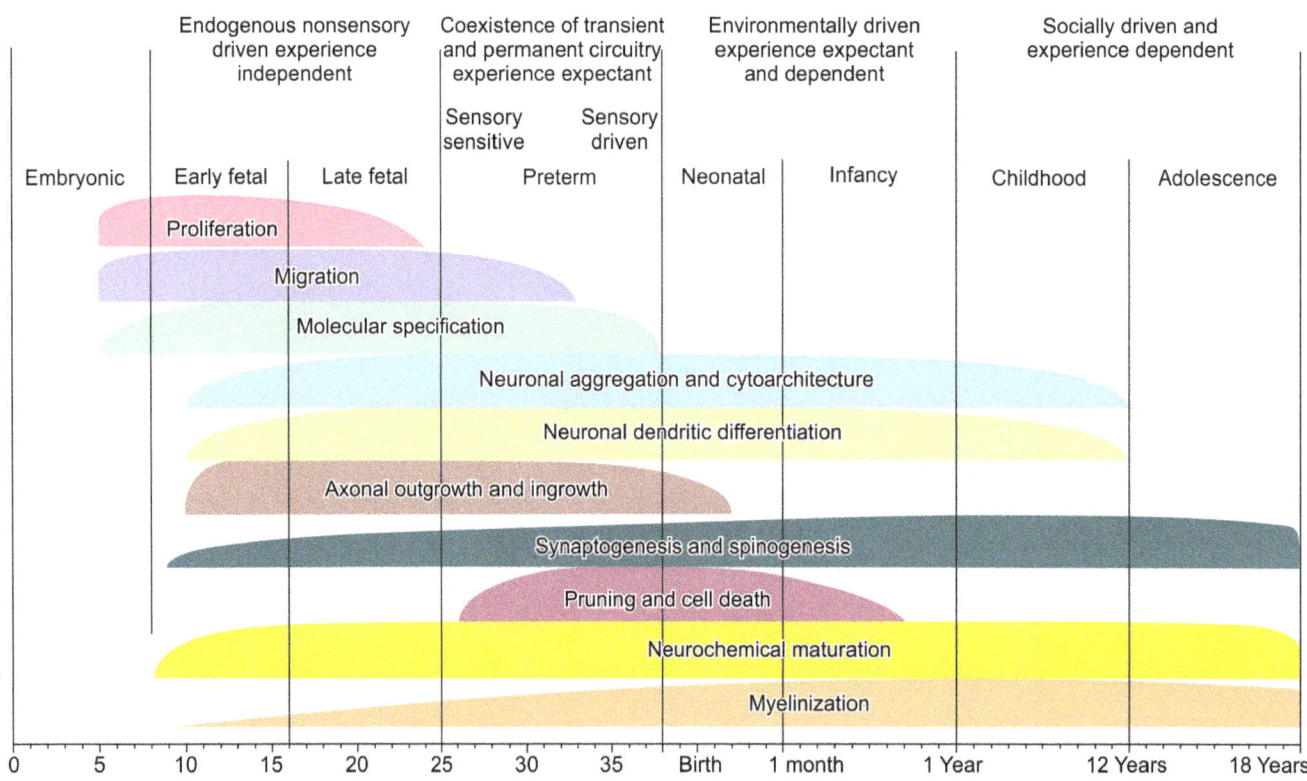

Fig. 1.1: Timing and sequence of neurogenetic events in neocortical development from embryonic period to adolescence.
Source: With permission from Elsevier.[5]

with intensive occurrence of events may show increased vulnerability to adverse extrinsic and intrinsic pathogenetic influence and are usually described as sensitive or critical or vulnerable periods.

DEVELOPMENT BETWEEN 22 DAYS TO 7 POSTCONCEPTUAL WEEKS

Cerebral cortex originates from the neuroepithelial cells in the wall of the paired telencephalic (endbrain) vesicles which develops on the each side of prosencephalon (forebrain) as early as 22 day postconception (2 mm length, stage 10), as shown in Figure 1.2 from the Zagreb Neuroembryological Collection. The telencephalic vesicle becomes visible during 4th embryonic week, 28 days (4 mm, stage 13, Fig. 1.3). During this period, thin wall of telencephalic vesicle consists of only one embryonic zone or lamina, the ventricular zone.[27-29] This zone is known as matrix or germinal epithelium or "primitive" ependyma. Ventricular zone is composed of immature neuroepithelial cells (neuroepithelial stem cells), which display elongated prismatic, polarized shape, radial orientation, and form single-layered neuroepithelium with cell nuclei positioned at the different distances from the cell pole (pseudostratified epithelium). One pole of this elongated neuroepithelial cells is in contact with ventricular (apical), ectodermal surface, while the other cell pole extends to the external mesodermal (basal) surface which is covered with basal membrane. These cells proliferate intensively and mitotic figures can be easily identified even on routinely stained histological sections. During the cell mitotic cycle, nuclei show characteristic "to and from" movement. More precisely, progenitor cells of VZ divide asynchronously during the DNA replication phase, and their nuclei move away from the ventricular surface and then move back to undergo another mitotic cycle.[27] This process is called interkinetic nuclear movement. The neuroepithelial cells in the VZ (neuroepithelial stem cells) divide symmetrically, that is, after every division new proliferative cells are produced and number of proliferative neuroepithelial cells increases with concomitant growth of telencephalic vesicles. It is important to emphasize that neuroepithelial cells of VZ communicate and exchange signaling molecules via intercellular junctions at the apical (ventricular) pole. Two types of intracellular junctions are seen:[37]

1. Complex tight junction in tortuous configuration
2. Adherence junction.

During the 5th week there is an increase in number of cells and thickening of VZ with further expansion of telencephalic vesicle. At this point, forebrain primordium and VZ are thicker in humans than in rodents.[27] The most important cellular event at this period is the onset of asymmetrical division of some neuroepithelial stem cells—one cell remains progenitor, the other is a postmitotic cell destined to become neuron or glia.[27] This is considered to be the beginning of neurogenesis! During this period, postmitotic neurons detach their apical pole from the VZ and together with most superficial processes of

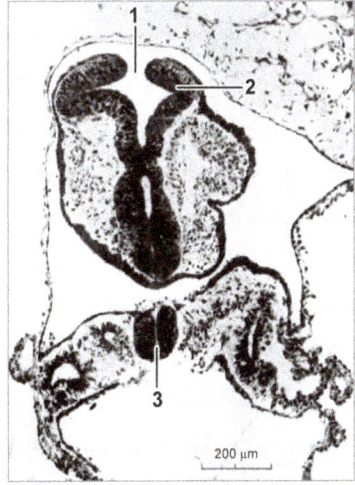

Fig. 1.2: Longitudinal section through the human embryo at 22nd postconceptional day (2 mm, stage 10) from the Zagreb Neuroembryological Collection. 1-Rostral neuroporus; 2-prosencephalon; 3-spinal cord.
Source: With permission from Springer-Verlag.[29]

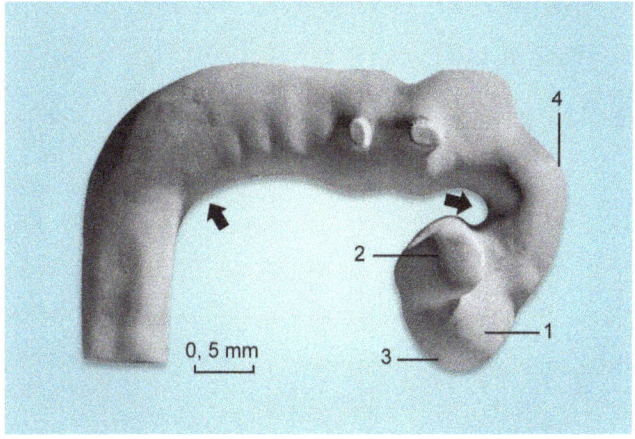

Fig. 1.3: The telencephalic vesicle becomes visible during 4th embryonic week, 28 days (4 mm, stage 13) 1- telencephalon; 2-optic vesicle; 3-lamina terminalis; 4-mesencephalon.
Source: With permission from Springer-Verlag.[29]

ventricular cells form a new cell-less densely packed zone which was originally called the intermediate zone (Fig. 1.4).[12,28,29] However, due to the newly introduced concept of the "preplate" (Fig. 1.5), this zone is considered as a forerunner of preplate.[5,27] Term "marginal zone" from this new terminology is reserved for the most superficial zone after formation of the CP (Fig. 1.5). The current neuroembryological studies have shown that elongated neuroepithelial stem cells have changed their property during neuroepithelial production. The most important cells generated by neuroepithelial cells are radial glial cells. This process is regulated by specific genes, such as *Foxg1*, *Lhx2*, *Pax6* and *Emx2*.[27] Radial glia serves two functions:

1. As progenitor cells for production of neurons and glia
2. As radial glia guide for neuronal migration.[38]

The next phase of embryonic development corresponds approximately to 6 postconceptual weeks (stages 17, 18, 19). In this phase, different portions of the cerebral wall show differences in thickness and cellular compositions. At this point, basic subdivisions of the telencephalic wall are much better macroscopically pronounced (Fig. 1.6) than in the earlier stages and first subdivision between thinner dorsal neuroepithelial wall (pallium) and basal portion (subpallium) is seen. The narrow portion of the telencephalon in the midline which is situated between two vesicles is very thin and is called telencephalon impar. In the dorsal wall (pallium), it is visible that medial telencephalon is thinner than the lateral telencephalon. In the medial telencephalic wall, the most interesting feature is the most ventral marginal part of the pallium where cerebral wall is slightly curved and shows clear enlargement of the marginal zone. This medial marginal (limbic) portion of telencephalon will differentiate into allocortex and curved part with the wide marginal zone (MZ) will

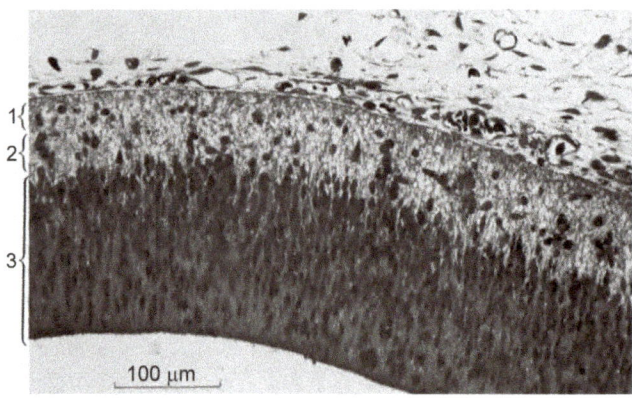

Fig. 1.4: Cross-section through the telencephalic vesicles of human embryo at 16 mm—1-marginal zone; 2-intermediate zone; 3-ventricular zone.
Source: With permission from Springer-Verlag.[29]

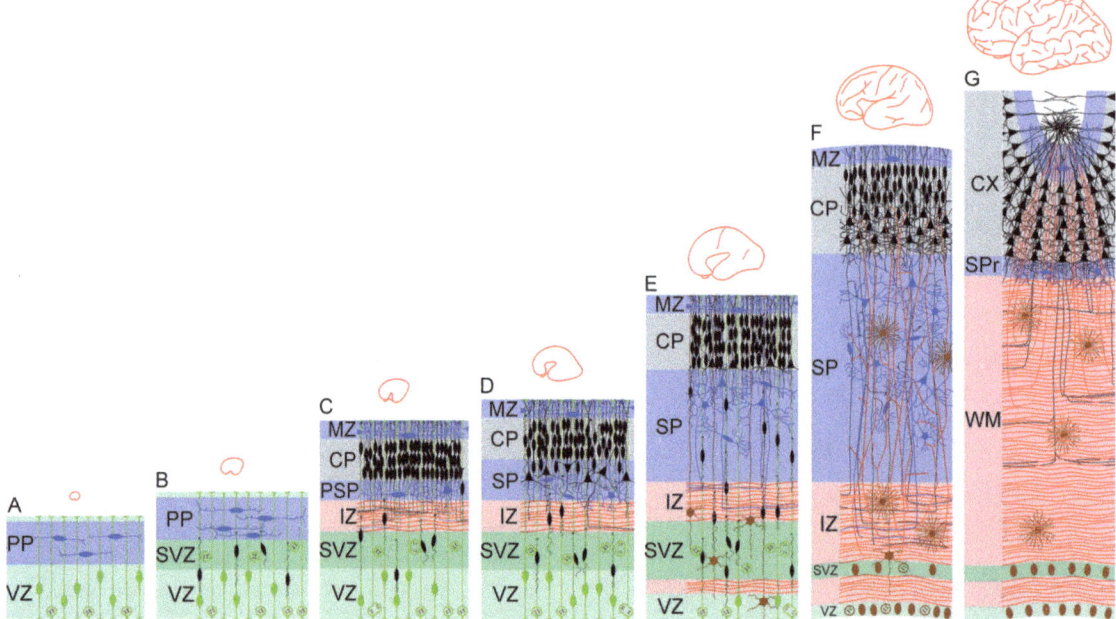

Fig. 1.5: Transient patterns of lamination in the neocortical cerebral wall from embryonic (A, B) to late fetal period (G).
[VZ: ventricular zone; SVZ: subventricular zone; PP: preplate; SP: subplate zone; MZ: marginal zone; CP: cortical plate; IZ: intermediate zone (fetal "white" matter)]
Source: With permission from Elsevier.[5]

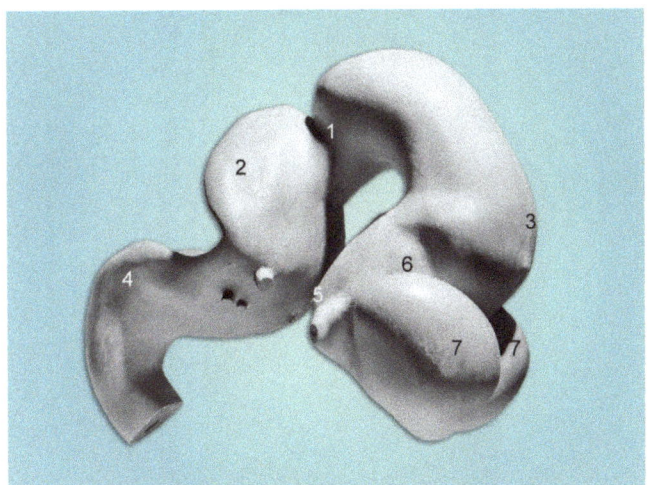

Fig. 1.6: Reconstruction model of the CNS of the 6th postconceptual week embryo (11 mm, stage 17). 1-isthmus rombencephali; 2-cerebellar plate; 3-epiphysis; 4-myelencephalon; 5-corpus mamillare; 6-sulcus telodiencephalic; 7-telencephalic vesicles.

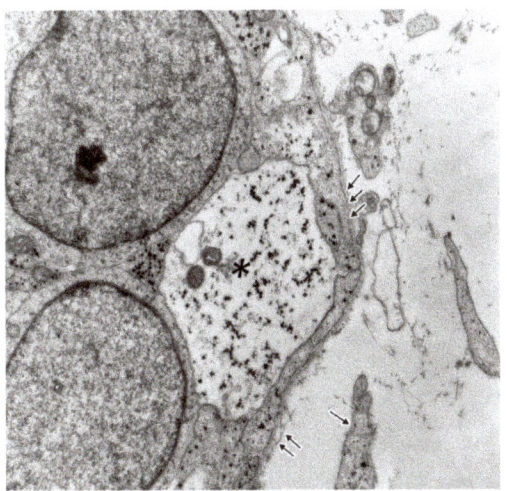

Fig. 1.7: Electron micrograph of the human superficial fetal cortex, after formation of the CP, at 9 PCW showing EM-lucent glycogen-loaded end feet of specialized (radial) glia. At the interface of neuroepithelium and mesenchyma, following elements can be seen: glia (asterisk), basal membrane (three arrows), collagen fibrils (two arrows) and fibroblasts (one arrow).

differentiate into hippocampus. Anlage of hippocampus is characterized by enlargement of MZ, which remains characteristic throughout development.

At the very limbus, the cerebral wall is transformed into thin epithelial lamellae (area epithelialis of lamina tectoria), which stretches from one telencephalic vesicle to another. At the transitional zone between margin of pallium (of telencephalic vesicles) and area epithelialis, one single-layer portion of lamina epithelialis invaginates in the cavity of ventricles and forms anlage of plexus choroideus. First primitive blood vessels appear outside the epithelia. Since there are no blood vessels within telencephalic portion of the neuronal tube, it was proposed that metabolically necessary nutrients have access to neuroepithelium from the liquor inside neural tube—telencephalic anlage or via extracellular fluid outside the neuroepithelium.[37,39] During the 6th week, mesenchyme envelops of the telencephalic vesicle differentiates into pia mater. Primitive vessels penetrate through pia mater in the neuroepithelial wall of the telencephalic vesicles. As a first step in this process, there is an accumulation of collagen fibrils at the external surface of the basal membrane and primitive blood vessels become aligned on the external surface of the telencephalic vesicles. In the second phase, fibroblasts appear between basal membrane—collagen layer on the side of neuroepithelium and blood vessels sheet on the other (mesenchymal) side. In the third phase, blood vessels covered with basal membrane and collagen fibrils penetrate into the wall of telencephalic vesicles.

Thus, by the end of embryonic period all structures of pia mater are developed: basal membrane, layer of collagen fibrils, layer of fibroblasts and blood vessels. Below the basal membrane, there are end feet of neuroepithelial cells which are poorly differentiated. At this early developmental point, it is difficult to answer whether these immature end feet below basal membrane and around vessels belong to the universal type of neuroepithelial cells or do they belong to glia. At the end of embryonic period and the beginning of fetal period, end feet became well differentiated, show electron microscopy (EM)-lucent features, may be filled with glycogen-rich granules, and belong to specialized glia cells (Fig. 1.7).

During this phase of embryonic period (6 postconceptual weeks), many postmitotic cells lose their attachments to apical (ventricular) surface in order to move–migrate toward pial (basal) surface and form a new embryonic zone, properly described by His,[12] called mantle layer or *Mantelschicht, Zwischenschicht* or intermediate zone.[12,28,29] However, due to the concept of preplate, currently, this zone is known as the term "preplate".[5,27] After formation of the preplate, telencephalic wall consists of VZ and preplate (two-laminar composition). However, preplate can be further divided in the mantle layer and marginal zone, and this phase can be described as three-laminar cerebral wall. At this point, we would like to point out to general rules of neurogenesis—all neurons are produced (born) on places which are different than their final position in the adult brain. That means that all cells must migrate in order to reach their final position. The distances for migration of neurons during embryonic period are much shorter and mechanisms of neuronal detachment and migration were not described for human cortex. In fetal period, when the distances for migration are extremely long (more than 1 cm), mechanisms of radial migration along radial glia were documented in 1972 by Rakic.[38]

Formation of the next zone, proliferative SVZ, during the end of 6 PCW is a crucial event for human cortical histogenesis. The SVZ is composed of proliferative progenitor cells which have lost attachment with ventricular surface and moved outward in basal (pial) direction. Some of the cells from VZ move tangentially and show polymorphic shape, while other maintained connection with basal surface. SVZ is particularly well developed in primate cortex and seems to be as a fountainhead of some neuronal population, such as projection neurons and calretinin interneurons which are characteristic for primate—human brain organization. The importance of SVZ zone as a second proliferative zone in a primate cortex was first described by Rakić.[40] In current developmental neurobiology, SVZ of midgestational fetal human cerebrum is considered as an essential fountainhead of cortical neurons and a key player in the production of complex, large gyrencephalic human brain.[41,42] It is very likely that neuron production in SVZ begins already in embryonic period. However, we have proposed that the real impulse for the neuronal production in the SVZ begins in the early fetal life (between 8 PCW and 10 PCW) when major afferent system from thalamus and basal forebrain interact with progenitor cells in SVZ.[43]

Histogenetic Events and Cytoarchitectonic Organization of Embryonic Brain at 20 mm Crown-rump Length

At 7th week, telencephalic vesicles have increased in their size and dominate the picture of external morphology of the embryo (Fig. 1.8). Please note gradual thinning of cerebral wall from thick basolateral portion to the thin dorsolateral portion (Figs. 1.9 to 1.11). Analysis of these semi-thin sections therefore reveals the following regions of the lateral telencephalon:
- Dorsolateral
- Midlateral
- Basolateral.

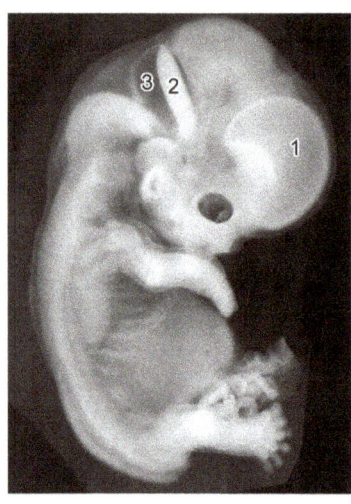

Fig. 1.8: Whole embryo at 22 mm CRL. Please note increased size of telencephalic vesicle (1). Rhombencephalon is still exposed and cerebellar plate (2) is clearly seen. (3) Marks fourth (IV) ventricle. *Source*: With permission from Springer-Verlag.[29]

The most important histogenetic event is the enlargement of the preplate (mantle layer) in the basolateral portion (Fig. 1.9C). Preplate shows two different sublaminas with different orientation and packing density of the cells. Deeper portion close to SVZ is characterized by the high density of cells, and superficial portion appears more fibrillar with lower cell density. The organization of preplate in two laminas is less obvious at:
- Dorsolateral
- Midlateral level (Figs. 1.9A and B).

Fine cytological analysis of one micron-thick plastic sections reveals large cells which are oriented parallel to pia matter, presumably immature Cajal–Retzius cells (Fig. 1.9B asterisk). Similar relationship is seen on more posterior level (Fig. 1.10). Please note enlarged blood vessels which form primordial plexus external of the basal membrane (Figs. 1.10A to C, arrows). These vessels are not regular arteries and veins, but form plexus resembling cavernous veins. There are also numerous vessels which start to form subventricular plexus within the telencephalic wall. Progressive diminishment in the preplate size is well seen in Figure 1.11. Proofs of intensive proliferative activity at this developmental period are numerous mitotic figures (Figs. 1.9A and B, arrows). The pale appearance in the ventricular zone close to ventricular surface is due to the densely packed apical processes of ventricular and eventually subventricular cells (Fig. 1.11, asterisk).

Neuronal communication and circuitry elements at 20 mm—synapses, axons, and postsynaptic elements. In our EM study, we have performed systematic analyses of

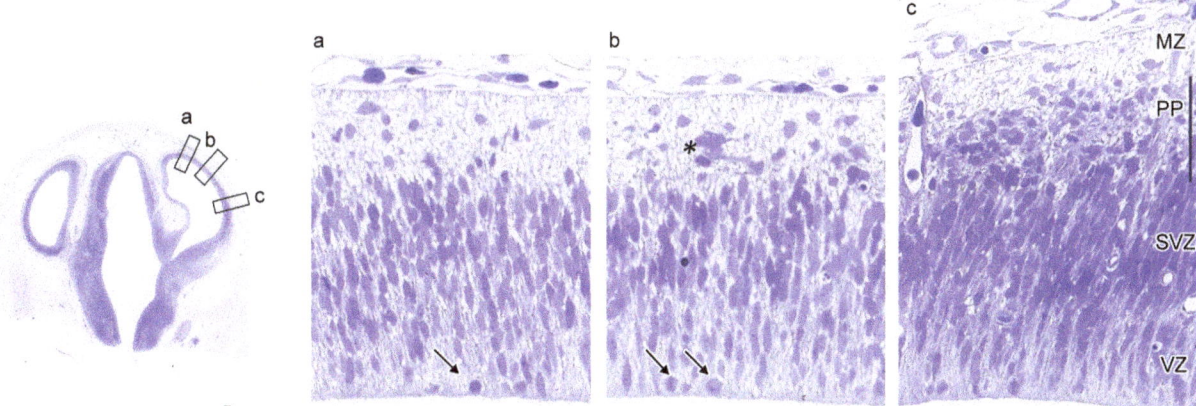

Fig. 1.9: Cross-section through the telencephalon, through the future foramen interventriculare, shows thick basal portion of subpallium with ganglionic eminence (low magnification on the left). Squares indicate position of large magnification shown in figures a, b, c. Arrows (a, b) indicate mitotic figures in the VZ. Asterisk marks prospective Cajal–Retzius neuron in the superficial portion of mantle-preplate layer. Scale bar = 100 μm.
(MZ: marginal zone; PP: preplate; SVZ: subventricular zone; VZ: ventricular zone)

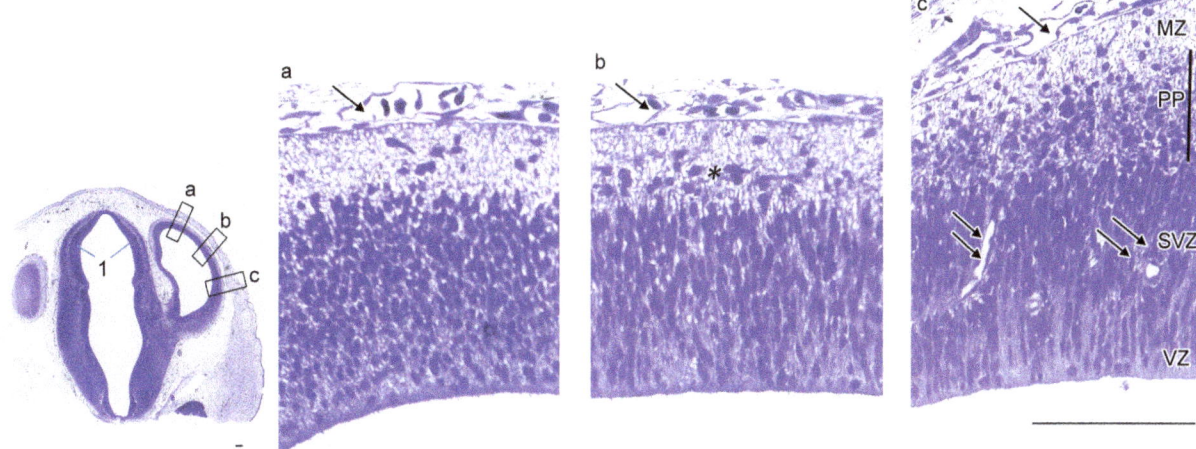

Fig. 1.10: Cross-section through the telencephalon on more posterior level than in Figure 9, showing thick basal portion of subpallium with ganglionic eminence (low magnification on the left). Squares indicate position of large magnification shown in figures a, b, c. (1) marks diencephalon. One arrow indicates pial blood vessels; two arrows indicate SVZ blood vessels. Scale bar =100 μm.
(MZ: marginal zone; PP: preplate; SVZ: subventricular zone; VZ: ventricular zone)

the whole thickness of the telencephalic wall and we have not found typical synapses characterized by membrane-associated pre- and postsynaptic densities and synaptic vesicles.[44] Thus, we have not confirmed observation of Larroche[45] about presence of synapses in 7-week-old embryo. However, we have found numerous intercellular junctions through preplate-mantle layer, but very few gap junctions. Gap junctions are equivalent of electrical synapses[30,37] and are supposed to be ultrastructural bases of oscillatory nonsynaptic activity of the developing cortex. Based on the absence of synapses and paucity of gap junctions, it seems that other nontypical transient junction, as well as increased extracellular space or extracellular matrix are crucial substrate of Ca^{2+} signaling and communication via processes.[30-36,46-48]

The communication between preplate neurons and first differentiated glia may occur via classical transmitters, which are secreted and diffused through extracellular matrix and act on other cells without involvement of synapses and junctions.[49] The most likely source of early transmitter synthesis and release are prospective GABAergic neurons which begin to develop at the early fetal development.[50-54] The most remarkable population of early neurons are forerunners of large Cajal–Retzius cell,

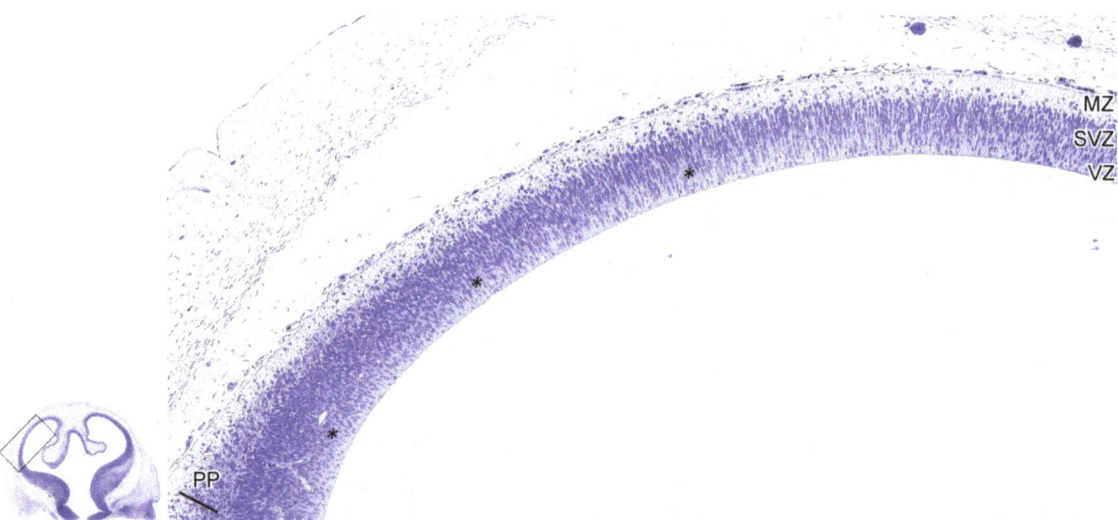

Fig. 1.11: Progressive diminishment of the preplate size is well seen along the hemispheric curvature. Asterisk marks tightly packed apical processes of proliferative cells. Scale bar = 100 μm.
(MZ: marginal zone; PP: preplate; SVZ: subventricular zone; VZ: ventricular zone)

which are reelin–positive and there are some evidence about their glutamatergic nature.[55] However, it is not clear at what exact moment do they become synapticly engaged, and what are their postsynaptic elements in the early fetal cortex. Furthermore, the data on early gliogenesis are incomplete; even though it was well documented that microglia were found in intracerebral structures as early as 6 weeks of gestation.[56] Other types of glia develop eventually early,[57] but the exact onset of their earliest appearance is not determined at this moment.

In conclusion, human embryonic cortex at 20 mm CRL displays remarkable human characteristic features of proliferative zones, presence of postmigratory neurons, and first nonsynaptic communication via intercellular junctions and/or extracellular matrix-rich environment. Morphologically, all parts of brain may be clearly recognized and prominent telencephalic vesicles are result of intensive proliferation in VZ and SVZ, and initial migration.

Formation of Cortical Plate at 22/24 mm, Transition between Embryonic and Fetal Period (8 PCW, Stages 22/23)

During transition between embryonic and fetal period, the first postmitotic and postmigratory neurons settle in the most superficial zone of the preplate and form one layer of densely-packed cells, so called CP. The CP formation is considered to be crucial event in histogenesis of cerebral cortex in both classical[12,14,58] and current literature.[29,52] CP appears in basolateral portion of telencephalic vesicle, in a form of disc-like shape, latter extends along the hemisphere and by 8.5-9 weeks of postconception, all parts of neocortex contain cell-dense CP. This event marks the beginning of the cortical gray matter development. Below the CP, there is a thin plexiform disrupted layer— presubplate (PSP) zone of Kostović and Rakic.[59] Above the CP, there is a cell-poor marginal zone which contains Cajal–Retzius cells, apical branching of CP cells and axons. Thus, after formation of the CP, at the end of embryonic period, cortex consists of three layers: MZ, CP, and PSP. At the very beginning, some neurons (pioneering) form initial pioneering CP.[52] The earliest formation of CP was described by His[12] and is also visible on the cross sections through the human telencephalon at 20 mm CRL embryos-fetuses shown in Hochstetter atlas[13] (Fig. 1.12). Neuronal organization of the CP was described by Kostović-Knežević et al.[60] CP is built by immature neurons which have bipolar shape of cell body, but they develop apical bouquet in the MZ and root-like arborization on their basal side. One of these processes of root-like arborization is an immature axon which is already directed toward IZ. Early CP cells are densely packed and form, so called, embryonic columns.[61]

Parallel with the formation of immature CP between 8 weeks and 8.5 weeks, there is a first appearance of synapses characterized by membrane-associated presynaptic and postsynaptic vesicles and synaptic vesicles.[1] This crucial event in the earliest human fetal cortex during transition between embryonic and fetal period

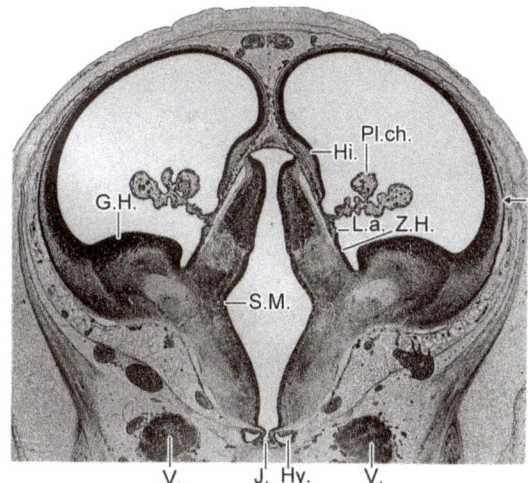

Fig. 1.12: Earliest formation of CP is seen on the cross sections though the human telencephalon at 20 mm CRL embryos-fetuses from Hochstetter atlas (1919). Arrow indicates CP in a form of initial disc in the basolateral portion of telencephalic vesicles. (Pl. ch.: choroid plexus; Hi.: hippocampus; L.a.: lamina affixa; Z.H.: diencephalon; S.M.: sulcus Monroi; G.H.: ganglionic eminence)

was emphasized by our group in many articles.[59,62] Here we emphasize the fact that this event marks the beginning of humans as cortical beings. From that point, human immature cortical compartments (MZ, CP, and PSP) are incorporated in early synaptic network. Significance of human fetus as a patient and early cortical functions were extensively discussed in numerous publications edited by Kurjak and Chervenak,[63] Chervenak, Kurjak and Comstock[64] and Pooh and Kurjak.[65] It is notable that synapses were found above and below CP and that cell-dense CP is synapse-free until 24 PCW. Significance of this bilaminar distribution of synapses (below and above CP) is not clear, but it obviously corresponds to the early maturing cells of presubplate and MZ, and apical bouquets of CP neurons. When early synapses were first described, they were interpreted as transient synapses[1,59] and their functional significance was not known. Transient early synapses may underlie different patterns of fetal behavior, which can show continuity throughout fetal life.[66,67] However, subsequent experimental studies have confirmed that early synapses are important constituents of early endogenous, spontaneous activity.[68-74] Impairment of spontaneous activity may have far-reaching consequences for the cortex development.[47,70]

CONCLUSION

- Second half of embryonic period (4–8 PCW) is a critical developmental window for telencephalic vesicles development, which is neuroepithelial fountainhead for development of human cortex. Three histogenetic processes dominate in this period of early development:
  - Proliferation of neurons and glia in the ventricular and subventricular zones ("factories" of the brain)
  - Early migration of postmitotic cells in the preplate (mantle) zone
  - Molecular specification with transient activity of different genes.

Telencephalic vesicles (anlage of cerebral vesicle) are composed of pluripotent neuroepithelial cells (stem cells), which are polarized and contact apical (ventricular) and basal (pial) surface during the earliest phases. At 20 mm CRL, two human-characteristic histogenetic events take place:
1. Formation of SVZ as a fountainhead of associative cortical neurons and interneurons
2. Formation of preplate as a forerunner of CP and subplate (SP).

Early embryonic cortical cells communicate through nonsynaptic junctions and extracellular space. First synapses are formed after formation of the CP, around 8 PCW, and show bilaminar distribution: deep synaptic stratum below CP, in the presubplate and superficial synaptic stratum in the MZ, above CP. Onset of synaptogenesis around 8 PCW marks the beginning of human life as cortical beings. Nonsynaptic and synaptic junctions of the embryonic or early fetal cortex underlie spontaneous endogenous activity and present basic framework for cortical development. Therefore, it can be predicted that if different extrinsic and intrinsic pathogenetic factors act during late embryonic period, it will cause major abnormalities of cerebral wall structure and laminar organization of the cerebral cortex.

REFERENCES

1. Molliver ME, Kostović I, Van Der Loos H. The development of synapses in cerebral cortex of the human fetus. Brain Res. 1973;50(2):403-7.
2. Kostović I, Judaš M. Prenatal and perinatal development of the human cerebral cortex. In: Kurjak A, Chervenak F (Eds). The fetus as a patient: advanced diagnosis and therapy. New York: The Parthenon Publishing Group; 1994. pp. 35-55.
3. Kostović I, Judaš M. Prenatal development of the cerebral cortex. In: Chervenak F, Kurjak A, Comstock C (Eds). Ultrasound and the fetal brain (Progress in obstetric and gynecological sonography series). New York: The Parthenon Publishing Group; 1995. pp. 1-26.

4. Kostović I, Judaš M. Maturation of Cerebral Connections and Fetal Behavior. In: Pooh R, Kurjak A (Eds). Fetal Neurology. New Delhi: Jaypee Brothers Medical Publishers;2009. pp. 440-52.
5. Kostović I, Judaš M. Embryonic and fetal development of the human cerebral cortex. In: Toga (Ed). Brain Mapping: An Encyclopedic Reference (volume 2): Anatomy and Physiology Systems. London: Elsevier Academic Press; 2015. pp. 167-75.
6. Kostović I, Judaš M, Kostović-Knežević L, et al. Zagreb research collection of human brains for developmental neurobiologist and clinical neuroscientist. Int J Dev Biol. 1991;35:215-30.
7. Judaš M, Šimić G, Petanjek Z, et al. The Zagreb Collection of human brains: a unique, versatile, but underexploited resource for the neuroscience community. Ann NY Acad Sci. 2011;1225(Suppl 1):E105-30.
8. Olivier G, Pineau H. Horizons de Streeter et age embryonnaire. Bulletin de l'Association des anatomists. 1962;47:573-6.
9. Tanaka H, Senoh D, Yanagihara T, et al. Intrauterine sonographic measurement of embryonic brain vesicle. Hum Reprod. 2000;15(6):1407-12.
10. Tanaka H, Hata T. Intrauterine sonographic measurement of the embryonic brain mantle. Ultrasound Obstet Gynecol. 2009;34(1):47-51.
11. Kurjak A, Pooh RK, Merce LT, et al. Structural and functional early human development assessed by three-dimensional and four-dimensional sonography. Fertil Steril. 2005;84(5):1285-99.
12. His W. Die Entwicklung des menschlichen Gehirns wahrend der ersten Monate. Leipzig: Hirzel; 1904.
13. Hochstetter F. Beitrage zur Entwicklungsgeschichte des menschlichen Gehirus. Wien: Franz Deuticke; 1919.
14. O'Rahilly R, Gardner E. The timing and sequence of events in the development of the human nervous system during the embryonic period proper. Z Anat Entwicklungsgesch. 1971;134(1):1-12.
15. O'Rahilly R, Müller F. Developmental stages in human embryos: revised and new measurements. Cells Tissues Organs. 2010;192(2):73-84.
16. Streeter G. Weight, sitting height, head size, foot length, and menstrual age of the human embryo. Contrib Embryol Carnegie Inst. 1921;11:143-70.
17. Streeter G. Developmental horizons in human embryos. Description of age group XI, 13 to 20 somites, and age group XII, 21 to 29 somites. Contributions to Embryology. Washington: Carnegie Institution of Washington publication. 1942;30(541):21-245.
18. Streeter G. Developmental horizons in human embryos. Description of age group XIII, embryos about 4 or 5 millimeters long, and age group XIV, period of indentation of the lens vesicle. Contributions to Embryology. Carnegie Institution of Washington publication. 1945;31(557):27-63.
19. Streeter G. Developmental horizons in human embryos. Description of age groups XV, XVI, XVII, and XVIII, being the third issue of a survey of the Carnegie Collection. Contributions to Embryology. Carnegie Institution of Washington publication. 1948;32(575):133-203.
20. Streeter G. Developmental horizons in human embryos. Description of age groups XIX, XX, XXI, XXII, and XXIII, being the fifth issue of a survey of the Carnegie Collection (prepared for publication by C. H. Heuser and G. W. Corner). Contributions to Embryology. Carnegie Institution of Washington publication. 1951;34(592):165-96.
21. O'Rahilly R, Gardner E. The initial development of the human brain. Acta Anat (Basel). 1979;104(2):123-33.
22. O'Rahilly R. Early human development and the chief sources of information on staged human embryos. Eur J Obstet Gynecol Reprod Biol. 1979;9(4):273-80.
23. Müller F, O'Rahilly R. The development of the human brain, the closure of the caudal neuropore, and the beginning of secondary neurulation at stage 12. Anat Embryol. 1987;176(4):413-30.
24. O'Rahilly R, Müller F. The Embryonic Human Brain. An atlas of Developmental Stages, 3rd edition. New York: John Wiley and Sons Inc; 2006.
25. Marin-Padilla M. Dual origin of the mammalian neocortex and evolution of the cortical plate. Anat Embryol (Berl). 1978;152(2):109-26.
26. Marin-Padilla M. Structural organization of the human cerebral cortex prior to the appearance of the cortical plate. Anat Embryol (Berl). 1983;168(1):21-40.
27. Bystron I, Blakemore C, Rakic P. Development of the human cerebral cortex: Boulder Committee revisited. Nat Rev Neurosci. 2008;9(2):110-22.
28. Embryonic vertebrate central nervous system: revised terminology. The Boulder Committee. Anat Rec. 1970;166(2):257-61.
29. Kostović I. Zentralnervensystem. In: Hochstetter F (Ed). Humanembryologie-Lehrbuch und Atlas der vorgeburtlichen Entwicklung des Menschen. New York: Springer-Verlag; 1990. pp. 381-448.
30. Dermietzel R, Spray DC. Gap junctions in the brain: where, what type, how many and why? Trends Neurosci. 1993;16(5):186-92
31. Araque A, Parpura V, Sanzgiri RP, et al. Tripartite synapses: Glia, the unacknowledged partner. Trends Neurosci. 1999;22(5):208-15.
32. Elmariah SB, Oh EJ. Astrocytes regulate inhibitory synapse formation via Trk-mediated modulation of postsynaptic GABAA receptors. J Neurosci. 2005;25(14):3638-50.
33. Sutor B, Hagerty T. Involvement of gap junctions in the development of the neocortex. Biochmi Biophys Acta. 2005;1719(1-2):59-68.
34. Eroglu C, Barres BA. Regulation of synaptic connectivity by glia. Nature. 2010;468(7321):223-31.
35. Faissner A, Pyka M, Geissler M, et al. Contributions of astrocytes to synapse formation and maturation-Potential functions of the perisynaptic extracellular matrix. Brain Res Revi. 2010;63(1-2):26-38.
36. Allen NJ. Synaptic plasticity: Astrocytes wrap it up. Curr Biol. 2014;24(15):697-9.
37. Mollgard K, Balslev Y, Lauritzen B, et al. Cell junctions and membrane specializations in the ventricular zone (germinal matrix) of the developing sheep brain: a CSF-brain barrier. J Neurocytol. 1987;16(4):433-44.

38. Rakić P. Mode of cell migration to the superficial layers of fetal monkey neocortex. J Comp Neurol. 1972;145(1):61-83.
39. Mollgard K, Jacobsen M. Immunohistochemical identification of some plasma proteins in human embryonic and fetal forebrain with particular reference to the development of the neocortex. Brain Res. 1984;13(1):49-63.
40. Rakić P. Timing of major ontogenetic events in the visual cortex of the rhesus monkey. In: Buchwald N, Brazier M (Eds). Brain mechanisms in mental retardation. New York: Academic Press; 1975. pp. 3-40.
41. Hansen DV, Lui JH, Parker PR, et al. Neurogenic radial glia in the outer subventricular zone of human neocortex. Nature. 2010;464(7288):554-61.
42. Ortega JA, Memi F, Radonjic N, et al. The Subventricular Zone: A Key Player in Human Neocortical Development. Neuroscientist. 2018;24(2):156-70.
43. Žunić Išasegi I, Radoš M, Krsnik Ž, et al. Interactive histogenesis of axonal strata and proliferative zones in the human fetal cerebral wall. Brain Struct Funct. 2018;223(9):3919-43.
44. Kostović I, Molliver ME. A new interpretation of the laminar development of cerebral cortex: synaptogenesis in different layers of neopallium in the human fetus. Anat Record. 1974;(178):95.
45. Larroche JC. The marginal layer in the neocortex of a 7 week-old human embryo. A light and electron microscopic study. Anat Embryol (Berl). 1981;162(3):301-12.
46. Demarque M, Represa A, Becq H, et al. Paracrine intercellular communication by a Ca^{2+} and SNARE independent release of GABA and glutamate prior to synapse formation. Neuron. 2002;36(6):1051-61.
47. Moore AR, Zhou WL, Sirois CL, et al. Connexin hemichannels contribute to spontaneous electrical activity in the human fetal cortex. Proc Natl Acad Sci USA. 2014;111(37):3919-28.
48. Bruzzone R, Dermietzel R. Structure and function of gap junctions in the developing brain. Cell Tissue Res. 2006;326(2):239-48.
49. Spitzer NC. Electrical activity in early neuronal development. Nature. 2006;444(7120):707-12.
50. Al-Jaberi N, Lindsay S, Sarma S, et al. The early fetal development of human neocortical GABAergic interneurons. Cereb Cortex. 2015;25(3):631-45.
51. Zecevic N, Hu F, Jakovcevski I. Interneurons in the developing human neocortex. Dev Neurobiol. 2011;71(1):18-33.
52. Meyer G, Schaaps JP, Moreau L, et al. Embryonic and early fetal development of the human neocortex. J Neurosci. 2000;20(5):1858-68.
53. Jakovcevski I, Mayer N, Zecevic N. Multiple origins of human neocortical interneurons are supported by distinct expression of transcription factors. Cereb Cortex. 2011;21(8):1771-82.
54. Bystron I, Rakic P, Molnar Z, et al. The first neurons of the human cerebral cortex. Nat Neurosci. 2006;9(7):880-6.
55. Kirischuk S, Sinning A, Blanquie O, et al. Modulation of neocortical development by early neuronal activity: physiology and pathophysiology. Front Cell Neurosci. 2017;11:379.
56. Monier A, Evrard P, Gressens P, et al. Distribution and differentiation of microglia in the human encephalon during the first two trimesters of gestation. J Comp Neurol. 2006;499(4):565-82.
57. Jakovcevski I, Zecevic N. Sequence of oligodendrocyte development in the human fetal telencephalon. Glia. 2005;49(4):480-91.
58. Bartelmez G, Dekaban A. The early development of the human brain. Contrib Embryol Carnegie Inst. 1962;37:13-32.
59. Kostović I, Rakić P. Developmental history of the transient subplate zone in the visual and somatosensory cortex of the macaque monkey and human brain. J Comp Neurol. 1990;297(3):441-70.
60. Kostović-Knežević L, Kostović I, Krmpotić-Nemanić J, et al. The cortical plate of the human neocortex during the early fetal period (at 31-65 mm CRL). Verh Anat Ges. 1978;(72):721-3.
61. Rakić P. Specification of cerebral cortical areas. Science. 1988;241(4862):170-6.
62. Kostović I, Judaš M. Transient patterns of cortical lamination during prenatal life: Do they have implications for treatment? Neurosci Biobehav Rev. 2007;31(8):1157-68.
63. Kurjak A, Chervenak F. The Fetus as a Patient: Advances in Diagnosis and Therapy. New York-London: The Parthenon Publishing Group; 1994.
64. Chervenak F, Kurjak A, Comstock C. Ultrasound and the fetal brain (Progress in obstetric and gynecological sonography series). London-New York: The Parthenon Publishing Group; 1995.
65. Pooh R, Kurjak A. Fetal neurology. New Delhi: Jaypee Brothers Medical Publishers; 2009.
66. Kurjak A, Stanojevic M, Andonotopo W, et al. Behavioral pattern continuity from prenatal to postnatal life–a study by four-dimensional (4D) ultrasonography. J Perinat Med. 2004;32(4):346-53.
67. Kurjak A, Stanojevic M, Andonotopo W, et al. Fetal behavior assessed in all three trimesters of normal pregnancy by four-dimensional ultrasonography. Croat Med J. 2005;46(5):772-80.
68. Friauf E, Shatz CJ. Changing patterns of synaptic input to subplate and cortical plate during development of visual cortex. J Neurophysiol. 1991;66(6):2059-71.
69. Khazipov R, Sirota A, Leinekugel X, et al. Early motor activity drives spindle bursts in the developing somatosensory cortex. Nature. 2004;432(7018):758-61.
70. Khazipov R, Luhmann HJ. Early patterns of electrical activity in the developing cerebral cortex of humans and rodents. Trends Neurosci. 2006;29(7):414-8.
71. Kanold PO. Subplate neurons: crucial regulators of cortical development and plasticity. Front Neuroanat. 2009;3:16.
72. Moore AR, Filipovic R, Mo Z, et al. Electrical excitability of early neurons in the human cerebral cortex during the second trimester of gestation. Cereb Cortex. 2009;19(8):1795-805.
73. Moore AR, Zhou WL, Jakovcevski I, et al. Spontaneous electrical activity in the human fetal cortex in vitro. J Neurosci. 2011;31(7):2391-8.
74. Kanold PO, Luhmann HJ. The subplate and early cortical circuits. Ann Rev Neurosci. 2010;33:23-48.

CHAPTER 2

Morphogenetic and Differentiation Powers of the Human Embryo

Srećko Gajović

INTRODUCTION

The current advancements of biomedical technologies resulted with a surprising outcome, that nowadays the embryo can be considered not only as a patient, but as well as a potential cure. Together with taking care and monitoring the normal sequence of developmental events, the medical interventions are possible and some of them are already in the everyday medical practice. Furthermore, new emerging technologies are envisaged to generate the embryo-derived cells and organs, aimed for innovative medical treatments of the adult patients, in particular in the regenerative medicine.[1]

There is no doubt that the whole process of arising of the adult human from a single cell of the fertilized egg is extraordinary. The embryo period is when these transformations are the most prominent and fastest. The goal to be accomplished for the human embryo to reach the stage of the fetus is rather complex and demanding even in the sense of normal development. Although embryo is mostly hidden during this period and the changes occur very fast, still the new technologies provide very detailed insight in the events going on.

In this chapter, I am introducing the concept of embryo powers, which is distinct from the embryo potentials and their realization, but complementary to them. When we consider the embryo potential at the time of fertilization, it is indeed the whole new being, but in sense of realization, it is still a single-cell zygote. Together with following how the stepwise realization of the potential in the developing structures leads to the healthy baby, I would consider as well the powers of the embryo. The embryo powers describe what embryo is capable at each stage. These powers determine quite directly the possibilities for medical intervention in case of "embryo as a patient", and as well enable the controversial enhancement of the embryo status in the "embryo as a cure".

The embryo in the current society is much more than a target of medical intervention. Through the powers exercised during this profound transformation, there are as well the societal powers of the embryo. The technologization of the embryo in the current society raises a wide array of controversies, not limited to the question when the embryo would start to be a little human.[2] The possibility to create an embryo through in vitro fertilization, to keep it frozen and use it not only for creation of new being, but as well for the embryonic stem cells, and the recent possibility of creation of human-animal chimeras, all these are some of the examples leading to the previously unimaginable situations with the human embryo in the focus. Conceiving a new life is central for the human species and for the human society. Therefore, the embryo had already a special place in society long before recent technological advances. Still, these technological advances bring new discourses to the old topics in consideration, which are frequently not possible to be solved and would remain opened for the future. These controversies, although important, would not be the topic of this chapter, as I would like to concentrate on the biological sequence of developmental events and the biological powers embryo has during this process. Nevertheless, the new individual experiences of the pregnancies, which would be generated by the emerging technologies, would influence the public debates and create new discourses, which eventually could solve some current, but in the same time generate new controversies in relation to the human embryo.[3]

FROM THE FERTILIZATION TO THE ACTIVATION OF THE NEW GENOME

At the moment of fertilization, the half of the genome of the new human being is contributed by the sperm cell and half by the egg cell. This completes new set of chromosomes having all genes necessary for the new being. In sense of the potential, it is at its maximum and the abilities written in the genome of the new human are assembled and defined. However, in sense of the realization, the embryo is a single cell, zygote, which would immediately start its first mitotic division. If we would like to discuss the powers of the embryo and of its new genome, contrary to its potential, at this moment it is completely powerless. The new set of the chromosomes is located in the egg cell provided completely by the mother. The new embryo-specific set of genes would need several days after fertilization to be activated, transcribed to mRNA, and create new proteins generated by the new genome. During this period, the cell components apart from the set of chromosomes are those of the egg cell, generated by the mother through the process of oogenesis. There is as well a substantial amount of the stored mRNA from the mother, which serves as a template for the new proteins needed for the development to start. The activation of the egg cell is achieved by the fertilization, when at the moment of fusion of the plasma membranes of the sperm and egg cells, calcium ions enter from the extracellular space in the oocyte and activate the sequence of developmental events. Subsequently, after calcium ions start the developmental sequence, the first period is not dependent on the embryo genome, but it is completely executed by the maternal genome, and RNA and proteins provided by the mother during oogenesis.[4]

The proteins of the mother will take care in the next days of the embryo genome. This actually implies that the mother will power-up the initially powerless embryo genome and help it to achieve the functioning state. This switch between functional proteins provided by the mother and new ones being generated by the embryo itself occurs gradually, and it is estimated that 3 days after fertilization the embryo has more of its own proteins than those of the mother, implying that the embryo starts to take over its own destiny.[5]

Together with taking care of the new genome, the mother-provided proteins start the first developmental phase, cleavage. The cleavage involves a series of mitotic divisions and creates new daughter cells, blastomeres, assembled in the morula. This first developmental phase is focused on the embryo genome, with the aim to generate, in a short time, new cells—each one with the additional genome copy. There is neither growth nor other noticeable activities during this period, to give maximum priority to the cell divisions, but as well due to the lack of space, embryo being encapsulated in the zona pellucida.

As the embryo genome is powerless at this stage, and in the caring hands of the mother, it is easy to understand that the outcome of this period is not at all dependent on the embryo quality, nor it is predictor of the embryo quality. Subsequently, neither chromosomal nor genetic anomaly of the embryo will be influencing the morula formation, and no prediction about embryo genome is possible by morulas obtained during in vitro fertilization.

The action of the embryo genome is present and visible in the following stage of development, compaction. The rounded blastomeres of the morula change their shape to polygonal and create intercellular junction characteristic for the epithelial tissue. Before compaction, whatever was present around blastomeres, (e.g. molecules of water, ions, and sugars) could not be assigned to be either inside or outside the embryo. After compaction, the cells create a superficial layer of tightly connected cells and this clearly separates the center of the embryo (now being "inside"), from the surface of the embryo (being "outside"). The process is dependent on the activity of the cytoskeleton changing the shapes of the cells and formation of the intracellular junction sealing the spaces between the cells to make the layer impermeable. The compaction is a sign of the activated embryo genome and the compacted embryos have higher probability to start pregnancy during in vitro fertilization.[6]

The embryo at compaction stage has some distinguished powers, as it is not powerless any more. It has already active genome, and it has generated its first form, the superficial layer of the epithelial cells. It is not any more a loose aggregation of blastomeres generated by the cleavage, but a compact mass of connected cells. Compaction represents a milestone between two stages. Before it, the loose blastomeres could be removed from the morula without damaging the embryo, which is used in preimplantation diagnostics. The isolated cells of morula serve to get the insight in the embryo genome, and diagnose gene alterations. Taking cells for preimplantation diagnostics after compaction is theoretically possible, but it would require the removal of the intracellular junctions and "uncompacting" the embryo in order to remove a cell or two. The biopsies are again possible at the blastocyst stage explained in the next chapter, where thin layer of trophoblast offers this possibility.[7]

In the same way as the cells can be taken out of the morula, they can be added to it, and the additional cells would be incorporated in the embryo by compaction process. This is widely used in animal experiments on mice and rats as "morula aggregation". This technique enables creating one animal from multiple embryos, or merging embryonic stem cells with the host embryo to generate animals derived from embryonic stem cells. Human embryos are not subject of these types of the experiments, but the human embryonic stem cells could be used to merge with animal embryos, (e.g. pigs or cows). These human-animal chimeras are not produced only due to scientific curiosity, but as well by intention to eventually generate human organs ready for transplantation, (e.g. human kidney growing in the body of the pig).[8]

How the Embryo Escapes the Imminent Dangers Threatening its Survival

The compaction is a prerequisite for the following stage of development, blastocyst stage. The fact that the embryo has the superficial epithelial sheet allows the liquid to accumulate in its center. This creates the rapidly expanding hollow structure, blastocyst, with liquid in its central cavity, blastocoel. The surface epithelium, trophoblast, differs from the small group of cells protruding in the blastocoel, inner cell mass.

As embryo with compaction acquires the power of compartmentalization using its newly formed epithelial sheet at the blastocyst stage it uses this power for its own undertakings. Embryo needs to escape two imminent dangers and this would be its first priority during the following days. Just to mention, the embryo does not consider anything close to "building a new human" at these early stages as any of its activities. This is because embryo has bigger concerns, which threaten him and it needs to use its powers to counteract them first.

The first danger is zona pellucida, which is an inert capsule, made by glycoproteins. The zona pellucida does not provide any space for the embryo growth and it isolates embryo completely from the eventual contacts with surrounding tissues. This could be beneficial, as eventual contacts between oviduct epithelium and the embryo can cause it to stay in the oviduct and eventually start extrauterine pregnancy. However, as the embryo approaches uterus it would need to free itself before implantation. During blastocyst formation, the liquid accumulates fast inside the embryo, and puts the pressure to break zona pellucida. This makes minute lacerations of the zona pellucida resulting with a tiny hole through which water filled blastocyst can easily exit out (what would not be possible if it would be a solid structure made by cells only). This "hatching" of the blastocyst makes it exit to the uterus and establish cell-to-cell contacts with uterine endometrium necessary for implantation.[9] The explained power of the embryo, to form epithelial sheets, accumulate water and easily expand, is used later for creating spaces for the unhindered baby development, i.e. amniotic and chorionic cavities.

The second imminent danger for the embryo is menstrual bleeding, which would shed not only uterine endometrium but as well the embryo itself. To cancel the menstrual bleeding the embryo would need to interfere with the hormonal regulation of the mother, which implies it needs somehow to get access to the maternal blood. This is achieved through the process of implantation, which in addition allows the embryo to use the maternal blood as well to get nourishment and to get rid of the waste products. Although combining this with release of embryo-derived hormones to the blood is very convenient, the embryo at this stage gets all necessary nourishment by simple diffusion through the endometrial epithelium and from the secretions of the uterine glands. Therefore, at the implantation stage, the first priority for the embryo is cancelling menstrual bleeding, and all other handy advantages of ingredients' exchange with maternal blood would become important later, during the period of the fetal growth.

To achieve the task of the implantation, the embryo will develop a new power, power of differentiation. By the use of its activated genome among its cells organized as the epithelial layer, it will create first type of cells with dedicated function. The final product of differentiation process is fully functional cells, which are difficult to reverse in another type of the cells. Therefore, every differentiation comes on the cost of losing potential. The reason for this is accumulation of many long-lasting proteins specific for the given function, and eventual dedifferentiation and redifferentiation would be costly process of getting rid of these high quality proteins and in the meantime synthesizing new proteins for some other function. Subsequently, although dedifferentiation is possible, it is an exception achieved mostly in experimental conditions, and not something a living being would consider as an appropriate option. Therefore, the embryo at this stage needs to dedicate a group of cells to be differentiated, but as well to keep another group of cells in undifferentiated state in order to use them later on for all other differentiation purposes. As the danger of menstrual bleeding is indeed very serious, the embryo will dedicate actually around 90% of its cells for the task of differentiation, and keep only around 10% in the undifferentiated state. The differentiation takes place in the trophoblast layer generating highly specialized cells, syncytiotrophoblast. The undifferentiated cells stay loosely attached to the trophoblast as a bulge of cells toward blastocoel, inner cell mass.

Syncytiotrophoblast is a very potent and highly active cell type. It disrupts the epithelium of the uterine endometrium, dissolves the extracellular matrix underneath, and aggressively erodes the closest capillaries. Upon reaching the blood, it releases a hormone, chorionic gonadotropin, which instead of luteinizing hormone (LH) of the mother, supports corpus luteum in the ovary to produce progesterone, and evade menstrual bleeding by keeping endometrium healthy and active. As syncytiotrophoblast is so complex and versatile cell type, differentiating well-functioning syncytiotrophoblast requires activity of many genes dispersed across almost all chromosomes. Therefore, achieving high quality syncytiotrophoblast, which would generate enough of chorionic gonadotropin, represents a major checkpoint of the embryo quality.[10] In case of chromosomal anomalies or some major genetic anomaly, the embryo would not be able to secrete necessary amounts of chorionic gonadotropin to the maternal blood and subsequently the necessary levels of progesterone would not be maintained leading to the spontaneous abortion. This is an "all or nothing" principle, the embryo will either escape the danger of endometrial shedding and survive, or it would not be able to cope with the task and perish. There are no malformations at this stage as there is no body plan yet.

In case of in vitro fertilization, mothers are treated frequently by progesterone to provide some advantages for the embryo during the implantation. Still, in case of major chromosomal anomalies the external progesterone would not help to maintain the pregnancy.[11] The levels of chorionic gonadotropins increase and can be measured in the maternal blood to assess the embryo vitality, and the slow increase can indicate chromosomal anomalies, e.g. Down syndrome.

Providing Extraembryonic Membranes as a Necessary Infrastructure for the Development

The inner cell mass of the blastocyst is a small group of undifferentiated cells within the blastocyst. Although epithelial, these cells lack polarity due to their arrangement expanding toward the blastocoel. Their characteristics are very similar to blastomeres, but those centrally located, which did not turn into the trophoblast. The undifferentiated state is reflected in their gene expression being protected not to activate the syncytiotrophoblast program. Human blastocysts are possible to be obtained by in vitro fertilization, and they are the last stage of human embryo available for manipulation as after implantation the embryo would be hidden somewhere in the uterine endometrium. Therefore the inner cell mass was taken as an ideal source for embryonic stem cells. Compared to the morula stage embryo, their potential to make trophoblast is significantly reduced, they are undifferentiated, and due to the lack of epithelial polarity, still easy to be removed from the blastocyst and grown further in the culture.

Just opposite to that, the blastocyst is as well the last stage when something can be added to the embryo, which is widely used in animal experiments to add embryonic stem cells and generate chimeric animals. For human embryo, this could represent an entry level for genetically modified stem cells with corrected genome to cure the embryo, but these experiments were not considered yet. This is as well, the stage where human cells can be added to the animal embryo creating human-animal chimeras.

Following the implantation, the inner cell mass goes through the process similar to compaction and its cells acquire polarity. It results in accumulation of liquid inside the inner cell mass in the same way it has accumulated during formation of the blastocysts.[12] The new lumen generating by this process is amniotic cavity and the epithelium divides in the two domains. The outside domain consists of two epithelia, the epithelium of the amnion consisting of the amnioblasts, and the epithelium of the hypoblast destined to make yolk sac. The inside-facing domain is epiblast, which is present only near the hypoblast, creating bilaminar embryonic disk. The epiblast keeps the undifferentiated state, while the outside epithelia are involved in generating extraembryonic membranes.

The implantation marks the end of the first week of development after fertilization, and the formation of the extraembryonic membranes will take the complete second week. This is a long period still without any body plan, but the extraembryonic membranes are necessary infrastructure to be provided for the embryo development. Together with the power of differentiation, the embryo would add the ability to combine different cell types in the specific forms, morphogenesis. In addition to the epithelial tissue, the primitive connective tissue or mesenchyme would appear as extraembryonic mesoderm. This as well allows the different types of cells to influence each other through so-called epithelial-mesenchymal interactions. The new structures evolving include amnion, chorion, yolk sac, and allantois. The amnion would supply the isolated, but ample space for the embryo body to develop. Chorion would create the interface with the uterine endometrium, now referred as decidua, which would contribute to the placenta and the amniochorionic membrane. The yolk sac in human embryo represents the first sight for vasculogenesis and hematopoiesis, and allantois contributes with its blood vessels to the formation of the umbilical cord. Through this process, the extraembryonic membranes provide roomy compartments within the endometrium, while uterine cavity obliterates. The connection between mother and embryo stabilizes in a form of placenta and umbilical cord. Still, parallel to this extensive extraembryonic morphogenesis, epiblast would stay in the undifferentiated form until the 3rd week of development.

The Formation of the Body Plan and Organogenesis

At the beginning of the 3rd week, the embryo has collected and exerted already significant powers. It has activated its genome and tested its quality through the implantation process, it is able to form two types of tissues, epithelium and mesenchyme, and it can differentiate fully functional cells, which can be combined in the definite forms through the process of the morphogenesis. All this helped embryo to create a comprehensive setup to activate finally its ultimate power—the power of creating the body plan. In case of molar pregnancy, most of the powers described previously were achieved, but there is no body plan, highlighting the distinguished property of this crucial power. Moreover, not only the embryo without body can be made like in molar pregnancy, but, opposite to that, the embryo with two or multiple bodies could be created in form of the monozygotic twins. The monozygotic twins arise through the division of the undifferentiated group of cells either at the stage of morula, inner cell mass or epiblast, highlighting the undifferentiated state of these structures.[13]

The body plan appears in the epiblast by formation of the primitive streak and the process of gastrulation. The primitive streak defines the major axes of the embryo, cranial-to-caudal and lateral-to-lateral.[14] As primitive streak is formed the epiblast cells start to migrate through the primitive streak and change their positions in relation to each other.

The human, similar to other vertebrate embryos, does not follow determined development, where the sequences of events are predetermined and follow in hierarchical order. At the first sight, the determinate (mosaic) development seems as the best way to control the intricate process. Although it serves well for simple organisms (like nematode *Caenorhabditis elegans*), it is not appropriate in case of the complex organisms. Therefore, at some point of evolution it was replaced in higher organisms by regulative development, where the developmental plan is executed by interactions among cells, in particular different types of cells. The regulative development offers necessary flexibility to achieve increased complexity. By adapting to different situations, it reduces the developmental mistakes and speeds-up the evolution.[15]

Gastrulation process uses the principle of regulative development at its best. It provides the axial orientation for the cells by establishing the primitive streak, and subsequently lets cells to pass through it and end at the different locations across newly formed trilaminar embryonic disk. This achieves two goals, first to bring different types of cells to interact with each other at the different parts of the newly formed structure, and second it primes them with their future tasks by the process of invagination through the primitive streak. The nature of cell priming by the primitive streak is still speculative, but the information they get is the location along the primitive streak and the timing.[16] The cells entering first would end more cranially and those that follow would take positions more caudally. The migration through the primitive streak would result, instead of epiblast, in three new germ layers, ectoderm, mesoderm, and endoderm. The hypoblast layer would be pushed away to be part of the yolk sac. The three germ layers are the representations of the established body plan and the interactions between germ layers and different cell types within the layer will lead to establishing the organ primordia during next step of development, organogenesis.[17]

The in vitro experiments using embryonic stem cells or the parts of the embryo, (e.g. epiblast and hypoblast) could recreate the powers of the embryo present before gastrulation including differentiation of functional cells and morphogenesis of the simple structure, but they did never recreate the power of generating the body plan, present specifically during gastrulation. Subsequently, although the gastrulation process seems quite free-formed and based on seemingly random migration, it is indeed a very complex and demanding process, which represents a key event during embryo development. This is the ultimate power of the embryo, to generate the body plan, the power lacking in all in vitro stem cells systems. The body plan appearance needs all prerequisites generated during two previous weeks of human development and only in this particular setting the epiblast is capable for gastrulation process.[18]

Although stem cells, in particular embryonic stem cells and induced pluripotent stem cells, lack the ability to generate body plan by themselves, when introduced in the embryo, they could obey the host embryo cells and together with them generate the body plan. The embryonic stem cells as well as induced pluripotent stem cells, corresponding to the inner cell mass of the blastocyst, by themselves lack the spatial relations of the epiblast. When introduced in the embryo, and reaching the epiblast stage, the body plan is generated and subsequently it makes stem cells capable for the normal organogenesis. All other types of the differentiating cells and partial organogenesis achieved in vitro from the stem cells, can supply by specific stem cells the eventual needs for therapy within the scope of regenerative medicine, but are (at least currently) not possible to recreate the full organogenesis, where organ is formed in accordance and integrated with all surrounding structures.[19]

This issue, how to create a fully functional organ suitable for transplantation, depends on the embryo power to create a body plan. Therefore, the evolving strategy to create the organs for transplantation is with the help of the embryos, but using animal embryos instead of human.[8] The strategy envisages the use of human-animal chimeras, where the host embryo is animal. The pig is chosen as the most suitable to be host according to the size and anatomy. If the human stem cells could be added at morula or blastocyst stage to the pig embryo, they would contribute to the body plan of the pig during the gastrulation process (using the power of the pig embryo to generate a body plan). As the organ with only human cells is needed for transplantation, the pig embryo should be genetically deficient, not to be able to produce the organ in question, (e.g. kidney). Consequently, the human cells will replace pig cells in this particular task and the pig will have all organs chimeric (pig and human origin), but the kidney will be human only. One can imagine the clean facility, where these specific pigs will be grown with human organs, generated by induced pluripotent cells to match exactly the patient in the need for transplantation.

Extreme ethical issues burden the technique described, and one of the most difficult to predict would be the levels of humanizing the pig by this procedure. As the contribution of the cells to the chimeric organs can vary, one can imagine the pig with mostly human-derived brain, which could then have the human-like mind. At the other hand, the humanized brain of such an embryo at the fetal stage can serve as a source of human fetal neural stem cells, which could provide an alternative source of the cells to be applied in the possible therapy of the neurodegenerative diseases.[20]

CONCLUSION

The morphogenetic and differentiation powers of the human embryo described here show how powerful and how flexible is the human embryo. The early development starts with maximum potential of the human embryo upon fertilization, which is realized gradually by developing powers of the embryo. They include the activation of the new genome, creation of the epithelial tissue and later on mesenchyme, functional differentiation of the specific cell types, and morphogenesis based on inductive interactions between different groups of cells. These powers are supplemented by the power of generating body plan, which appears in the epiblast at the gastrulation, and enables all other powers to start the concerted action of organogenesis.

Before generating body plan, the embryo is occupied by many important tasks to prepare the scene for the gastrulation. The developing powers are used to achieve these tasks and they are necessary proof that the new genetic set is capable to make a new living being. Through the "all or nothing" principle, most of the chromosomally and genetically anomalous embryos would not reach the body plan stage and would be spontaneously aborted due to the inadequate connection with the mother. As during these preparatory stages no body plan is present, the embryo appears to be flexible for various interventions, twin formation being the example of natural one. Adding or removing cells is possible throughout this time period, which could serve to treat the embryo as a patient, or use the embryo cells as a cure for other patients. Whatever intervention envisaged, it is highly ethically controversial. The embryo is one of the most controversial bio-objects, defying the existing classification and definitions.[21] As the evolving technologies would change the experience of the pregnancy, this would influence as well the societal debate on the embryo issues, and eventually redefine the current concepts. The unpredictable process of technical challenges and ethical controversies makes the developing powers of the embryo one of the most intriguing medical and social concerns.

REFERENCES

1. Angelos MG, Kaufman DS. Pluripotent stem cell applications for regenerative medicine. Curr Opin Organ Transplant. 2015;20(6):663-70.
2. de Miguel Beriain I. What is a human embryo? A new piece in the bioethics puzzle. Croat Med J. 2014;55(6):669-71.
3. Svenaeus F. Phenomenology of pregnancy and the ethics of abortion. Med Health Care Philos. 2018;21(1):77-87.
4. Rossant J, Tam PPL. Exploring early human embryo development. Science. 2018;360(6393):1075-6.
5. Ortega NM, Winblad N, Plaza Reyes A, Lanner F. Functional genetics of early human development. Curr Opin Genet Dev. 2018;52:1-6.
6. Le Cruguel S, Ferré-L'Hôtellier V, Morinière C, et al. Early compaction at day 3 may be a useful additional criterion for embryo transfer. J Assist Reprod Genet. 2013;30(5):683-90.
7. Minasi MG, Fiorentino F, Ruberti A, et al. Genetic diseases and aneuploidies can be detected with a single blastocyst biopsy: a successful clinical approach. Hum Reprod. 2017;32(8):1770-7.
8. Suchy F, Nakauchi H. Interspecies chimeras. Curr Opin Genet Dev. 2018;52:36-41.
9. Seshagiri PB, Sen Roy S, Sireesha G, et al. Cellular and molecular regulation of mammalian blastocyst hatching. J Reprod Immunol. 2009;83(1-2):79-84.
10. Fox C, Morin S, Jeong JW, et al. Local and systemic factors and implantation: what is the evidence? Fertil Steril. 2016;105(4):873-84.
11. Wahabi HA, Fayed AA, Esmaeil SA, et al. Progestogen for treating threatened miscarriage. Cochrane Database Syst Rev. 2018;8:CD005943.
12. Taniguchi K, Shao Y, Townshend RF, et al. Lumen Formation Is an Intrinsic Property of Isolated Human Pluripotent Stem Cells. Stem Cell Reports. 2015;5(6):954-62.
13. Gardner RL. The timing of monozygotic twinning: a pro-life challenge to conventional scientific wisdom. Reprod Biomed Online. 2014;28(3):276-8.
14. Stern CD. Evolution of the mechanisms that establish the embryonic axes. Curr Opin Genet Dev. 2006;16(4):413-8.
15. Morgani S, Nichols J, Hadjantonakis AK. The many faces of Pluripotency: in vitro adaptations of a continuum of in vivo states. BMC Dev Biol. 2017;17(1):7.
16. Mulas C, Chia G, Jones KA, et al. Oct 4 regulates the embryonic axis and coordinates exit from pluripotency and germ layer specification in the mouse embryo. Development. 2018;145(12):dev159103.
17. Shahbazi MN, Scialdone A, Skorupska N, et al. Pluripotent state transitions coordinate morphogenesis in mouse and human embryos. Nature. 2017;552(7684):239-43.
18. Turner DA, Girgin M, Alonso-Crisostomo L, et al. Anteroposterior polarity and elongation in the absence of extra-embryonic tissues and of spatially localised signaling in gastruloids: mammalian embryonic organoids. Development. 2017;144(21):3894-906.
19. Simunovic M, Brivanlou AH. Embryoids, organoids and gastruloids: new approaches to understanding embryogenesis. Development. 2017;144(6):976-85.
20. Sawai T, Hatta T, Fujita M. Public attitudes in Japan towards human-animal chimeric embryo research using human induced pluripotent stem cells. Regen Med. 2017;12(3):233-48.
21. Metzler I, Webster A. Bio-objects and their boundaries: governing matters at the intersection of society, politics, and science. Croat Med J. 2011;52(5):648-50.

CHAPTER 3

Sonoembryology

Ritsuko K Pooh

INTRODUCTION

Recent revolution of assisted reproductive technology (ART) and advanced technologies of experimental magnetic resonance (MR) microscopy of embryos[1-4] and computer graphics[5] have marvelously elucidated the beginning of human life. "Sonoembryology" was first described by Timor-Tritsch et al. in 1990[6] after the introduction of high-frequency transvaginal transducer in obstetrical field. Combination of transvaginal approach and three-dimensional (3D) ultrasound has been establishing "3D sonoembryology", producing more objective and accurate information of early embryonal and fetal development and natural history of fetal abnormalities.[7] Although 3D sonoembryology has been approaching modern high-tech embryology, it still cannot demonstrate internal organs of embryos as clearly as by embryonal magnetic resonance (MR) microscopy. However, a great advantage in sonoembryology, which human embryology cannot possess, is "demonstration of living embryos with circulation in vivo". Human embryology is based on dead embryos which had been well-preserved. 3D sonoembryology has a remarkable potential to discover new findings of living embryos and fetuses in utero. In this chapter, we introduce up-date embryology and 3D sonoembryology. Although "gestational age" usually used in obstetrical field based on menstrual period or crown lump length, has been criticized in the embryological point of view,[8] it is used in this chapter on description of sonograms.

MODERN EMBRYOLOGY

Carnegie stages, well-known embryonal staging system till 8 weeks after conception, were named after the famous institute which began collecting and classifying embryos in the early 1900s. An embryo is assigned a Carnegie stage (numbered from 1 to 23) based on its external morphological features. Age and size proves a poor way to organize embryos. It is very difficult to accurately age an embryo, and it could shrink a full 50% in the preserving fluids. Therefore, this staging system is neither dependent on the chronological age nor the size of the embryo. The stages, are in a sense, arbitrary levels of maturity based on multiple physical features. Embryos that might have different ages or sizes can be assigned the same Carnegie stage based on their external appearance because of the natural variation which occurs between individuals. Table 3.1 shows the Carnegie stages from stage 1 to 23.

The recent advance in MR microscopic technology has made it possible to scan and visualize relatively small samples, including mammalian embryos.[1] MR microscopy demonstrates tomographic imaging of small objects, and the digitized data can be manipulated to achieve 3D reconstruction of the samples.[1] Although the resolution and long imaging speed were initial problems in MR microscopy, those have been solved by invention of a super-parallel MR microscope.[2] Additionally, recent advanced computer graphic techniques combined MR microscopy have produced detailed 3D images of human embryos. Yamada et al.[5] successfully constructed a series of 3D images of human embryos, based on the MR microscopy data of human embryo specimens in the Kyoto Collection, with the aid of CG techniques, to illustrate 3D structures and morphogenetic movements in human embryos. In addition, they produced movies using these 3D images to show the entire process of morphogenesis in human embryos from fertilization to the completion of organogenesis.[5]

Normal Embryo Visualization by three-dimensional Sonoembryology

Since the introduction of high frequency transvaginal transducer, ultrasonographic visualization of embryos and fetuses in early stage has been remarkably progressed and sonoembryology[6] has been established. In addition, recent introduction of three-dimensional and four-dimensional ultrasounds combined with the transvaginal approach has

Table 3.1: Carnegie stages.

Stage	Days after conception (approximately)	Size (mm)	Events
1	1 (week 1)	0.1–0.15	Fertilized oocyte, pronuclei
2	2–3	0.1–0.2	Cell division with reduction in cytoplasmic volume, formation of inner and outer cell mass
3	4–5	0.1–0.2	Loss of zona pellucida, free blastocyst
4	5–6	0.1–0.2	Attaching blastocyst
5	7–12 (week 2)	0.1–0.2	Implantation
6	13–15	0.2	Extraembryonic mesoderm, primitive streak
7	15–17 (week 3)	0.4	Gastrulation, notochordal process
8	17–19	1.0–1.5	Primitive pit, notochordal canal
9	19–21	1.5–2.5	Somite number 1–3 neural folds, cardiac primordium, head fold
10	22–23 (week 4)	2–3.5	Somite number 4–12 neural fold fuses
11	23–26	2.5–4.5	Somite number 13–20 rostral neuropore closes
12	26–30	3–5	Somite number 21–29 caudal neuropore closes
13	28–32 (week 5)	4–6	Somite number 30 leg buds, lens placode, pharyngeal arches
14	31–35	5–7	Lens pit, optic cup
15	35–38	7–9	Lens vesicle, nasal pit, hand plate
16	37–42 (week 6)	8–11	Nasal pits moved ventrally, auricular hillocks, footplate
17	42–44	11–14	Finger rays
18	44–48 (week 7)	13–17	Ossification commences
19	48–51	16–18	Straightening of trunk
20	51–53 (week 8)	18–22	Upper limbs longer and bent at elbow
21	53–54	22–24	Hands and feet turned inward
22	54–56	23–28	Eyelids, external ears
23	56–60	27–31	Rounded head, body and limbs

produced more objective and accurate information on embryonal and early fetal development.[7,9]

The 3D/4D ultrasound has improved our knowledge regarding the normal and abnormal development of the embryo and fetus.[10] The great achievement in the field of 3D/4D ultrasound is HDlive technology. This technology is a novel ultrasound technique that improves the 3D/4D images. HDlive ultrasound has resulted in remarkable progress in visualization of early embryos and fetuses and in the development of sonoembryology.[11] With HDlive ultrasound, both structural and functional developments can be assessed from early pregnancy more objectively and reliably and indeed, those new technologies have moved embryology from postmortem studies to the in vivo environment.[12] In obstetrical ultrasound, HDlive could be used during all three trimesters of pregnancy. There have been several reports on HDlive demonstration of fetal surface.[13-15] Furthermore, the advanced 3D technology had produced exciting new applications of HDlive silhouette and HDlive flow, released at the end of 2014. The algorithm of HDlive silhouette creates a gradient at organ boundaries, fluid-filled cavity and vessels walls, where an abrupt change of the acoustic impedance exists within tissues.[16-18] By HDlive silhouette mode, an inner cystic structure with fluid collection can be depicted through the outer surface structure of the body and it can be appropriately named as *"see-through fashion".*[16,18] The examiner can adjust HDlive silhouette percentage with controlling threshold and gain simultaneously for visualizing target organs of interest.

Figures 3.1A to C show development of gestational sac between 4 weeks and 5 weeks of gestation. At 4 weeks (2 weeks after conception) of gestation, 3D reconstructed image demonstrated early gestational sac. At the beginning of 5 weeks, yolk sac is detectable inside gestational sac and an embryo is detectable with yolk sac at the end of 5 weeks.

Figures 3.2A and B show an embryo at 6 weeks of gestation by high definition imaging and silhouette ultrasound imaging with high-frequency transvaginal transducer (Voluson® E8 with 12 MHz/256 element vaginal probe, GE Healthcare, Milwaukee, USA). Early neural tube and premature spinal cord are successfully demonstrated in a small embryo on Figures 3.3A and B. From 1990s, the development of the embryonic circulation became visualized by 3D power Doppler imaging technology.[19,20] Figure 3.4 shows intrauterine vascularity with the rich vascularity of embryo and chorionic villi inside gestational sac. At 7 weeks of gestation, embryonal vascularity and cord blood supply become clearly depictable (Figs. 3.5A and B). Figure 3.6 shows 3D vascularity of 8-week embryo. The premature brain vessel to the midbrain is clearly visualized.

During the early embryonic period, the central nervous system anatomy rapidly changes in appearance.

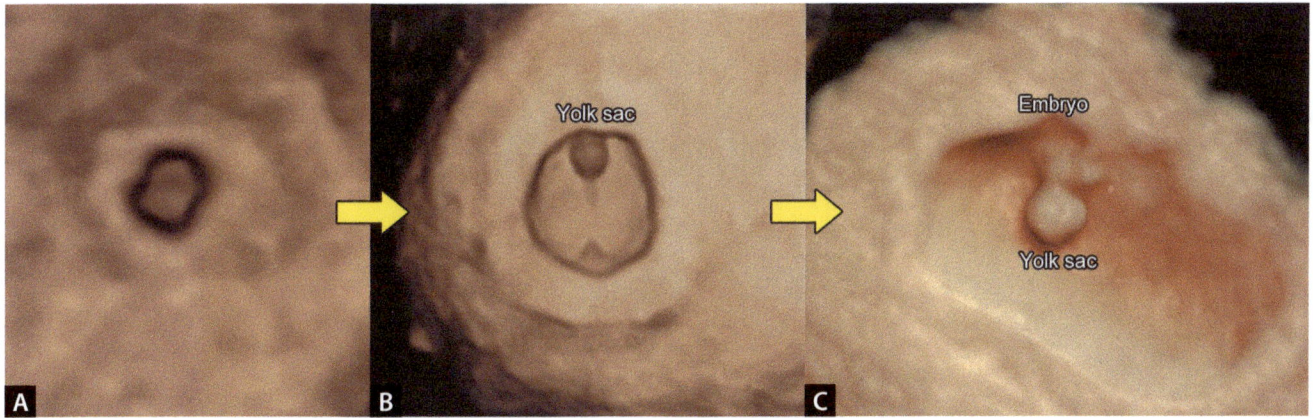

Figs. 3.1A to C: Development of gestational sac between 4 weeks and 5 weeks of gestation. (A) 4 weeks (2 weeks after conception) of gestation. 3D reconstructed image demonstrated early gestational sac; (B) The beginning of 5 weeks, yolk sac is detectable inside gestational sac; (C) Embryo is detectable with yolk sac at the end of 5 weeks.

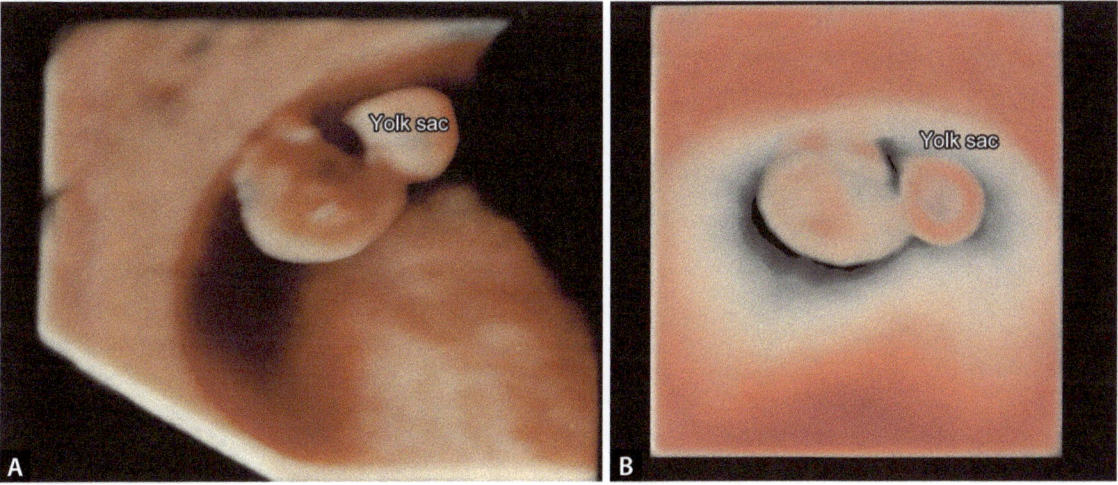

Figs. 3.2A and B: Embryo and yolk sac at 6 weeks of gestation. (A) High definition mode; and (B) Silhouette mode.

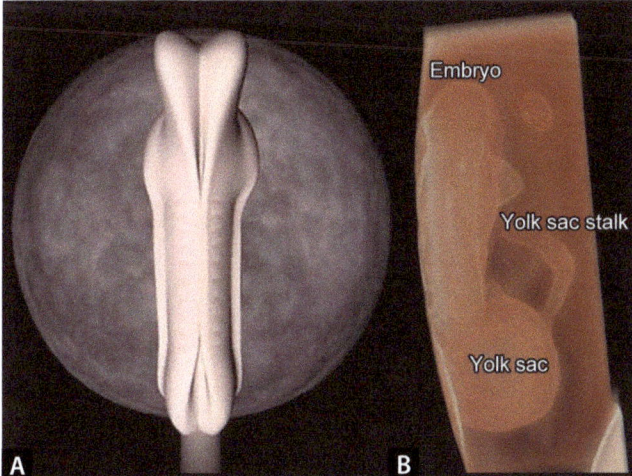

Figs. 3.3A and B: Embryo and yolk sac at 6 weeks and 6 days of gestation. (A) Computer graphics; (B) Silhouette ultrasound image of the embryo (posterior view).
Courtesy for Figure A: Professor Yamada, Kyoto University, Japan.

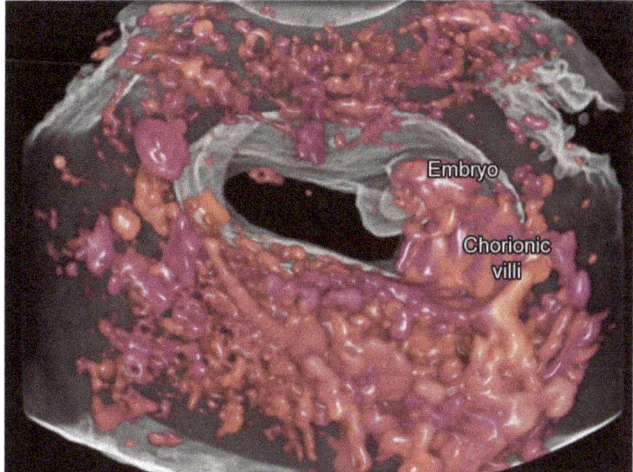

Fig. 3.4: Intrauterine vascularity at 6 weeks of gestation. Note the rich vascularity of embryo and chorionic villi inside gestational sac.

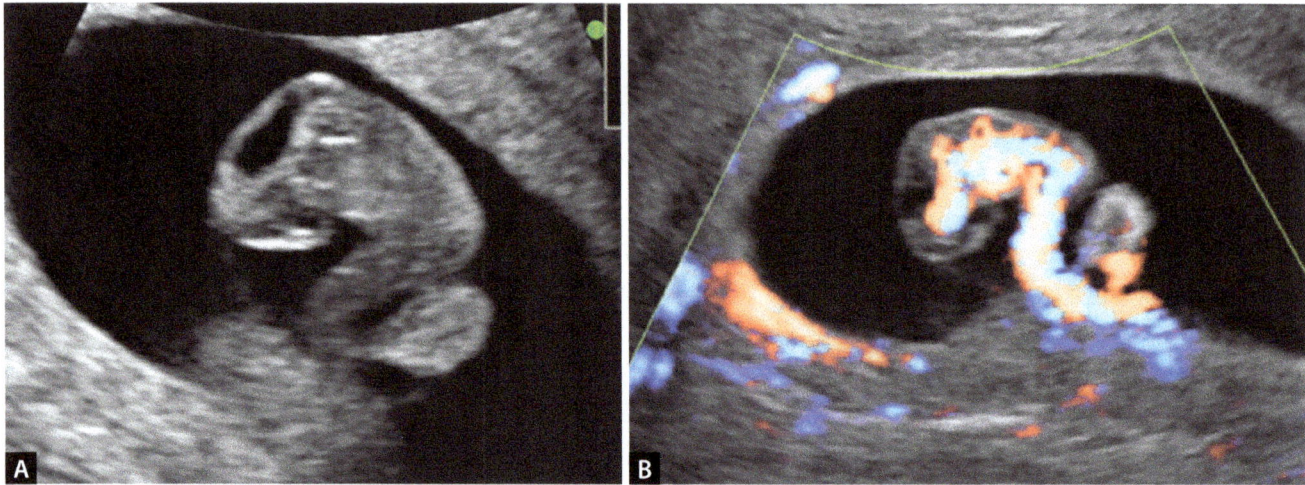

Figs. 3.5A and B: Embryo and embryonal vascularity at 7 weeks of gestation. (A) Two-dimensional image of embryo; (B) Power Doppler image of embryo and umbilical cord.

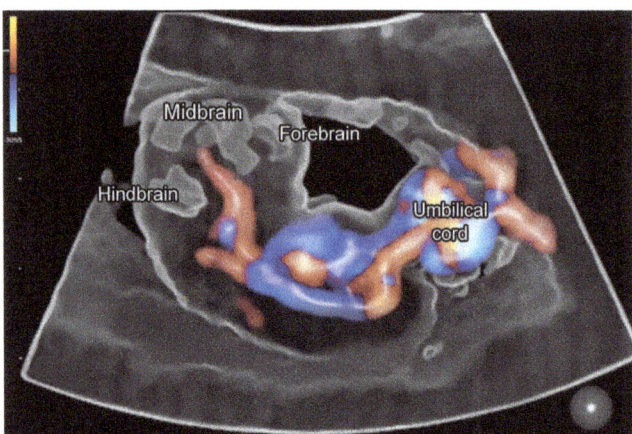

Fig. 3.6: Embryonal vascularity at 8 weeks of gestation (lateral view). Note the premature brain vascularity to the midbrain.

The 3D sonography using transvaginal sonography with high-resolution probes allows imaging of early structures in the embryonic brain. Embryonic brain contains three parts of forebrain (prosencephalon), midbrain (mesencephalon) and hindbrain (rhombencephalon). The forebrain (prosencephalon) includes the telencephalon containing cerebral hemispheres and diencephalon containing thalamus, hypothalamus, epithalamus and subthalamus. The midbrain (mesencephalon) is the most rostral part of the brainstem and located above the pons, and adjoined rostrally to the thalamus. The hindbrain (rhombencephalon) is the posterior of the three primary divisions and includes metencephalon containing pons and cerebellum and myelencephalon containing medulla oblongata. In 1998, Blaas et al.[21] sensationally demonstrated early human brain vesicles in different colors and measured their volumes by 3D scanning embryos ranged between 9.3 mm and 39 mm and performed post-processing procedure. Thereafter, embryonic brain structure was demonstrated by advancing 3D technology of inversion-rendering mode,[22,23] and sonoembryology has become more sophisticated and objective. Advancing imaging techniques allow the definition of invivo anatomy including visualization of the embryonic features that could not be characterized in fixed specimens.[24]

Figures 3.7 and 3.8 show the early brain vesicles in an embryo at 7 weeks of gestation by Silhouette ultrasound imaging. Figures 3.9 and 3.10 show frontal view and lateral view of the brain at 8 weeks. Changing appearance of the premature brain structure between 7 weeks and 8 weeks of gestation is shown in Figures 3.11A to C. Thus, embryonal brain is rapidly developing day by day during embryonal stage.

ABNORMALITIES AT EMBRYONAL STAGE

The yolk sac plays an important role in embryonal hemopoiesis and fetomaternal transportation of nutritive properties before establishment of fetoplacental circulation. The primary yolk sac forms at around 3rd week of the menstrual age, then following the formation of the extraembryonic coelom, and the secondary yolk sac is formed. From the 5th week of gestation, it appears as a spherical and cystic structure covered by numerous superficial small vessels merging at the basis of the vitelline duct. This connects the yolk sac to the ventral part of the embryo, the gut and main blood circulation. During the

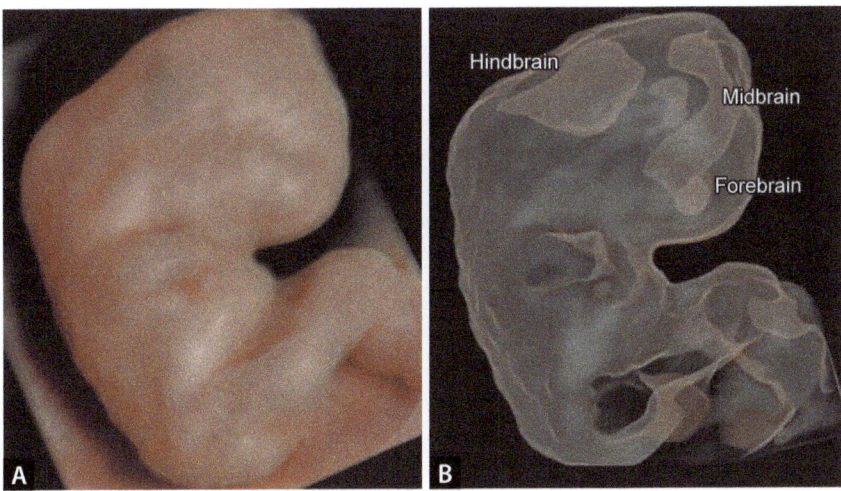

Figs. 3.7A and B: Embryo at 7 weeks of gestation. (A) High definition image of embryo; (B) Silhouette ultrasound image from the same volume dataset of the left. Note clear depiction of the brain vesicles.

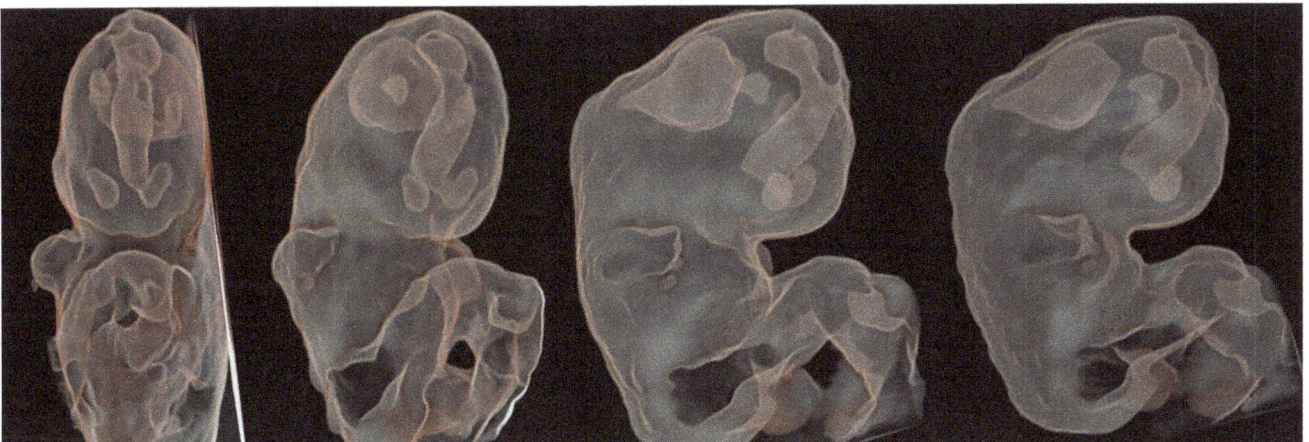

Fig. 3.8: Embryo at 7 weeks of gestation (Silhouette images). Rotated images of embryo. The forebrain, midbrain, and hindbrain are clearly demonstrated.

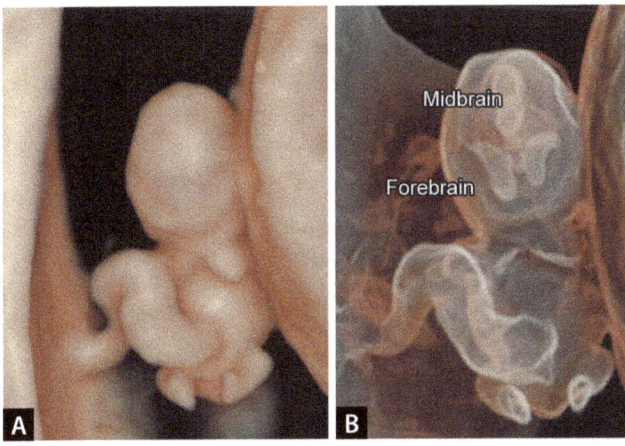

Figs. 3.9A and B: Embryo at 8 weeks of gestation (frontal view). (A) High definition image of embryo; (B) Silhouette ultrasound image from the same volume dataset of the left. Note clear depiction of the brain vesicles.

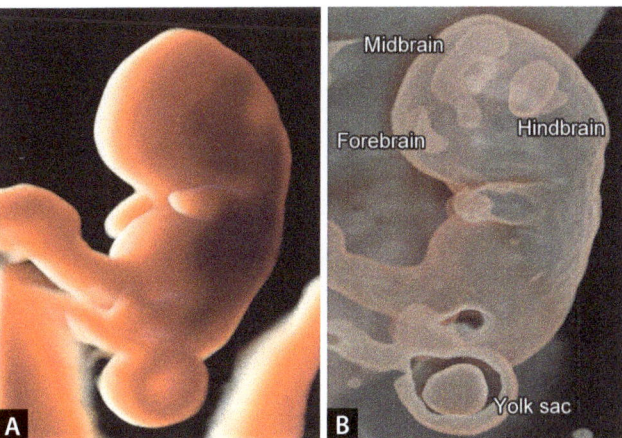

Figs. 3.10A and B: Embryo at 8 weeks of gestation (lateral view). (A) High definition image of embryo; (B) Silhouette ultrasound image from the same volume dataset of the left. Note clear depiction of the brain vesicles.

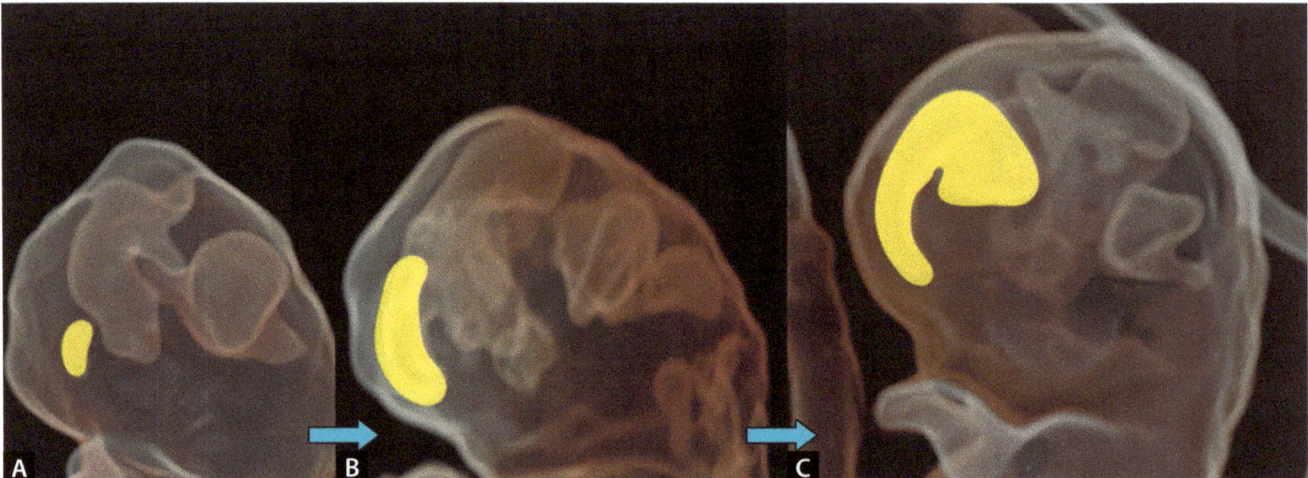

Figs. 3.11A to C: Changing appearance of the brain between 7 weeks and 8 weeks of gestation. (A) Silhouette ultrasound images from different embryonal stages at 7 weeks. The beginning of 8 weeks (B) and middle of 8 weeks (C). Yellow color area indicates the forebrain. Note the rapid development of forebrain at these stages.

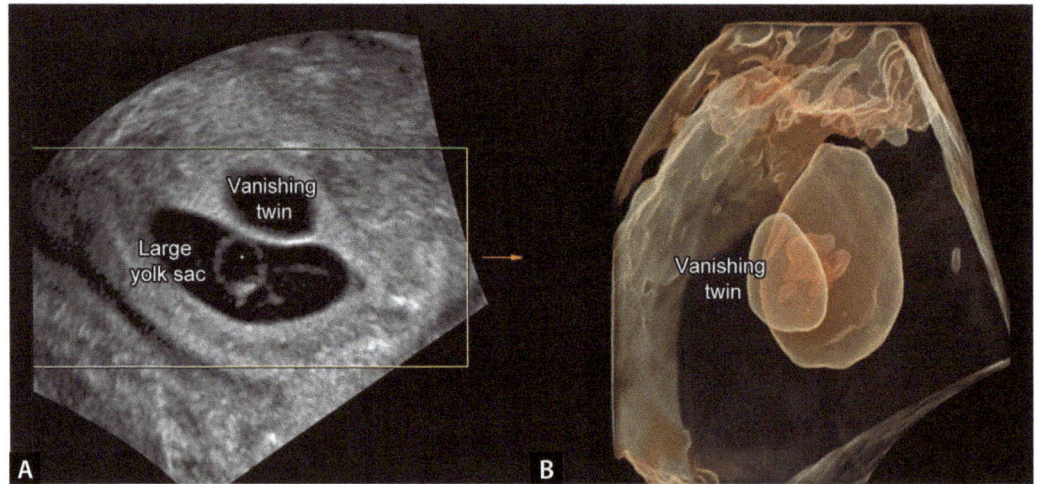

Figs. 3.12A and B: Early intrauterine fetal death with large yolk sac, with vanishing twin at 8 weeks of gestation. (A) Two-dimensional image; and (B) Silhouette image. Chromosomal examination of villi resulted in trisomy 15.

10th week of gestation, the yolk sac begins to degenerate and rapidly ceases to function.[25]

It has been reported that abnormal size and/or shape of yolk sac may be associated with ominous pregnant outcome.[25] Large yolk sac is defined more than two standard deviations above the mean, which indicates over 5.6 mm of diameter at less than 10 weeks menstrual age.[26,27] Large yolk sac is strongly associated with chromosomal aberration of autosomal trisomy (Figs. 3.12 to 3.14). Figures 3.15A and B show a case of large yolk sac with normal karyotype and normal single nucleotide polymorphism microarray result but congenital abnormalities were detected thereafter. Echogenic yolk sac is also related to adverse pregnant outcome with autosomal trisomy as shown in Figures 3.16A to C.

Embryonal pleural effusion is often seen in early pregnancy. Hashimoto et al.[28] investigated the incidence of embryonic/fetal pleural effusion between 7 weeks and 10 weeks. They reported the incidence is 1.2%, chromosomal aberration was confirmed in 84% including 67% of Turner syndrome (45,X). According to the other recent study,[29] all three cases with pleural effusion at 7–8 weeks of gestation were associated with Turner syndrome. Majority of early pleural effusion may be Turner syndrome as shown in Figures 3.17A to C but autosomal trisomy is occasionally confirmed as shown in Figures 3.18A to C.

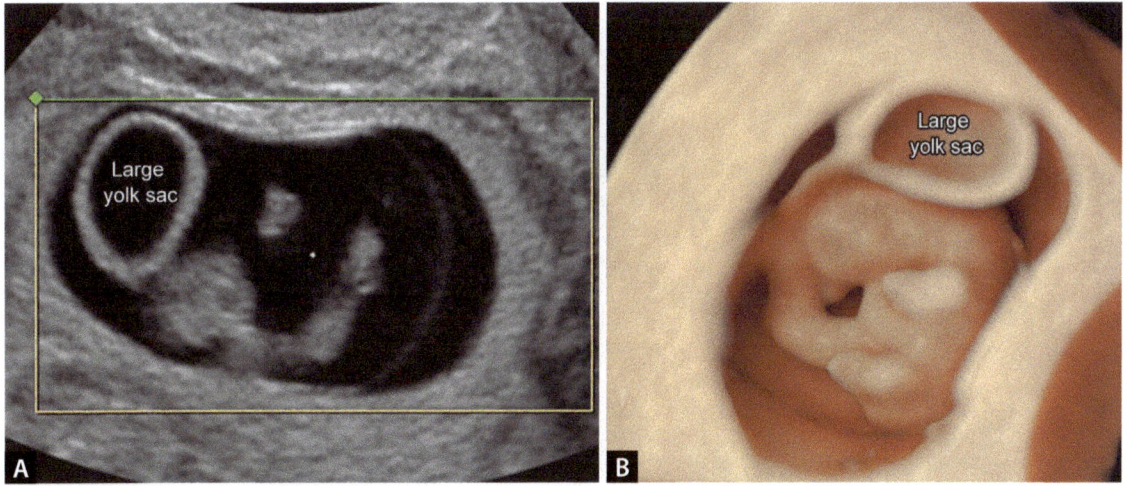

Figs. 3.13A and B: Large yolk sac at 8 weeks of gestation. (A) Two-dimensional image; and (B) High-definition image. Villous chromosomal examination resulted in trisomy 22.

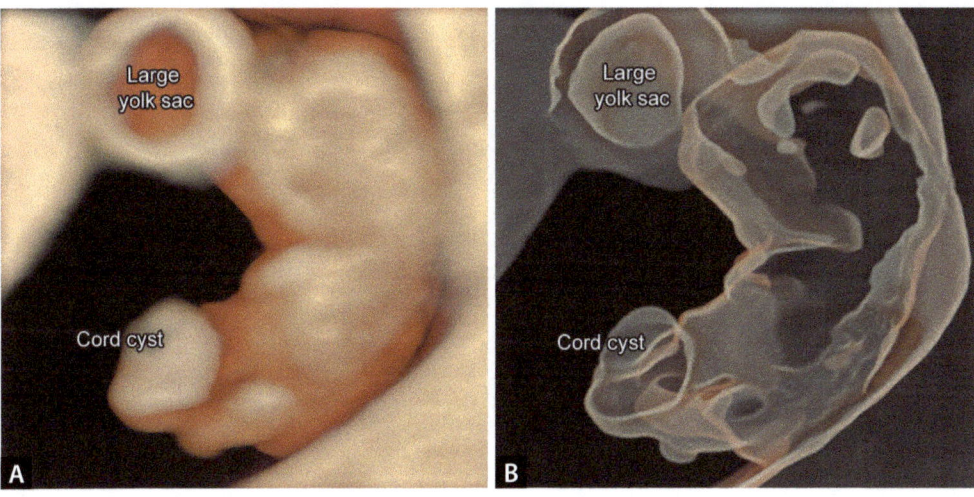

Figs. 3.14A and B: Large yolk sac and cord cyst at 8 weeks of gestation. (A) High-definition image; and (B) Silhouette ultrasound image. Villous chromosomal examination resulted in trisomy 22.

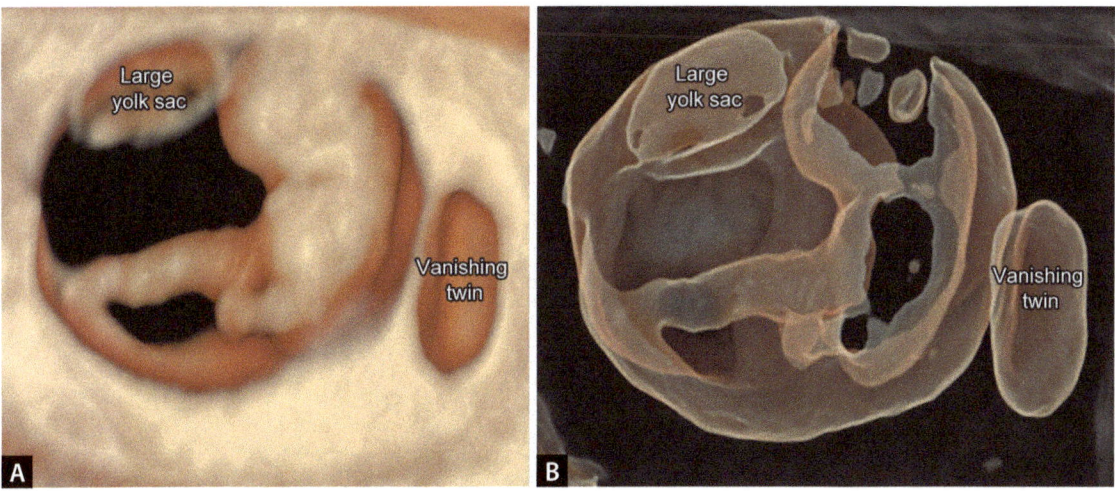

Figs. 3.15A and B: Large yolk sac, with vanishing twin at 8 weeks of gestation. (A) High-definition image; and (B) Silhouette ultrasound image. Normal single nucleotide polymorphism microarray but thereafter cleft lip was detected at 10 weeks and progressive hydrocephalus was detected from 15 weeks of gestation.

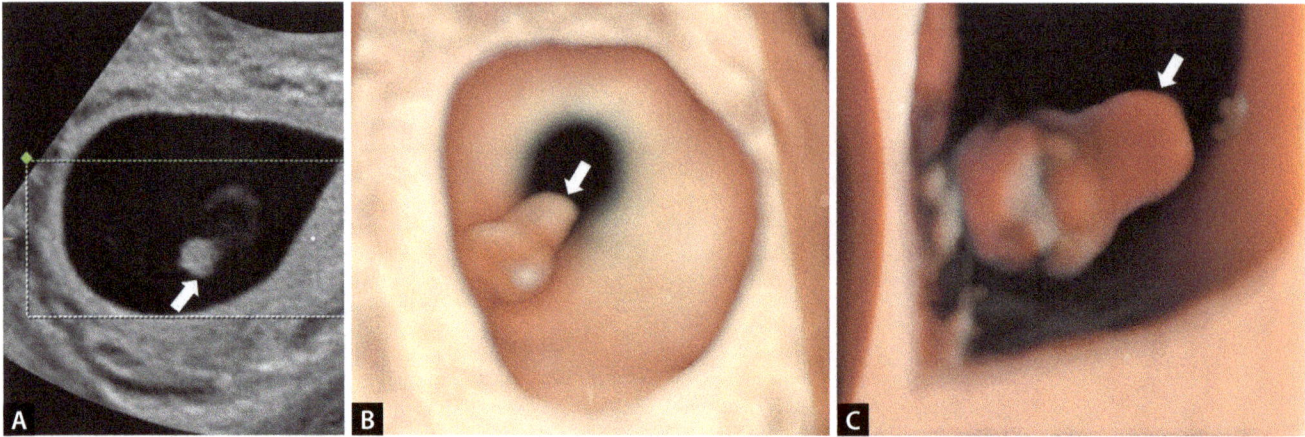

Figs. 3.16A to C: Early intrauterine fetal death with echogenic shrunk yolk sac (arrows) at 8 weeks of gestation. (A) Two-dimensional image; (B) High-definition image; and (C) Silhouette image. Villous chromosomal examination resulted in trisomy 22.

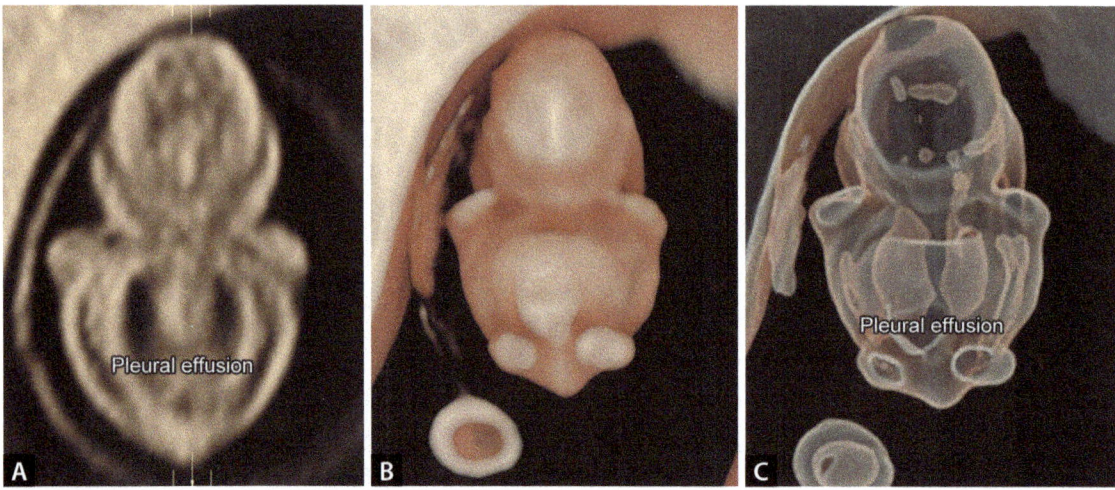

Figs. 3.17A to C: Intrauterine embryonal death with bilateral pleural effusion at the end of 8 weeks of gestation. (A) Coronal cutting image; (B) Frontal views of high-definition image; and (C) Silhouette image. Note bilateral pleural effusion. Villous chromosomal examination resulted in Turner syndrome (45,X).

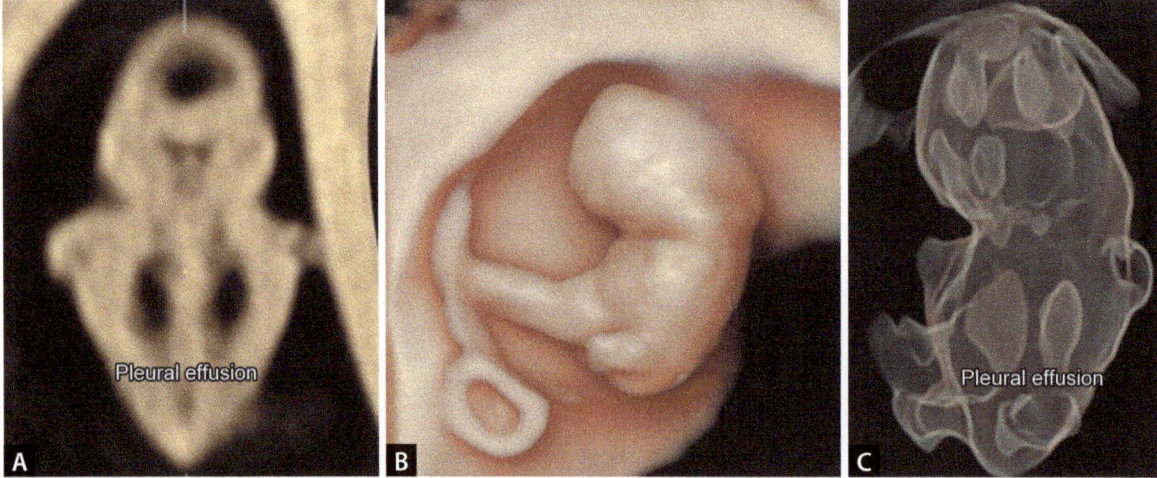

Figs. 3.18A to C: Bilateral pleural effusion at 8 weeks of gestation. (A) Coronal cutting image; (B) Lateral view by high definition imaging; and (C) Oblique view by Silhouette imaging. Note bilateral pleural effusion. Embryonal death was confirmed five days later and villous chromosomal examination resulted in trisomy 15.

CONCLUSION

Recent advances of imaging technologies have greatly contributed to the fields of sonoembryology before the end of 8 weeks. There has been an immense acceleration in understanding early human development. The anatomy and physiology of embryonic development in vivo may open fascinating aspects of embryonic differentiation. In near future, further new findings will be discovered by technological advances. We must recognize *"the embryo as a patient"* as well as "the fetus as a patient".

REFERENCES

1. Smith BR, Huff DS, Johnson GA. Magnetic resonance imaging of embryos: an Internet resource for the study of embryonic development. Comput Med Imaging Graph. 1999;23(1):33-40.
2. Matsuda Y, Utsuzawa S, Kurimoto T, et al. Super-parallel MR microscope. Magn Reson Med. 2003;50(1):183-9.
3. Shiota K, Yamada S, Nakatsu-Komatsu T, et al. Visualization of human prenatal development by magnetic resonance imaging (MRI). Am J Med Genet A. 2007;143A(24):3121-6.
4. Otake Y, Handa S, Kose K, et al. Magnetic resonance microscopy of chemically fixed human embryos at high spatial resolution. Magn Reson Med Sci. 2015;14(2):153-8.
5. Yamada S, Uwabe C, Nakatsu-Komatsu T, et al. Graphic and movie illustrations of human prenatal development and their application to embryological education based on the human embryo specimens in the Kyoto collection. Dev Dyn. 2006;235(2):468-77.
6. Timor-Tritsch IE, Peisner DB, Raju S. Sonoembryology: an organ-oriented approach using a high-frequency vaginal probe. J Clin Ultrasound. 1990;18(4):286-98.
7. Benoit B, Hafner T, Kurjak A, et al. Three-dimensional sonoembryology. J Perinat Med. 2002;30(1):63-73.
8. O'Rahilly R, Muller F. Prenatal ages and stages-measures and errors. Teratology. 2000;61(5):382-4.
9. Pooh RK, Shiota K, Kurjak A. Imaging of the human embryo with magnetic resonance imaging microscopy and high-resolution transvaginal three-dimensional sonography: human embryology in the 21st century. Am J Obstet Gynecol. 2011;204(1):77.
10. Kurjak A, Pooh RK, Merce LT, et al. Structural and functional early human development assessed by three-dimensional and four-dimensional sonography. Fertil Steril. 2005;84(5):1285-99.
11. Bonilla-Musoles F, Raga F, Castillo JC, et al. High definition Real-Time Ultrasound (HDlive) of embryonic and fetal malformations before week 16. Donald School J Ultrasound Obstet Gynecol. 2013;7(1):1-8.
12. Grigore M, Cojocaru C, Lazar T. The role of HD Live Technology in Obstetrics and Gynecology, Present and Future. Donald School J Ultrasound Obstet Gynecol. 2014;8(3):234-8.
13. Kagan KO, Pintoffl K, Hoopmann M. First-trimester ultrasound images using HDlive. Ultrasound Obstet Gynecol. 2011;38(5):607.
14. Hata T, Hanaoka U, Tenkumo C, et al. Three- and four-dimensional HDlive rendering images of normal and abnormal fetuses: pictorial essay. Arch Gynecol Obstet. 2012;286(6):1431-5.
15. Pooh RK, Kurjak A. Novel application of three-dimensional HDlive imaging in prenatal diagnosis from the first trimester. J Perinat Med. 2015;43(2):147-58.
16. Pooh RK. 'See-through Fashion' in Prenatal Diagnostic Imaging. Donald School J Ultrasound Obstet Gynecol. 2015;9(2):111.
17. Pooh RK. Brand new technology of HDlive silhouette and HDlive flow images. In: Pooh RK and Kurjak A (Eds). Donald School Atlas of Advanced Ultrasound in Obstetrics and Gynecology. New Delhi: Jaypee Brothers Medical Publishers Private Limited; 2015. pp. 1-39.
18. Pooh RK. Novel Application of HDlive Silhouette and HDlive Flow - Clinical Significance of the 'See-Through Fashion' in Prenatal Diagnosis. Donald School J Ultrasound Obstet Gynecol. 2016;10(1):90-8.
19. Kurjak A, Zudenigo D, Predanic M, et al. Recent advances in the Doppler study of early fetomaternal circulation. J Perinat Med. 1993;21:419-39.
20. Pooh RK, Aono T. Transvaginal power Doppler angiography of the fetal brain. Ultrasound Obstet Gynecol. 1996;8:417-21.
21. Blaas H-G, Eik-Nes SH, Berg S, et al. In-vivo three-dimensional ultrasound reconstructions of embryos and early fetuses. Lancet. 1998;352:1182-6.
22. Kim MS, Jeanty P, Turner C, et al. Three-dimensional sonographic evaluations of embryonic brain development. J Ultrasound Med. 2008;27:119-24.
23. Hata T, Dai SY, Kanenishi K, et al. Three-dimensional volume-rendered imaging of embryonic brain vesicles using inversion mode. J Obstet Gynaecol Res. 2009;35(2):258-61.
24. Pooh RK. Neurosonoembryology by three-dimensional ultrasound. Semin Fetal Neonatal Med. 2012;17(5):261-8.
25. Jaumiaux E, Gulbis B, Burton GJ. The human first trimester gestational sac limits rather than facilitates oxygen transfer to the foetus-a review. Placenta. 2003;24(17):S86-S93.
26. Kucuk T, Duru NK, Yenen MC, et al. Yolk sac size and shape as predictors of poor pregnancy outcome. J Perinat Med. 1999;27:316-20.
27. Lindsay DJ, Lovett IS, Lyons EA, et al. Yolk sac diameter and shape at endovaginal us: predictors of pregnancy outcome in the first trimester. Radiology. 1992;183:115-8.
28. Hashimoto K, Shimizu T, Fukuda M, et al. Pregnancy outcome of embryonic/fetal pleural effusion in the first trimester. J Ultrasound Med. 2003;22(5):501-5.
29. Kosinski P, Ismail M, Abramowicz JS. Early 2D/3D ultrasound diagnosis of pleural effusion in fetuses with Turner syndrome. J Clin Ultrasound. 2018;46(9):585-7.

CHAPTER 4

Controversies on the Beginning of Human Life

Asim Kurjak, Lara Spalldi Barišić

INTRODUCTION

This golden era of medicine, science, and technology stimulates our endless drive to push medical evolution even more forward. State of the art medicine requires cutting-edge technology used by individuals who continually invest in their knowledge, improve and embrace innovations to improve the quality of patient life.

As mentioned earlier, technology opens a range of possibilities which are all produced by science, but often are still missing adequate evaluation as well as understanding of different alternatives and possible consequences.

Our life is far more richer than it can be illustrated only by science and cannot be always proven through logical deduction. Other insights are necessary to get the whole picture. The views of the great religions certainly must be taken into consideration.

Nowadays, we are witnessing a general increase of interest in the relationship between the science and religion. It is subject of persistent debate and polemic in philosophy and theology.

The dispute is still not ended on question to what extent are religion and science compatible. Over the years, science and religion had to adopt the new findings and required some integration and reinterpretation on their views on certain important subjects. These blending of theory and principle in science and religion will endure in the future.

What is Science and what is Religion?

Following the old Chinese proverb that: *"the path to wisdom begins by calling things by their right names"*, we focus on some common terminology and several definitions. For better understanding of the extent of *science and religion* and their interaction, we have to acknowledge that both are complex and not constant and the interpretation of each has changed through the time and across the different cultures.[1]

The etymological Latin roots of both science (*scientia*) and religion (*religio*), in the ancient and medieval times, were understood as inner qualities of the individual or virtues, rather than actual sources of knowledge.[2]

The term "religion" meaning the belief and worship (controlling power, especially a personal God or Gods). This term was barely used before the 17th century.[1]

The considerably broader meaning and systematically used term for world religions was used by some anthropologist like EB Taylor (1871).

The term "science" has become more common from 19th century and emerged from "natural philosophy" which studied the nature and universe and was antecedent to evolution of modern science.[2-5]

Science differs from the religion in the way that its truth must be experimentally verified and its methodological knowledge can be learned.[6] With other words, there is a hypothesis that has to be tested by experiments and with the gained knowledge, one must form the theories that best apply the observed evidence (evidence based). The theories and all scientific knowledge can be adjusted, added, or even rejected by new insight or evidence.[7]

Religion is dominated by irrational moment and science by rational moment. Intellectual knowledge in science is expressed in the form of mathematical formulas and equations (quantitatively), but religion on the other hand uses the form of metaphors and abstractions (qualitatively).[6,8,9]

The other way of explaining it is that science concerns of natural world and does not use supernatural entities such as Gods, angels, or Karma, whereas religion concerns both natural and supernatural.

Natural philosophers such as Isaac Newton, Robert Hook, Johannes Kepler, and Robert Boyle, preferred the naturalistic explanations but sometimes also appealed to supernatural agents in their natural philosophy (now known as science). Later on there where others, like T Huxley and friends (1864) who tried to promote a science that would be free from religious dogmas.[5]

Albert Einstein (1940)[10] states in his book on religion and science: "For science can only ascertain what is, but not what should be, and outside of its domain value judgments of all kinds remain necessary. Religion, on the other hand, deals only with evaluations of human thought and action; it cannot justifiably speak of facts and relationships between facts".[10]

"Now, even though the realms of religion and science in themselves are clearly marked off from each other, nevertheless there exist between the two strong reciprocal relationships and dependencies. Though religion may be that which determine the goals, it has, nevertheless, learned from science, in the broadest sense, what means will contribute to the attainment of the goals it has setup".[10]

A systematic study of science and religion started in the 1960s. Until than, predominant view was that science and religion were either in fight against each other or indifferent to each other. Barbour (1966)[11] and Torrance (1969)[12] try to argue on this by comparing the methodology and theory in both fields. Since that time, science and religion is recognized field of study. The first specialist journal on science and religion was founded and published in 1966 by the name: *Zygon*.

Speaking in general about "science" and "religion" and discussing their interference and relationship in general may be pointless since the "science and religion" try to ignore the definitions. Kelly Clark (2014)[13,14] proposes that we can only sensibly inquire into relationship between a widely accepted claim of science (quantum mechanics or findings in neuroscience) with the specific claim of particular religion (such as Islamic understanding of divine providence or Buddhist views of the no-self).[5] In the modern public circles, the most dominant debate between science and religion involve *the evolutionary theory and creationism—intelligent design*.[5]

In the last several decades, conciliatory public statement has been issued by the Church leaders on *the statement on evolutionary theory*. Pope John Paul II (1996) affirmed the evolutionary theory in his message to the Pontifical Academy of Sciences. However, he rejected it from the "human soul", which he saw as the result of a separate, special creation.[5]

As noted, up until recently, most studies and investigation on the relationship between science and religion have focused mainly on Christian religion and tradition. Nowadays, we investigate all other non-Christian traditions and religions such as Judaism, Hinduism, Buddhism, and Islam contributing on the richer picture of interactions.

SCIENCE AND RELIGION: MODELS OF THE INTERACTION

According to Stenmark[1] characterizing the relationship between science and religion, we can identify three different views:
1. *The independence view*: There is no overlap between science and religion
2. *The contact view*: There is some overlap between the fields of science and religion. This one can be further subdivided into conflict or harmony
3. The union of domains of science and religion.

According to Barbour[15] (2000), most widely accepted, the best model of the interaction of science and religion is:

- *The Independence model*: Science and religions explore different domains and ask distinct questions. In the SJ Gould model with his nonoverlapping magisteria *(NOMA) principle* he states that: the lack of conflict between science and religion arises from the lack of overlap between their respective domains of professional expertise[16]
- *The Conflict model*: Science and religion are in principal and everlasting conflict. This relays on two historical narratives: (1) *the Trial of Galileo*[17] and (2) *the Reception of Darwinism*.[18] The conflict is found because they discuss the same domain

    This model is in contemporary spheres present in minority. The majority of authors believe that this model relies on a shallow and biased reading of the historical record[5]
- *The Dialogue model*: Science and religion have mutual relationship. Even though these two fields stay separate, they communicate. There is a common ground in both fields, mainly in their belief (theories), methods, and concepts. In this context, science and religion can be in graceful duet according to their epistemological overlaps[19]
- *The Integration model*: More extensive unification of science and theology.

THE SCIENTIFIC STUDY OF THE SCIENCE AND RELIGION

Throughout history, science and religion are even more investigated in the "scientific study of the religion" which can be traced back to the 17th century. In the 19th and early 20th centuries, some of the authors focused on newly emerging scientific disciplines (anthropology, sociology, and psychology) and tried to investigate and explain diverse religious beliefs across cultures.[5]

Divergence of the assumptions is colorful. For example, the sociologist Émile Durkheim (1915)[20] considered "religious beliefs as social glue" that helped to keep society together. Sigmund Freud (1927),[21] a psychologist, known on his bizarre explanations, saw "religious belief as an illusion", a child-like yearning for a fatherly figure. These two authors along with the Karl Marx and Max Weber proposed the version of secularization thesis in which the religion would decline in the face of modern technology, science, and culture. Later on, several authors stated that the religious beliefs were more diverse than was previously assumed.[5]

The contemporary advancements in the scientific study of religion are *the cognitive science of religion*. This includes multidisciplinary fields, among others, developmental psychology, anthropology, philosophy, and cognitive psychology.[5]

ACADEMIA AND RELIGIOUS BELIEFS

Up to the 19th and early 20th century, it was very prevalent for the scientist to have religious beliefs which guided their work. Natural philosopher Isaac Newton held his strong somewhat unorthodox beliefs.

On contrary, modern scientists are less religious in comparison to the general population. Prominent exception to this statement is geneticist, Francis Collins, former leader of *the Human Genome Project*. In his book: "The Language of God" (2006)[22] and the BioLogos Institute, he presents and advocates compatibility between science and Christianity.

Atheism and agnosticism are widespread among the academics, even more among those working in elite institutions. However, the most recent findings indicate that academics are not opposed to religion and are more religiously diverse than has been popularly assumed.

It remains still unclear whether religious beliefs and scientific views are cognitively incompatible.

There are studies that suggest that religion draws more upon an intuitive style of thinking, which is well-defined from the analytic reasoning style characterized by science.[23]

THE DEFINITION OF "LIFE"

There is no straightforward answer to the everlasting question of how to define the life.

Answer is rather complex and needs multidisciplinary approach from different fields such as biology, theology, philosophy, sociology, law, and politics. They all give their view from different perspectives to form useful answer.

There are authors that argue that "life" as such does not exist, because no one has ever seen it. According to them, the noun "life" has no significance, there is no such thing as "life" says Szent-György.[24]

When trying to define life, we should take into consideration also the facts what life might have been in the past in its primordial form to the extent how life evaluated so far today and speculate to what life could develop in the future. What we do know until now mainly thanking to incredible revolution in science, anthropology, and technology. The most popular theory of our universe's origin—The Big Bang Theory—centers on a cosmic cataclysm unmatched in all of history.[25]

This theory reflects the observation that other galaxies are moving away from the earth at great speed and in all directions, as if they had all been propelled by an ancient explosive force. The oldest known planet in the Milky Way, the ancient planet is thought to be about 13 billion years old, more than twice as old as earth and a mere billion years younger than the estimated age of the universe.[25] However, some philosophers debate and argue against this interpretation that universe has a temporal beginning.[26]

The Big Bang Theory was first suggested by the Belgian priest G Lemaître in the 1920s when he theorized that the universe began from a single primordial atom.[25] Several questions are still not answered. Why "the big bang" happened? What exactly happened after "the big bang" is still unknown. Scientist propose and believe that as time passed and matter cooled, more diverse kinds of atoms began to form, and they eventually condensed into the stars and galaxies of our present universe.[25]

All present forms of life appear as something completely new. *Life*, then, is transferred and not conceived in each new generation. *The phenomenon of "life" has existed on the earth around 3.5 billion years old, as estimated*.[25] Having this in mind, although the genome of a new embryo is unique, the makeup of an embryo is not new. If "life" is observed through the cell, consequently, every life, also this one of human, is considered as continuum. Human cells and mankind have existed on earth since the appearance of the first man. Opposite to this, if "life" is observed as single human being or the present population, the statement that "human life is a continuum" is not acceptable.[6,8,9,24,27]

Life, in a true sense of the word, begins when the chemical matter gives rise, in a specific way, to an autonomous, self-regulating, and self-reproducing system. Life is connected with a living being, and it creates its own system as an indivisible whole—it forms its individuality. One of the most important characteristics of living beings is reproduction. *Reproduction* means creating a new life by transferring forms of an old one into newly formed human being. Therefore, variability, individual development, and harmony characterize human beings. *Individuality* is the most essential characteristic of human beings consisting of new life, but also all human life forms through evolution, characterized by phenotype, behavior, and the capability to recognize and adapt. Human embryo and fetus gradually develop into these characteristics.[28-30]

"Human life" poses a semantic problem. The placenta is "human life", as is every individual cell or organ of the human body, but "human life" is clearly not equivalent to "human being". It is, therefore, mandatory to differentiate between organic or vegetative human life and "potential personal human life". The latter term allows various groups to identify a point of the continuum between abortion and birth to which they can ascribe appropriate values and rights.[31]

Although we should not forget that in the same way today's research is tomorrow's benefit,[32] concerning human life, conclusions should not be treated one-sidedly from one perspective. This reality should be regarded in all its richness: the embryo gives the biologist and geneticist substance for consideration, but talking about the beginning of a human life requires philosophical/anthropological consideration, as well as theological and social sciences. In its protection, we have to include ethics and law. This approach leads to the conclusion that it is necessary to reject reductionism as well as integration, and to find a "golden middle" between these two methodologies.[30]

To have a good and lucid debate, even polemic, it is necessary to identify precisely what are the key questions that require a multidisciplinary approach, considering biology, anthropology, ethics, and other fields.[33]

What is Biological Point of View?

Biology characterizes human beings by the dynamics of the system and its self-control (homeostasis), excitability (response to stimuli of different nature and origins), self-reproducibility, the heredity of the characters, and the evolutionary trend.[30] For biologists, it is important to specify which form of life phenomena we are referring to: cell, organism, population, or species.

The basic level of organization and the simplest form of life is the cell. Biologically speaking, human cellular life never stops or if it did, the extinction of the human species would result and is passed on from one generation to another. Human individual organismic life is defined within its life cycle, which is temporarily limited, i.e. it has a beginning and an end.[34,35] It is obvious that life is a highly dynamic phenomenon that could be described and explained through the careful study of life processes and interactions by interdisciplinary approach. In human, spermatozoa and oocyte are two essential cells involved in creating human life (Figs. 4.1 and 4.2). It is clear that

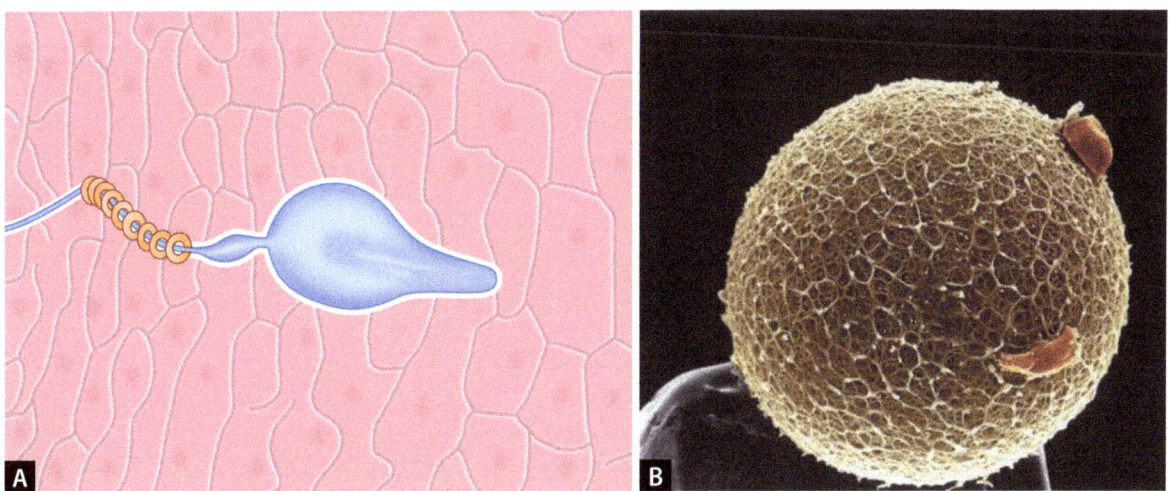

Figs. 4.1A and B: Schematic presentation of spermatozoa and oocyte.[8]

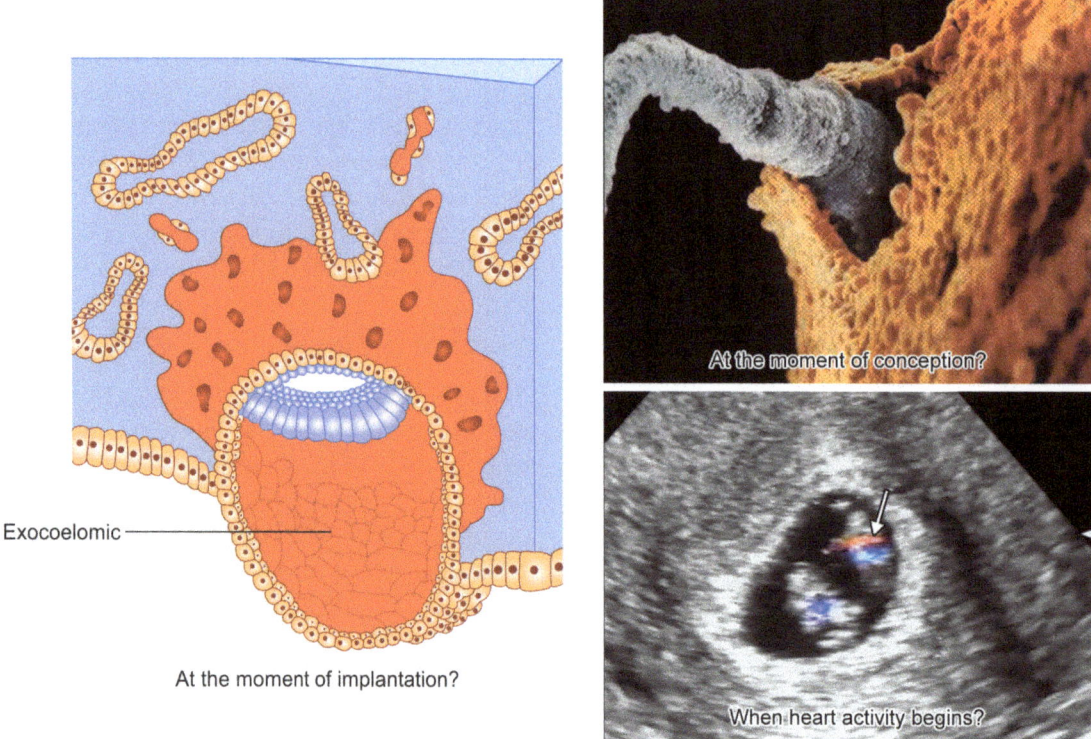

Fig. 4.2: Some possible questions on the beginning of human life.

biologists are most qualified to render judgment on the structure and function of cells. To quote Scarpelli,[36] the very broad scope of biological science (from molecular to behavioral biology, and from unicellular to multisystem forms) brings with it the justifiable understanding that the biological scientist knows and is able to define the state of being alive or "life". If not, the science fails.

The biological scientist, who may specialize within one or another domain of the broad scope, has particular and definitive knowledge and understanding of the living individual that is his specialty. If not, disorder will rise above failure.

Understanding of the beginning of human life and development of the embryo/fetus could provide definitive resolution. However, with the recent possibility of visualizing early human development virtually from conception, perinatologists should be those who by study, training, practice, and research are singularly qualified.[37]

While science provides us data about physical development of the human being, it does not provide information about its personality and personhood. These are philosophical, rather than scientific topics.

THE FACTS OF HUMAN EMBRYOGENESIS

The first reports ever recorded on the subject of *embryology* date back to the 5th century BC in the books of Hippocrates who studied the incubated chicken eggs. He noted that the nature of the bird can be likened to that of the man. Aristotle studied, a century later, a chick and other embryos and assumed incorrectly that they arose from the menstrual blood in combination with the semen. Later on in 1677, with the help of microscopes, Hamm and Leeuwenhoek observed spermatozoa, and thought that they contained miniature humans. It was not known until the Spallanzani showed in 1775 that both oocyte and the sperm were necessary to create a human.

Finally, in the focus of *the cell theory* developed in 1839 by Schleiden and Schwann, it was stated that the embryo develops from the single-celled zygote.[37-39]

According to Moore (1974),[39] development is continuous process that begins when ovum is fertilized by the sperm and it ends at death. In 2008, he added that development does not end by the birth but extends into early adulthood.[40]

Only proper understanding of the process of human embryogenesis enables answering scientifically the question of when the life cycle of a human individual starts. Therefore, in the following text, the main steps of the human developmental process are going to be briefly described, primarily during the first 15 days following fertilization.

A human being originates from two living cells: (1) *the oocyte and* (2) *the spermatozoon*, transmitting the torch of life to the next generation. The oocyte is a cell approximately 120 μm in diameter with a thick membrane, known as *the zona pellucida*. The spermatozoon moves, using the flagellum or tail, and the total length of the spermatozoon including the tail is 60 μm.[12]

Fertilization is the term which represents the initiation of life of a new human individual. This is an event that happens over the time and it starts when the ovum is penetrated by an spermatozoid.[33]

"Human development begins at fertilization, when a sperm fuses with an oocyte to form a single cell, the zygote. This highly specialized, totipotent cell (capable of giving rise to any cell type) marks the beginning of each of us as a unique individual."[40]

"All of us were once human embryos, so the study of human embryology is the study of our own prenatal origins and experiences."[41]

"Fertilization, the uniting of egg and sperm, takes place in the oviduct. After the oocyte finishes meiosis, the paternal and maternal chromosomes come together, resulting in the formation of a zygote containing a single diploid nucleus. Embryonic development is considered to begin at this point".[41]

Some embryologists consider the fertilization a 24-hour process. During this period, the cell membranes of a sperm and the ovum fuse together and the first cell division occurs.[33,42]

So, during these 24 hours, when does a new human life begin?

- During this first 24 hours, once the sperm and the ovum bind to each other and their membranes fuse, they create a *single hybrid cell: the zygote: one-cell embryo*.[43,44]
- To protect his/her body integrity, within the minutes, the zygote initiates changes in its ionic composition, releasing zinc in a spark that induces "ovum activation"—modifying the surrounding zona pellucida blocking further sperms to bind to the cell surface.
- Cooperation between sperm and the egg—achieve replication of DNA, cell division, and growth.[42]

Regarding the beginning of human, life as occurring around the end of this process (of 24 hours) is called syngamy.[38,40,45] *There are also others who believe that fusion of the cell membrane is the process of syngamy—the nuclear membranes of the pronuclei break down.*

After *syngamy*, the zygote undergoes mitotic cell division as it moves down the fallopian tube toward the uterus. A series of mitotic divisions then leads to the development of the pre-embryo. The newly divided cells are called *blastomeres*. From 1–3 days after syngamy, there is a division into two cells, then four cells. Blastomeres form cellular aggregates of distinct, totipotent, and undifferentiated cells that, during several early cell divisions, retain the capacity to develop independently into normal *pre-embryos*. As the blastocyst is in the process of attaching to the uterine wall, the cells increase in number and organize into two layers of cells. Implantation progresses as the outer cell layer of the blastocyst, the trophectoderm, invades the uterine wall and erodes blood vessels and glands. Having begun 5 or more days after fertilization with the attachment of the blastocyst to the endometrial lining of the uterus, implantation is completed when the blastocyst is fully embedded in the endometrium several days later. Even during these 5-6 days, modern medicine introduces the possibility of making preimplantation genetic diagnosis.[46,47] However, at this time, these cells are not yet totally differentiated in terms of their determination to specific cells or organs of the embryo.

The term pre-embryo, then, includes the developmental stages from the first cell division of the zygote through the morula and the blastocyst.

By approximately the 14th day after the end of the process of fertilization, all cells, depending on their position, will have become parts of the placenta and membranes or the embryo.

The embryo stage, therefore, begins approximately 16 days after the beginning of the fertilization process and continues until the end of 8 weeks after fertilization, when organogenesis is complete.[46]

The pre-embryo is the structure that exists from the end of the process of fertilization until the appearance of a single primitive streak. Until the completion of implantation, the pre-embryo is capable of dividing into multiple entities, but does not contain enough genetic information to develop into an embryo, it lacks of genetic material from maternal mitochondria and of maternal and parental genetic messages in the form of messenger RNA or proteins.

Therefore, during the pre-embryonic period, it has not yet been determined with certainty that a biological individual will result, or would be one or more (identical twins forming), so that the assignment of the full rights of an individual human person is inconsistent with biological reality.

One conclusion from this is that the pre-embryo requires the establishment of special rules in the society: it cannot claim absolute protection based on claims of personhood; although meriting respect, it does not have the same moral value that a human person has.

Today, one largely accepted opinion is that until the 14th day from fertilization or at least, until implantation—the human embryo may not be considered, from the ontological point of view, as an individual.

Genetic uniqueness and singleness coincide only after implantation and restriction have completed, which is about 3 weeks after fertilization.

Until that period, the zygote and its squeal are in a fluid process, are not physical individual, and therefore, cannot be a person.

It is well-known that high percentages of oocytes which have been penetrated never proceed on to further development, and that many oocytes which do, are thwarted so early in their development that their presence is not even recognized. It is suggested that 30% of conceptions detected by positive reactions to human chorionic gonadotropin (hCG) tests abort spontaneously before these pregnancies are clinically verified.

The newly conceived pre-embryo presents itself as a biologically defined reality. However, the status of the pre-embryo as an individual remains a great mystery. In the present scientific scene especially with the progress of ultrasound technologies, prenatal psychology and therapeutics opened a window into prenatal life of embryo and fetus confirming the evidence that the embryo/fetus is a true subject itself.[48,49]

INFLUENCE OF THE GENETICS AND EPIGENETICS

The work of Mendel concerning inheritance of maternal and paternal characteristics through the chromosomes and the discoveries of nucleus are the milestone in the history of human genetics.[33]

In the past several years, we became aware and found the secrets of human molecular basis of life and hereditary.

As we all know *the genome*: is the content of genetic material present in each human cell. It is made of molecular structure of the double helix DNA.[50] Each string of double strand of DNA is formed by subunits called nucleotides.

DNA is a simple but fascinating molecule that contains all the genetic information of an organism. This genetic information is hidden in specific particular order of the nucleotides in the DNA.

Human genome contains the nuclear and the mitochondrial genome.[33]

The nuclear genome is distributed over 46 human chromosomes, has approximately 25,000 genes and 3.2 billion nucleotides.[33]

The Human Genome Project recently provided us with the information about the sequencing of the whole *nuclear genome* and more than 21,000 genes of known functions (www.ornl.gov). The *mitochondrial genome*, which is found in the cytoplasm with the mitochondrion (energy forces), is much small (37 genes and 16,000 nucleotides) and is transmitted by the mother through the ovum.[33]

"As representatives of the 60 trillion cells that make a human body, a sperm and an egg meet, recognize each other, and fuse to create a new generation".

There are factors not found in the genes that are quite capable of interfering with the gene expression and function. These factors can come from within the organism or from the external environment. We call them *epigenetic factors*.

To conclude, the development of a new individual is a complex process in which both genetic and epigenetic factors intervene.[51]

Genotype (Genome + Epigenome) + Environment result in making *phenotype*.[52]

PERSONALITY

Defining personality is very complex. There is still no clear definition of personality. One dictionary offers "what constitutes an individual as distinct person", but does not define what the "what" is. Another dictionary asserts "the state of existing as a thinking intelligent being". This definition might lead to the inference that personality increases pro rata with intelligence, or that some people may not have a personality at all if we followed Bertrand

Russell's dictum that *"most people would rather die than think and many, in fact, do"*. Kenneth Stallworthy's Manual of Psychiatry is more helpful with the definition that *"personality is the individual as a whole with everything about him which makes him different from other people"*, because we can certainly distinguish fetuses from each other and from other people. With the next sentence—*"personality is determined by what is born in the individual in the first place and by everything which subsequently happens to him in the second"*—we are really in the field.[30,31]

Viewpoints on the nature of "personhood" and what it means ethically and legally varies widely. In his proposed Life Protection Act, Sass[53] acknowledges that a fetus with formed synapses is not a "person" in the usual sense of the word, connoting consciousness and self-consciousness.[53] Veatch sees the problem as defining the life that has full moral standing,[54] while Knutson[55] has noted that "those who employ spiritual or religious definitions of when life begins tend to place the beginning of life earlier than those who employ psychological, sociological, or cultural definitions".

Led by the truism, *"no insignificant person was ever born"*,[56] human beings should be valued from birth to natural death. It is hard to establish proper values and exact definitions. This becomes especially problematic when prenatal life is considered. The earlier stated truism opens an important question: "Is the person-unborn a person in the first place and, if so, is the person-unborn a "significant" person?"[30]

Let us evaluate further present controversies. There is no doubt that the embryo and fetus in utero are biologically human individuals prior to birth. The child who is born is the same developing human individual that was in the mother's womb. Birth alone cannot confer natural personhood or human individuality. This is confirmed by preterm deliveries of babies who are as truly human and almost as viable as those whose gestation goes to full term. All the known evidence supports the human fetus being a true ontological human individual and consequently a human person in fact, if not in law. A human person cannot begin before the appropriate brain structures are developed that are capable of sustaining awareness. The same applies to a grossly malformed fetus. It would still be a human individual even if its human nature was not perfect or its functions quite normal.

Nobody questions the humanity of a Down syndrome fetus or child. A fetus or child with severe open spina bifida is not less of a human being. The same should be said for the live anencephalic fetus or infant with only brainstem functions. It is a human individual even if it lacks a complete brain and usually survives birth by only a few hours or a day.[57,58]

"Person" and "personhood" are the legally operational terms in the United States and many other countries. Alternatively, "person" and "personhood" are replaced by terms such as "viable outside the uterus", "a woman's right to privacy", and "a woman's right to choose". In each case, viable, privacy, and choice, the life-support provider may legally order transfer of the dependent individual into a morbid environment. For this group, dilemma (which includes the stem cell, abortion, and cloning debates) is abated, but not resolved.[31]

Human society created several standards in defining "person" or "human being" based on what is familiar and easy recognizable.[30] For example, a human speaks, understands, and laughs. Absence of these characteristics (mutism, autism, and stoicism) does not disqualify. To the contrary, the conclusion is that the characteristics we have come to associate with being a person may not be applicable to each individual person. Therefore, it is necessary to establish criteria for a definition of "person" in society and in time (Figs. 4.3 and 4.4). Some prominent Italian professors[48] committed themselves to caring for the embryo in such a way, giving the same dignity to every patient, and the human conditions to grow and develop, to educate others inside and outside the specialty, and to carry out research involving all the components of society.

EMBRYO AS A PATIENT

Bioethical Aspects

The idea of the embryo/fetus as a miniaturized infant or adult is true to the extent that the embryonic/fetal physiologist must be able to apply knowledge of every system after birth, yet quite untrue in failing to recognize the many ways in which life before birth differs fundamentally from life after birth.[6,32] The newly conceived form presents itself as the biologically defined reality: it is an individual that is completely human in development that autonomously, moment by moment without any discontinuity, actualized its proper form in order to realize through intrinsic activity, and a design present in its own genome (Figs. 4.5 to 4.10).[48]

The embryo as a patient is best understood as the subset of the concept of the fetus as the patient. These

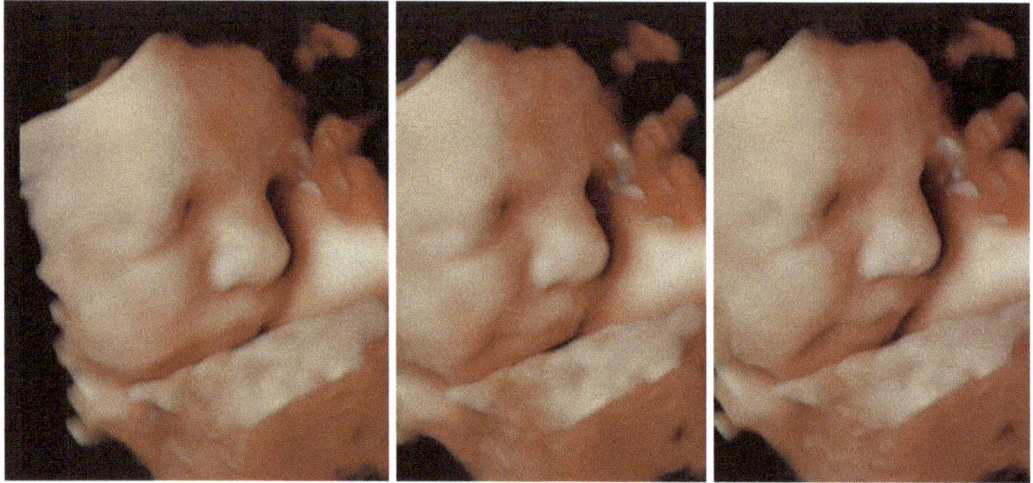

Fig. 4.3: When do we become a person?

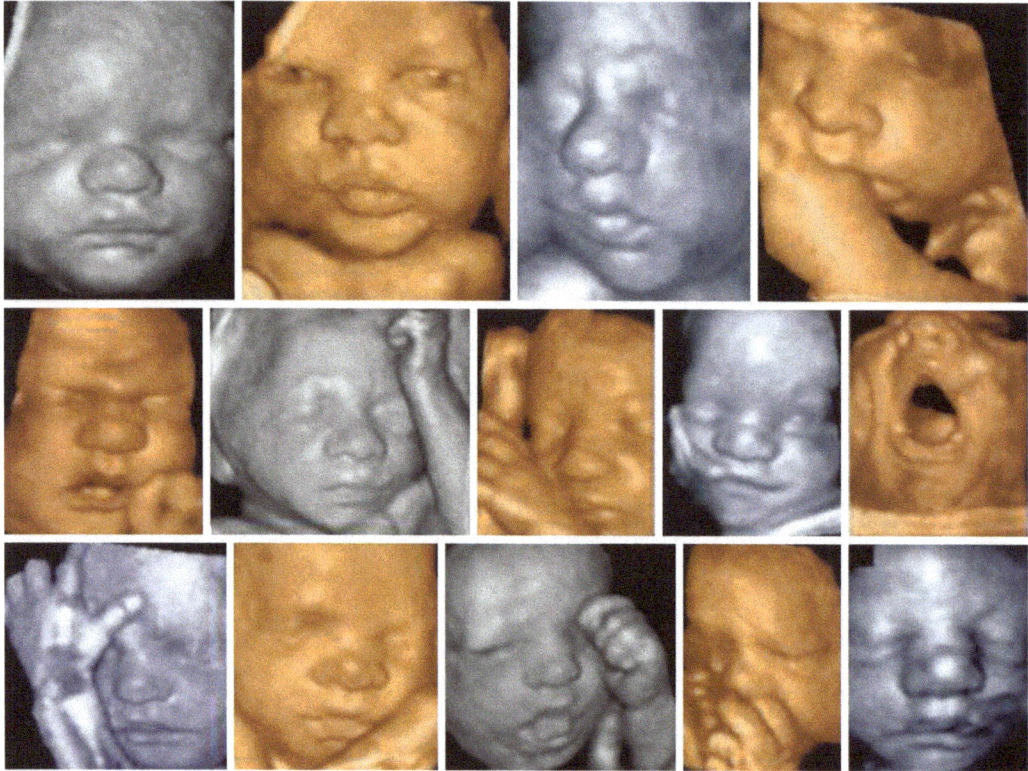

Fig. 4.4: Different behavioral patterns of the fetuses in second half of pregnancy. Are they different personalities?[8]

two concepts opened a whole set of questions regarding ethical problems. The embryo as the patient is indivisible from its mother. However, balance is needed in protecting the interests of the embryo/fetus and the mother. One prominent approach to understanding the concept of the embryo/fetus as a patient has involved attempts to show whether or not the embryo/fetus has independent moral status, or personhood.[59-61] Independent moral status for the fetus would mean that one or more of the characteristics possessed either in, or of the embryo/fetus itself, and, therefore, independently of the pregnant woman or any other factor, generate, and, therefore, ground obligations

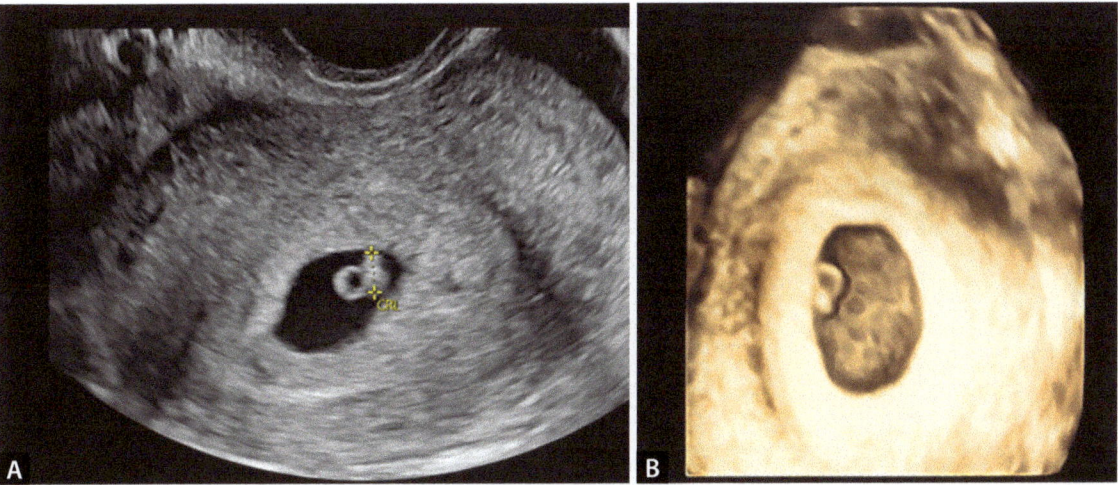

Figs. 4.5A and B: (A) Two-dimensional (2D) transvaginal sonography of the 6 weeks embryo with the yolk sac in utero; and (B) Three-dimensional (3D) transvaginal sonography of the same fetus as in the previous picture. The embryo and the yolk sac are visible.

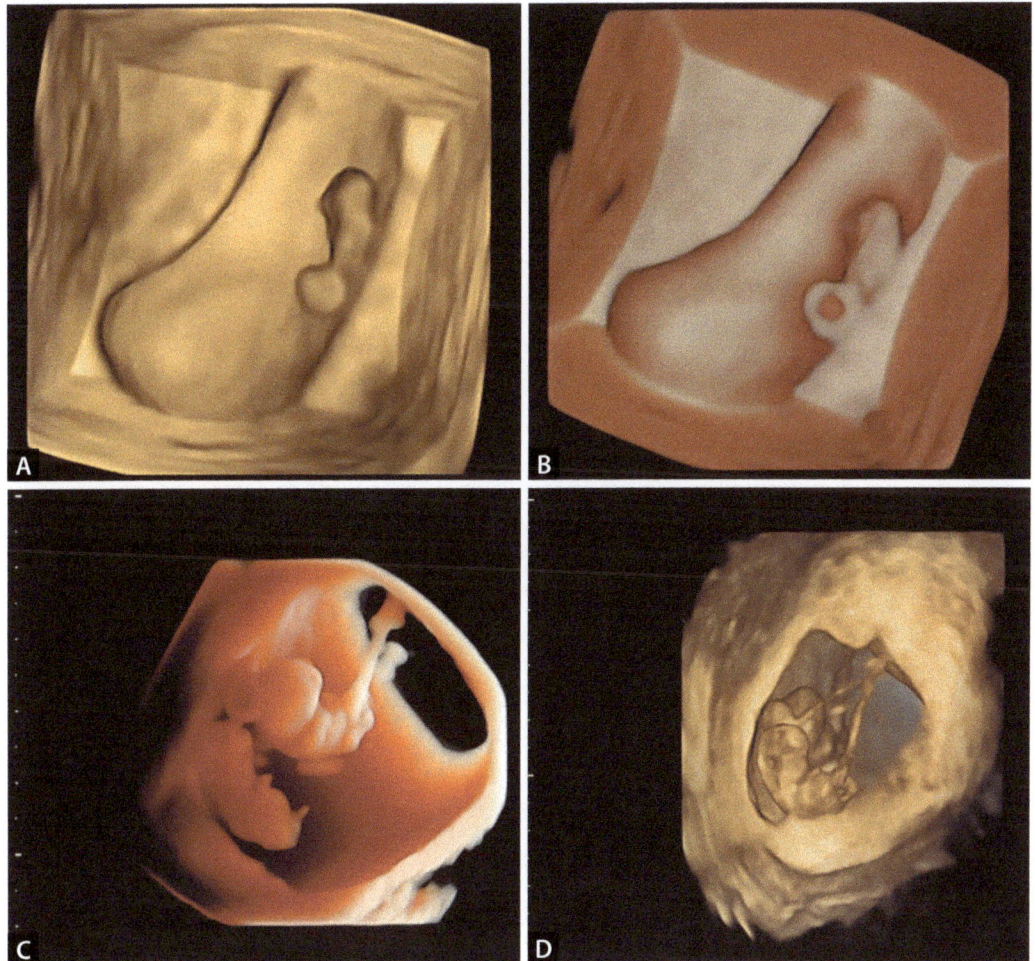

Figs. 4.6A to D: 7 weeks and 2 days of gestation. With the three-dimensional (3D) ultrasound imaging: (A) Surface; (B) HDlive rendering modes used to visualize the gestational sac in the utero, within the sac, there is embryo and the yolk sac; (C) 9 weeks and 4 days old twins gestation visualized by 3D HDlive rendering sonography; (D) 9 weeks and 4 days old twins gestation visualized by 3D surface mode rendering sonography (notice clearly visible two embryo's, umbilical cords, and yolk sac).

to the embryo/fetus on the part of the pregnant woman and her physician.

A wide range of intrinsic characteristics has been considered for this role, e.g. moment of conception, implantation, central nervous system development, quickening, and the moment of birth.[62] Given the variability of proposed characteristics, there are many views about when the embryo/fetus does or does not acquire independent moral status.

Some take the view that the embryo/fetus possesses independent moral status from the moment of conception or implantation. Others believe that the embryo/fetus acquires independent moral status in degrees, thus resulting in "graded" moral status. Still others hold, at least implicitly, that the embryo/fetus never has independent moral status so long as it is in utero.[61]

Being a patient does not require that one possesses independent moral status.[63]

Being a patient means that one can benefit from the application of the clinical skills of the physician.[64] Put more precisely, a human being without independent moral status is properly regarded as a patient when the following conditions are met: that a human being is presented to the physician for the purpose of applying clinical interventions that are reliably expected to be efficacious, in that they are reliably expected to result in a greater balance of goods over harms in the future of the human being in question.[62]

In other words, an individual is considered a patient when a physician has beneficence-based ethical obligations to that individual.

To clarify the concept of the embryo/fetus as the patient, beneficence-based obligation is necessary to be provided. *Beneficence-based obligations to the fetus and embryo exist when the fetus can later achieve independent moral status.*[64] This leads to the conclusion that ethical significance of the unborn child is in direct link with the child to be born—the child, it can become.

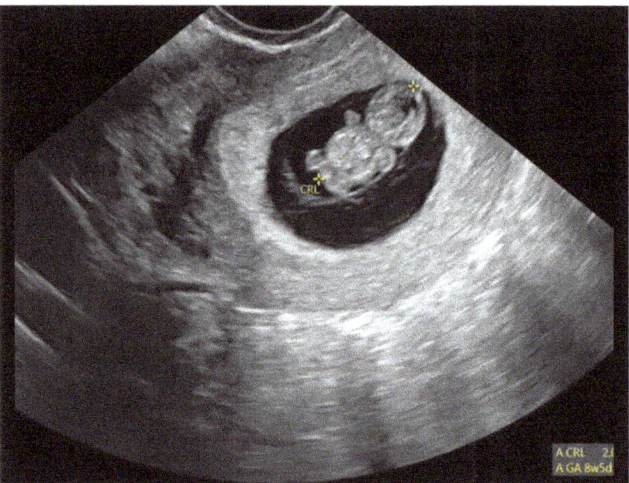

Fig. 4.7: Two-dimensional (2D) transvaginal sonography of the 8 weeks and 5 days old embryo (almost at the end of the embryonic period), with clearly visible head, body, and the limbs. Thin lines of the amniotic sac are visible around the embryo.

LEGAL STATUS OF THE EMBRYO

When discussing law, it should be always kept in mind that medicine is international, but law is not. Before the era of Aristotle, who taught that human life begins when

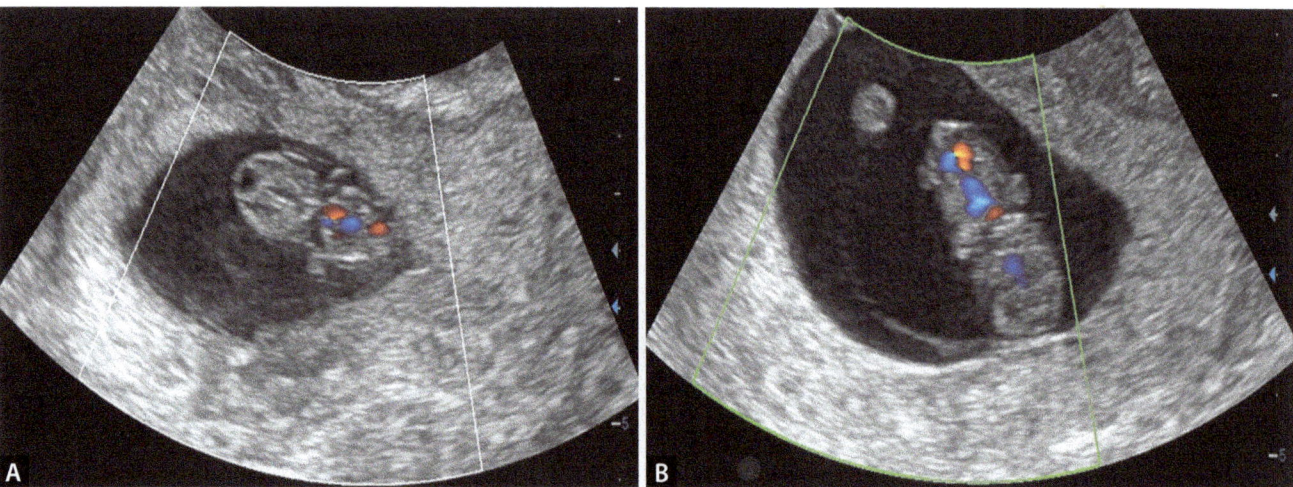

Figs. 4.8A and B: (A) Two-dimensional image with the color Doppler visualization of embryonic circulation at the 7th week of gestation; and (B) The same technique used by embryo at the 8 weeks and 5 days of gestation with clearly depicted brain circulation.

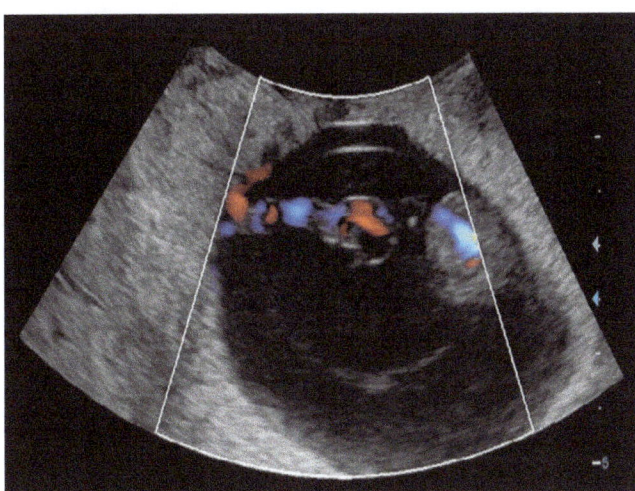

Fig. 4.9: Early visualization (9 weeks) of the circulation within the umbilical cord connecting the both ends; at the left side is the fetal part and at the right side is the placental side.

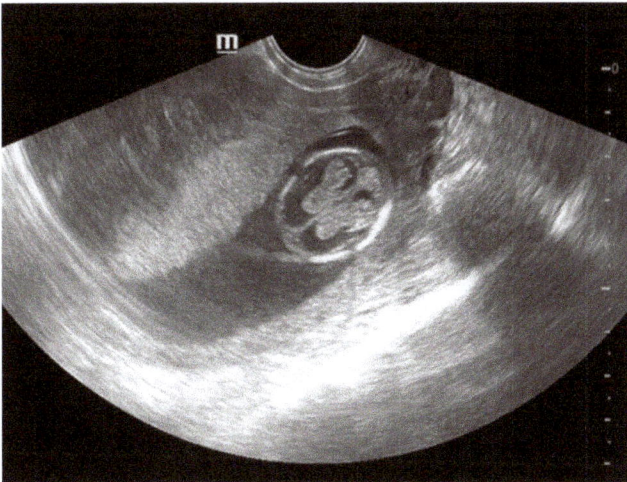

Fig. 4.10: Two-dimensional transvaginal imaging. Axial plane view of the fetal head at the 12 weeks and 5 days, within the skull hyperechoic structure: choroid plexus with typical shape, also called "butterfly sign".

the fetus is formed, human life was considered to begin at birth. Prior to birth, the fetus was not an independent human being but, like an organ, part of the mother.[65] Thus, the birth of a full-term infant has been used in the laws of various countries to signify the beginning of the human life that is to be protected.

Indeed, the status of the human embryo is not juridically defined and relies on the political, social, and religious influences in each country. Interestingly, nearly all countries of the Western world use the 12th week of pregnancy as the limit for legal abortion. It is not the end of the 1st trimester, which is 13.3 weeks, and there is no other particular biological event to justify this limit.

It is hard to answer the question when human life should be legally protected. At the time of conception? At the time of implantation? At the time of birth? In all countries (except Ireland and Liechtenstein), *juridical considerations are based on Roman law. Roman civil law says that the fetus has rights when it is born or if it is born nasciturus.*

Few countries agree with the definition of the beginning of human personality at the time of conception. The majority does not grant legal status to the human embryo in vitro (i.e. during the 14 days after fertilization). Thus, even in the absence of legal rights, there is no denying that the embryo constitutes the beginning of human life, a member of the human family. Therefore, whatever the attitude, every country has to examine which practices are compatible with the respect of that dignity and the security of human genetic material.[66]

ARGUMENTS FOR BEGINNING OF HUMAN LIFE AND HUMAN PERSON AT FERTILIZATION

The fundamental approaches of biomedical and social (secular) practice must begin with the understanding that the subject before birth is a person and that "personhood" is conferred by successful fertilization of the egg. To hide from this in silence or ignorance should be unacceptable to all, as stressed by Scarpelli.[67]

The view that human life begins when sperm and eggs fuse to give rise to a single cell-human zygote, whose genetic individuality and uniqueness remain unchanged during normal development, is widely supported. Because the zygote has the capacity to become an adult human individual, it is thought it must be one already. The same zygote organizes itself into an embryo, a fetus, a child, and an adult. By this account, the zygote is an actual human individual and not simply a potential one, in much the same way as an infant is an actual human person with potential to develop to maturity and not just a potential person. As Scarpelli[67] pointed out, outside the realm of religious dogma, there has been no one whose existence can be traced back to any entity other than the fertilized egg. The biological line of existence of each individual, without exception, begins precisely when fertilization of the egg is successful.[67]

The process of fertilization actually begins with conditioning of the spermatozoon in the male and female reproductive tracts. Thereafter, fertilization involves not only the egg itself, but also the various investments which surround the egg at the time it is released from the ovary or follicle.

Fertilization, therefore, is not an event, but a complex biochemical process requiring a minimum of 24 hours to complete syngamy, that is the formation of a diploid set of chromosomes.

During this process, there is no commingling of maternal and paternal chromosomes within a single nuclear membrane (prezygote); after this process, the parental chromosomes material is commingled (zygote).

Among the many other activities of this new cell, most important is the recognition of the new genome, which represents the principal information center for the development of the new human being and for all its further activities. For the better understanding of the very nature of the zygote, two main features are to be at least mentioned here.

The first feature is that the zygote exists and operates from syngamy on as a being, ontologically one, and with a precise identity.

The second feature is that the zygote is intrinsically oriented and determined to a definite development. Both identity and orientation are due essentially to the genetic information with which it is endowed.

That is why many do believe that this cell represents the exact point in time and space where a new human individual organism initiates its own life cycle.[30]

ARGUMENTS AGAINST THE BEGINNING OF HUMAN LIFE AT FERTILIZATION

Today, one largely accepted opinion is that until the 14th day from fertilization or at least, until implantation—the human embryo may not be considered, from the ontological point of view, as an individual. There are at least five main reasons in favor of this opinion:

1. *Before the formation of the embryonic disk, the embryo is* "a mass of cells, genetically human", "a cluster of distinct individual cells", which are each "distinct ontological entities in simple contact with the others".[68] The genetically unique, newly developed DNA, a genome, is not established until 48 hours after sperm penetration. The ovum and sperm lie side-by-side for more than 48 hours before they finally merge. In biological terms, this renders conception as a process that occurs overtime and not a specific point in time.[31]
2. Until approximately the 14th day after fertilization, all that happens is simply a preparation of the protective and nutritional systems required for the future needs of the embryo. *Only when the entity called embryonic disk is formed, the embryo develops into a fetus.*[69]
3. *The monozygotic twin phenomenon or chimeras can occur*. In fact, this seems to be the strongest reason why the embryo is denied the quality of individuality, and as a proof that the zygote cannot be an ontologically human being. In approximately one-third of cases, the embryo divides at about the two cells stage, and in the other two-thirds, the inner cell mass divides within the blastocyst from day 38. Occasionally, the division takes place from day 8 to day 12, but usually it is not complete, thereby forming conjoined identical twins or two-headed individuals. *The chimera*, resulting from the recombination of two individual to become one individual (and detectable through genetic testing), provides another argument against the equivalence of conception and the beginning of human life: no individuum has died, yet one has ceased to exist.
4. *Coexistence of the embryo with its mother is a necessary condition* for an embryo belonging to the human species, and this condition can be obtained only at implantation.[61] However, there is evidence that development of a human embryo in vitro can continue well beyond the stage of implantation, and that mouse embryos implanted under the male renal capsule can reach the fetal stage. It is also argued, or at least implied, that so many human embryos die before or after implantation that it would be lacking in realism to accept that the human individual begins before implantation.

It is well-known that high percentages of oocytes which have been penetrated never proceed on to further development, and that many oocytes which do, are thwarted so early in their development that their presence is not even recognized. Up to 50% of ovulated eggs and zygotes recovered after operations were found so grossly abnormal that it would be very unlikely that they would result in viable pregnancies.

It is also suggested that 30% of conceptions detected by positive reactions to HCG tests abort spontaneously before these pregnancies are clinically verified. The scientific literature is not unanimous on the incidence of natural wastage prior to, and during, implantation in humans, varying from 15% to as much as 50%. The vast majority of these losses are due to chromosomal defects caused during gametogenesis and fertilization.[68-70]

Genetic uniqueness and singleness coincide only after implantation and restriction have completed, which is about 3 weeks after fertilization. Until that period, the zygote and its sequelae are in a fluid process and are not a physical individual, and therefore, cannot be a person. Although in a set of twins, one individuum can disappear, genetic and individual identities are now more or less equivalent. Many eminent Catholic writers, among them the Australian priest Norman Ford, author of *"When Did I Begin?"* consider implantation to mark the beginning of human life; they maintain that the pre-embryo has only intrinsic potential and must be protected only from the time of implantation.[71]

5. *The product of fertilization may be a tumor, a hydatidiform mole, or chorioepithelioma.* Though the mole is alive and of human origin, it is definitely not a human individual or human being. It lacks a true human nature from the start and has no natural potential to begin human development.

A teratoma is another clear instance of cells developing abnormally that results from the product of fertilization, but which could not be considered to be a true human individual with a human nature. It has no potential to develop into an entire fetus or infant. Clearly, the fetus with the teratoma would be a human individual, but not the attached teratoma itself. Obviously, not all the living cells that develop from the conceptus, the early embryo, or the fetus form an integral part of a developing human individual.[30]

DIFFERENT RELIGIOUS TEACHINGS AND HISTORICAL ASPECTS

The Catholic Church's teachings are clearly described in the Introduction Donum Vitae: "A human creature is to be respected and treated as a person from conception and, therefore, from that same time his (her) rights as a person must be recognized, among which in the first place is the invaluable right to life of each innocent human creature".

In 1997, the Third Assembly of the Pontifical Academy for Life was held in Vatican City. It has been concluded that "at the fusion of two gametes, a new real human individual initiates its own existence, or life cycle, during which—given all the necessary and sufficient conditions—it will autonomously realize all the potentialities with which he is intrinsically endowed". The embryo, therefore, from the time the gametes fuse, is a real human individual, not a potential human individual. It was even added that recent findings of human biological science recognize that in zygotes resulting from fertilization, the biological identity of a new human individual is already constituted.[72,73]

In Western Europe and in North and South America, these opinions are mostly based on Judeo-Christian theology, in Arabian countries, in Africa, and in Asia prevails the influences of the Islamic and Buddhist religions. Although their approach to the beginning of human life is impressively similar, each of these religions has different attitudes to the problem of embryo research, infertility, and its therapy.

In a fact, while the Jewish attitude toward infertility is expressed in the Talmud sayings and in the Bible (synthesized in the first commandment of God to Adam "Be fruitful and multiply"), the Christian point of view establishes no absolute right to parenthood. According to the Islamic views, attempts to cure infertility are not only permissible, but also a duty.

Islamic teaching is based on prophet Mohammed description: "The creation of each of you in his mother's abdomen assumes a *"nufta"* (male and female semen drops) for 40 days, then becomes *"alaga"* for the same (duration), then a *"mudgha"* (like a chewed piece of meat) for the same, then God sends an angel to it with instructions. The angel is ordered to write the sustenance, lifespan, deeds, and whether eventually his lot is happiness or misery, then to blow the spirit into him".[110] The summary of this poetic and sacred description is: soul breathing "ensoulment" occurs at 120 days of gestation from conception.

To make this religious principle applicable to the practice, the Islamic Jurisprudence Council wrote a Fatwa in 1990 that said: "Abortion is allowed in the first 120 days of conception if it is proven beyond doubt that the fetus is affected with a severe malformation that is not amenable to therapy, and if his life, after being born, will be a means of misery to both him and his family, and his parents agree", so that there is no difficulty for either the prenatal diagnosis, or for the possible termination of pregnancy within the exposed limits.

Buddhism has imposed strict ethics on priests, but it has relatively lenient attitudes toward lay people, so if medical treatment for infertility is available, people should make use of it.

For about 2,000 years, the opinions of *Aristotle*, the great Greek philosopher and naturalist, on the beginning of the human being were commonly held. He argued that the male semen had a special power residing in it, *pneuma*, to transform the menstrual blood, first into a living being with a vegetative soul after 7 days, and subsequently into one with a sensitive soul 40 days after contact with the male semen.[74]

Aquinas adopted Aristotle's theory, but specified that rational *ensoulment* took place through the creative act of God to transform the living creature into a human being once it had acquired a sensitive soul. The first conception took place over 7 days, while the second conception, or complete formation of the living individual with a complete human nature, lasted 40 days.[68]

Hippocrates believed that entrance of the soul into the male embryo occurred on the 30th day of intrauterine life. It entered into the female embryo on the 40th day. Actually, this idea was a considerable improvement on the scheme found in the Book of Leviticus, where it is suggested that the soul does not enter the female until 40 days after the conception.[75]

In short, the rational soul enables the matter to become a human being, an animated body, an embodied soul, and a human person.

Harvey's experiments with deer in 1633 proved Aristotle's theory of human reproduction wrong, without himself finding a satisfactory explanation of human conception. After modern scientists discovered the process of fertilization, most people took for granted that human beings, complete with a rational soul, began once fertilization had taken place.

It is clear that the answer to the question *"When has the human being actually come to life?"* could only be given by combining the cognition of different religions, philosophies, and various biological scientific disciplines.

There is a very fine line between the competence of science and the one of metaphysics, and it greatly depends on the individual's philosophical principles. Those two, more or less autonomous, intellectual disciplines have very often tried dominating one another, or ignoring each other. It is only recently that the majority of scientists and some theologians have come to realize that the separate meanings of scientific and religious "truths" complement each other, thus representing methodologically independent entities. Current science is not interested in what nature is, but in the facts that could be stated regarding it, thus trying to explain the term, rather than inventing it.

The main difference between science and religion can be seen in the fact that scientific "truths", unlike religious postulates, can must be experimentally verified and the methods of scientific cognition can be easily explained and learnt. Whereas religion favors irrationality, science prefers an entirely rational approach to matters of importance. Intellectual cognition, when scientifically expressed, usually is in a form of mathematical formulas and presented quantitatively. Contrarily, religion tends to keep its truths in a form of metaphoric expressions, preferring qualitative.

Today, there is a tendency, on a higher level, to reopen the dialog between the science and religion, which was present at the very beginning of our culture. Religion had existed long before science came to life, but science is not to be thought of as a continuation of the religion.[6]

Each discipline should preserve its principles, its separate interpretations, and its own conclusions. In the end, both of them represent different components of the one and indivisible culture of mankind.

CLINICAL CONTROVERSIES

There are some clinical controversies pertinent in any discussion of when life begins. Spermatozoa are living cells. They present evidence that they are living by their motility. They are equipped with an effective mechanism for movement in the form of a tail that beats under the control of the cytoplasmic droplets within the head. These living cells, which have been manufactured in the testes, are released into the environment provided by the male reproductive tract. They are not yet capable of fertilization. The spermatozoon must first come under the influence of the male reproductive tract, where it acquires the ability to function in fertilization. Even after ejaculation, it is capable of penetrating the egg, and it is modified further by exposure to the female reproductive tract, taking on the ability or capacity to fertilize. The decision must be made as to whether the spermatozoon is a being (i.e. living and human with the potential for continued life once fertilization has occurred); albeit in another form, it is entitled to the right of protection as a person.

Those who deny right for life to the spermatozoon might argue that it is not a complete human cell chromosomally—it contains only the haploid number of chromosomes. Paradoxically, those who take that point of view would insist that an individual born with fewer or more chromosomes than normal is human and entitled to all the rights of "personhood". As Mastroianni stressed, the decision to base the definition of "human life" solely on the number of chromosomes in a given cell has far-reaching implications.[76]

Furthermore, life has been defined as being terminated when brain activity ends. If we were to say that life begins when brain activity starts, we would be admitting that the definition of the beginning of life is dependent upon technology and not upon ethics or morality.

Some suggested that the beginning of human life requires the neural fusion of the periphery with the center, as well as sufficient development of the brain itself.[77] Brody[78] formulated the so-called symmetry concept: *if the death of a human being requires the death of the brain, the beginning of human life shall correspond with the beginning of the life of the brain, considered to be at day 32 postconception (PC)*. However, Sass[79] has correctly pointed out that fusion is not established anatomically without neurons which form synapses, which would be expected from embryological development at 70 days (8 weeks) PC.[80]

In this light, let us take for example the accepted definition of birth, which some years ago was described as the complete expulsion of a fetus of 1,000 g or 28 weeks of pregnancy. With advances in perinatal and neonatal intensive care, the line was drawn at 500 g, or approximately at 22 weeks of gestation, some years later. This meant that a 20-week-old fetus was not born by definition, even if it was viable. This concept has changed. The same logic applies to a live fetus being accorded the term "life", if we use such definitions as the beginning of brain activity or ultrasonic proof of heartbeat and movement. The establishment of each of these parameters is shifted to an earlier stage year by year by improving technological refinements in electronic and ultrasonic equipment. This leads us to the conclusion that to follow this line of reasoning means to give life, birth, and viability definitions determined by technology. The more advanced the technology, the earlier life begins.

In any consideration of the beginning of human life, it helps to think about when life ends. Let us consider the following: a 2-week-old newborn is hospitalized with massive brain injury suffered in an automobile accident. Despite all measures, no electrical or other brain activity can be detected during the next 2 days and the child is pronounced dead. Its body parts may survive after its death, as after the death of every person of whatever age. Hair and nails grow for days. Kidneys, heart, liver, and other organs may go on living for years if transplanted into another individual. Cells were taken soon after death and cultured in a laboratory might live well beyond the 72 or more years; this child might have lived, although the life of the infant has ended. The conclusion reached in this case that death of the brain means the end of life, is generally accepted by physicians, courts, and the public.[32]

Returning to the question of when life begins, it is true that the DNA of the fertilized egg has the information necessary to form an individual, but so does virtually every other cell in the body. Nobody would claim full rights for the living cells of the infant killed in the accident, although each has a complete library of DNA. The same counts also for thousands of living skin cells we lose every time we wash our hands and faces.

Is there some stage in the development of the brain that is critical? Or is it the time at which the fetus can survive outside the womb, with or without the support of medical technology? Should we revert to a criterion used for many years, the time of quickening, when one can feel the fetus moving? These are questions still to be answered.

VISUALIZATION OF EARLY HUMAN DEVELOPMENT

Significant advances have been made in recent years in visualizing and analyzing the earliest human development. Most of them have been done by introduction of three-dimensional (3D) static and color Doppler and four-dimensional (4D) sonography. Many new parameters about early human development are now studied directly by new ultrasound techniques.

Considerable number of biochemical, morphological, and vascular changes occur within the follicle during the process of ovulation and luteinization and most of them can be studied by transvaginal ultrasound with color Doppler and 3D facilities.[79] If the oocyte is fertilized, the embryo is transported into the uterus where under favorable hormonal and environmental conditions, it will implant and develop into a new and unique individual. The introduction of transvaginal color Doppler improved the recognition of blood vessels enabling detailed examination of small vessels such as arteries supplying preovulatory follicle, corpus luteum, and endometrium.[69]

Perifollicular vascularization can help in identification of follicles containing high quality oocytes, with a high probability of recuperating, fertilizing, cleaving, and implanting, while 3D ultrasound enables accurate morphological inspection and detection of cumulus oophorus. Follicles without visualization of the cumulus by multiplanar imaging are not likely to contain fertilizable oocytes. This information is especially useful in patients undergoing ovulation induction (Figs. 4.11A to C).

Following ovulation, the corpus luteum is formed as the result of many structural, functional, and vascular changes in the former follicular wall. Color Doppler studies of the luteal blood flow velocities enable evaluation of the corpus luteum function in second phase of menstrual cycle and early pregnancy. When the placenta takes over the role of production of progesterone, the corpus luteum starts regressing.

After ovulation, there is a short period during which the endometrial receptivity is maximal. During these few days, a blastocyst can attach to the endometrium and provoke increased vascular permeability and vasodilatation at the implantation site. Trophoblast-produced proteolytic enzymes cause the penetration of the uterine mucosa and erode adjacent maternal capillaries. This results in formation of the intercommunicating lacunar network—the intervillous space of the placenta. A small intradecidual gestational sac can be visualized by transvaginal sonography between 32 days and 34 days (Figs. 4.12A to C).[81]

The secondary yolk sac is the earliest extraembryonic structure normally seen within the gestational sac in the beginning of the 5th gestational week. The yolk sac volume was found to increase from 5 weeks to 10 weeks of gestation. When the yolk sac reaches its maximum volume at around 10 weeks, it has already started to degenerate, which can be indirectly proved by a significant reduction in visualization rates of the yolk sac vascularity.[68] Therefore, a combination of functional and volumetric studies by 3D power Doppler helps to identify some of the most important moments in early human development.

The embryonic heart begins beating on about day 22–23, accepting blood components from the yolk sac and pushing blood into the circulation. The embryonic blood begins circulating at the end of the 4th week of development.

The start of the embryo-chorionic circulation changes the source of nourishment to all intraembryonic tissues. The survival and further development of the embryo become dependent on the circulation of embryonic/fetal blood. If the embryo-chorionic circulation does not develop, or fails, the conceptus is aborted. The embryo cannot survive without the chorion (placenta) and the

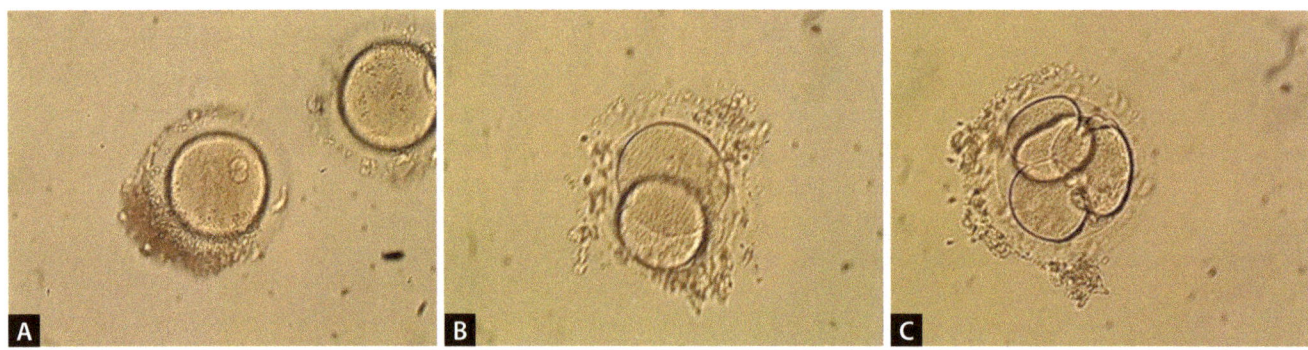

Figs. 4.11A to C: (A) Left: fertilized oocyte to zygote, and right: unfertilized oocyte; (B) Two-cell stage; and (C) Four-cell stage.
Courtesy: Dr S Tinjic.

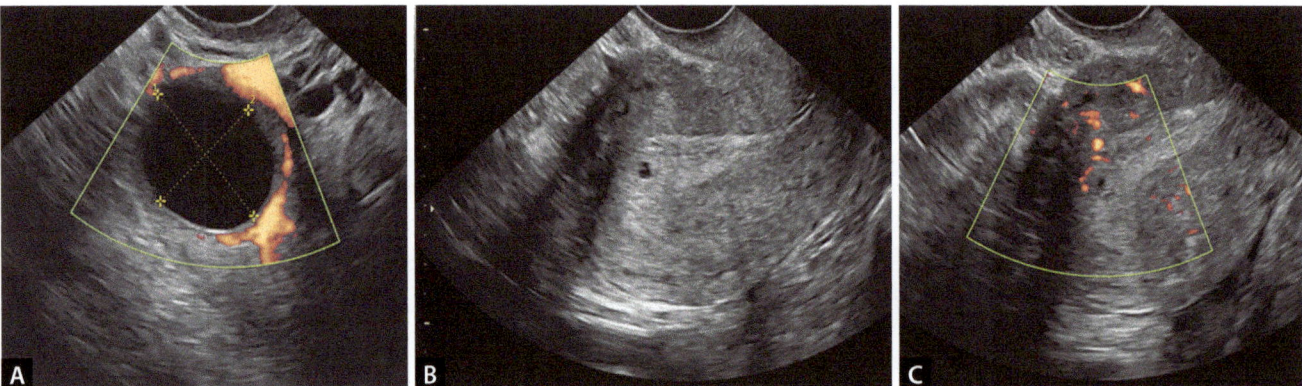

Figs. 4.12A to C: (A) Corpus luteum; (B) A small intradecidual gestational sac can be visualized by transvaginal sonography between 32 days and 34 days; and (C) During these few days, a blastocyst can attach to the endometrium and provoke increased vascular permeability and vasodilatation at the implantation site.

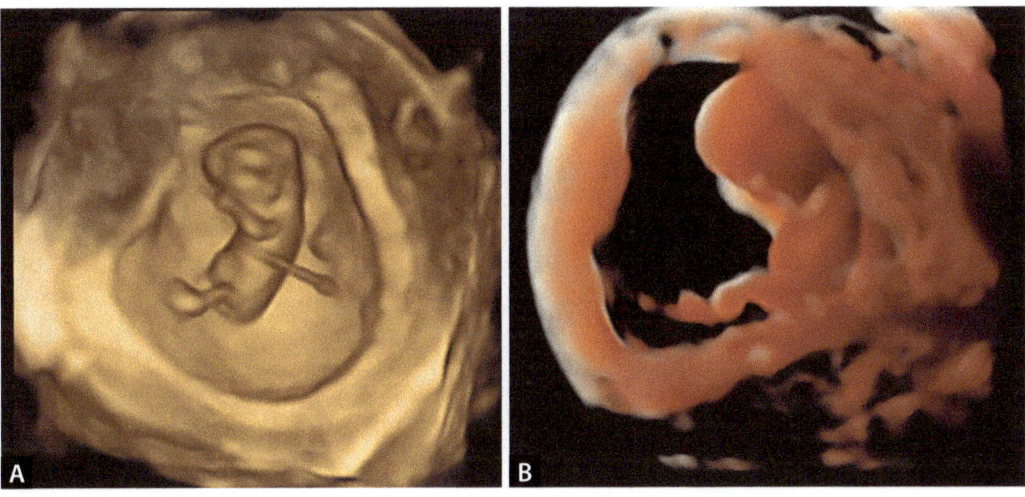

Figs. 4.13A and B: (A) 10 weeks and 4 days fetus, three-dimensional (3D) surface rendering, notice the arms with elbow and legs with knee are clearly visible as well as feet; and (B) The same fetus in 3D HDlive rendering.

chorion will not survive without the embryo. Avascular degenerated chorionic villi constitute the hydatidiform mole.

Within the embryo, there are three distinct blood circulatory systems:[47]
1. Vitelline circulation (from yolk sac to embryo)
2. Intraembryonic circulation (*see* Figs. 4.8 and 4.9)
3. Two umbilical arteries (from embryo to placenta—fetoplacental circulation) (*see* Fig. 4.9).

It is possible to visualize and assess them virtually from conception.[82-86]

- *At 5 weeks* from the maternal side of placenta, it is possible to obtain simultaneous 3D imaging of the developing intervillous circulation during the 1st trimester of pregnancy. 3D power Doppler reveals intensive vascular activity surrounding the chorionic shell starting from the first sonographic evidence of the developing pregnancy during the 5th week of gestation
- *At 7 weeks*, 3D power Doppler images depict aortic and umbilical blood flow. Initial branches of umbilical vessels are visible at the placental umbilical insertion
- *During the 8-9th weeks*, developing intestine is being herniated into the proximal umbilical cord (physiologic umbilical hernia)
- *At 9-10 weeks*, herniation of the midgut is present. The arms with elbow and legs with knee are clearly visible, while feet can be seen approaching the midline (Figs. 4.13A and B)
- *At 11 weeks*, 3D power Doppler imaging allows visualization of the entire fetal and placental circulation (Fig. 4.14)

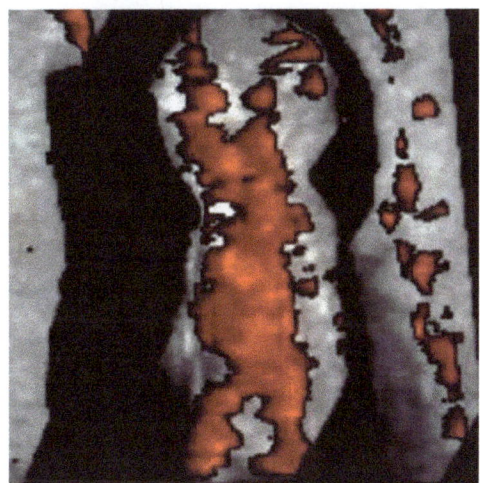

Fig. 4.14: A 14 weeks fetus. Complete visualization of fetal and placental circulation shown by three-dimensional (3D) power Doppler.[8]

- *During the 11-12th weeks* of pregnancy, development of the head and neck continues. Facial details such as nose, orbits, maxilla, and mandibles are often visible (Figs. 4.15 and 4.16). Herniated midgut returns into the abdominal cavity.

NEW POSSIBILITIES FOR STUDYING EMBRYONIC MOVEMENTS AND BEHAVIOR

The latest development of 3D and 4D sonography enables precise study of embryonic and fetal activity and behavior (Fig. 4.17).[6,9,86-109] With 4D ultrasound, movements of head, body, and all four limbs and extremities can be seen simultaneously in three dimensions.[6,9,87,88,91-109]

Therefore, the earliest phases of the human anatomical and motor development can be visualized and studied simultaneously. It is clear that neurologic development—early fetal motor activity and behavior needs to be re-evaluated by this new technique.[84-109]

Our group studied the development of the complexity of spontaneous embryonic and fetal movements.[89] With the advancing of the gestational age, the movements become more and more complex. The increase in the number of axodendritic and axosomatic synapses between 8 and 10, and again between 12 weeks and 15 weeks,[90] correlates with the periods of fetal movement differentiation and with the onset of general movements and complex activity patterns, such as swallowing, stretching, and yawning, seen easily by 4D technique.

By 7-8 weeks of pregnancy, gross body movements appear. They consist of changing the position of the head toward the body. By 9-10 weeks of pregnancy, limb movements appear. They consist of changing the position of the extremities toward the body without the extension or flexion in elbow and knee. At 10-12 weeks of pregnancy, complex limb movements appear. They consist of changes in the position of limb segments toward each other, such as extension and flexion in elbow and knee (Figs. 4.13 and 4.15 to 4.17).

Between 12 weeks and 15 weeks of pregnancy, *swallowing, stretching, and yawning activities appear*. In addition to these activities, it is now feasible to study by 4D ultrasound a full range of facial expression including smiling, crying, and eyelid movement (Figs. 4.15A and B).

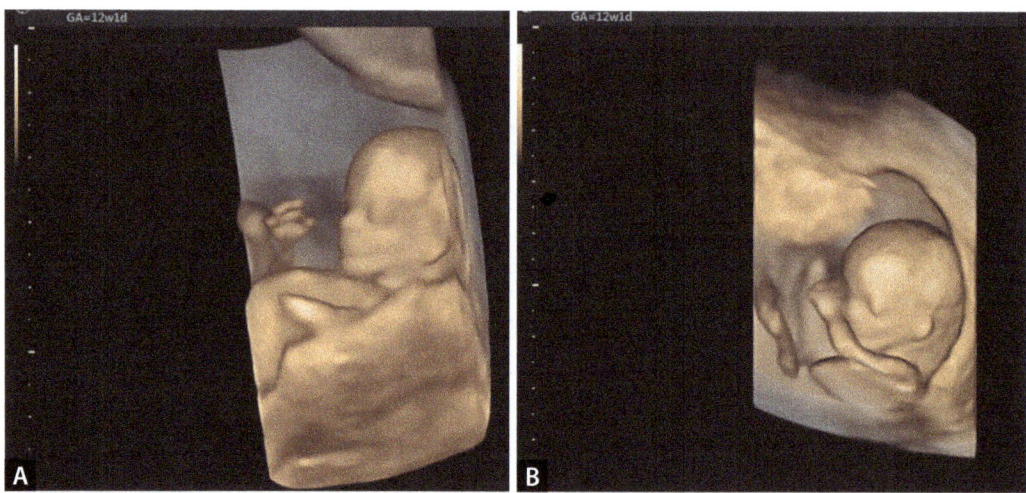

Figs. 4.15A and B: Fetus at the 12 weeks of gestation. Imaging: three-dimensional (3D) surface mode. Facial details such as nose, orbits, maxilla, and mandibles are clearly visualized.

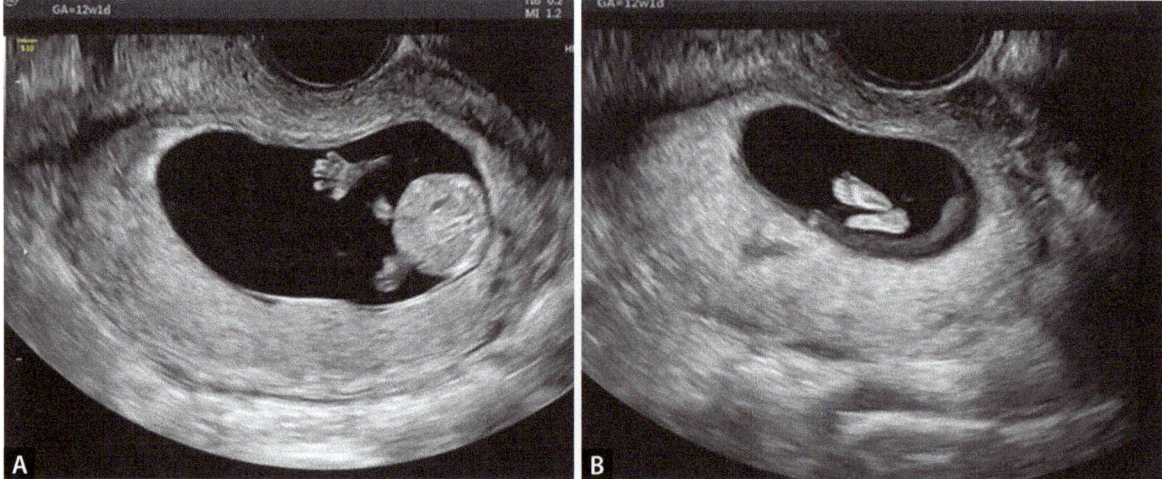

Figs. 4.16A and B: With two-dimensional (2D) imaging, visualization of the fetal fingers and toes at the 12 weeks and 1 day.

Chapter 4: Controversies on the Beginning of Human Life

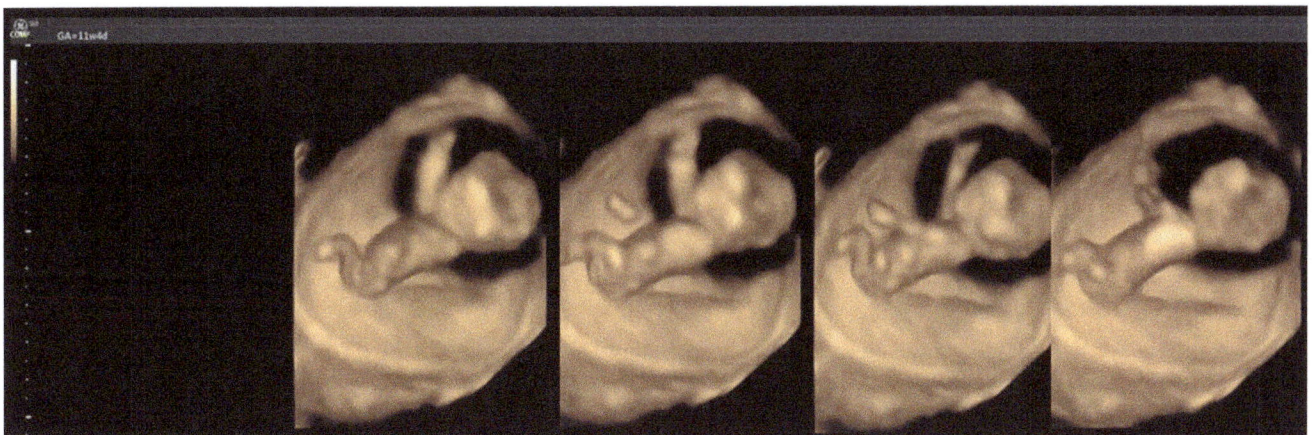

Fig. 4.17: 3D and 4D sonography enables precise study of fetal activity and behavior at 11 weeks and 4 days at the presented sequence of ultrasound images. (3D: three-dimensional; 4D: four-dimensional)

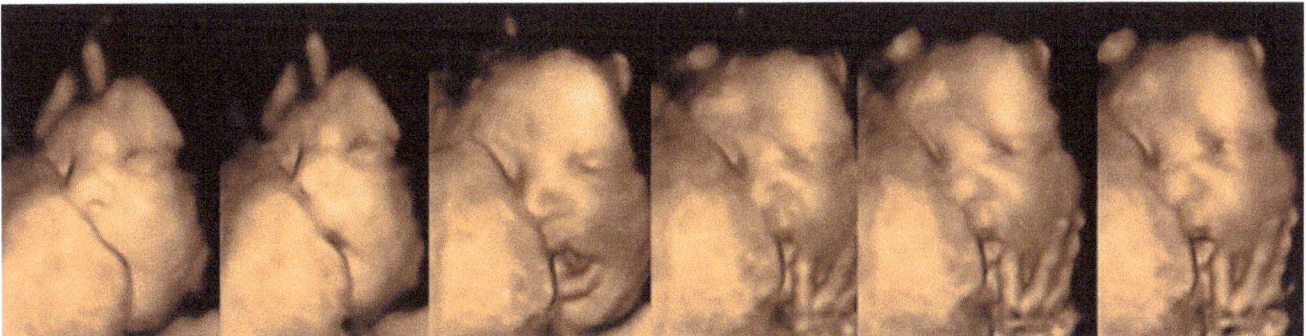

Fig. 4.18: Sequence of images recorded with the four-dimensional (4D) ultrasound, surface mode. Fetus at 33 weeks of pregnancy, Kurjak Antenatal Neurodevelopmental Test (KANET) was performed.[108] Notice how fetus explores the environment with the mouth, by the hand, and with the eyes.

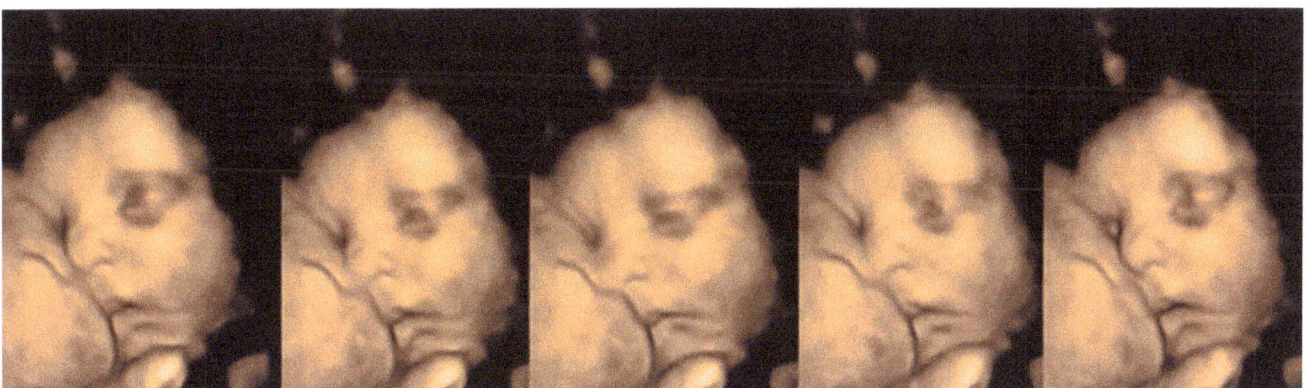

Fig. 4.19: The same fetus as in the Figure 18. Looking around in utero, exploring the environment.

It is hoped that the new 4D technique will help us to have a better understanding of both the somatic and motoric development of the early embryo. It will also enable the reliable study of fetal and even parental behavior (Figs. 4.18 and 4.19).[6,9,85-109]

There was recently number of papers on new attractive techniques for visualization of early human development. Interested reader can find more in the chapter of R Pooh.

CONCLUSION

The question of *when a human life begins and how to define it* could be answered only through the interconnecting pathways of history, philosophy, medical, science, and religion. It has not been easy to determine where to draw the fine line between the competence of science and metaphysics in this delicate philosophical field. To a large extent, the drawing of this line depends on one's fundamental philosophical outlook.

To quote Beller: *"The point at which human life begins will always be seen differently by different individuals, groups, cultures, and religious faiths. In democracy, there are always at least two sides, and the center holds only when the majority realizes that without a minority, democracy itself is lost. The minority, in turn, must realize its best chance lies in persuasion by reason and thoughtfulness rather than fanaticism".*[31]

REFERENCES

1. Mikael S. How to Relate Science and Religion: A Multi-dimensional Model. Grand Rapids, Michigan: William B Eerdmans Publishing Company; 2004.
2. Peter H. The Territories of Science and Religion. Chicago: University of Chicago Press; 2015.
3. David C. From Natural Philosophy to the Sciences: Writing the History of Nineteenth-Century Science. Chicago: University of Chicago Press; 2003.
4. Ronald N, David L. When Science and Christianity Meet. Chicago: University of Chicago Press; 2003.
5. Helen DC. Religion and science. In: Zalta EN (Ed). *The Stanford Encyclopedia of Philosophy*. Chicago: University of Chicago Press; 2018.
6. Kurjak A, Barišić LS, Ahmed B, et al. Beginning of human life: science and religion closer and closer. In: Kurjak A, Chernavak FA, McCullough LB, Hasanović A (Eds). Science and Religion: Synergy not Skepticism. New Delhi: Jaypee Brothers Medical Publishers (P) Ltd; 2018. pp. 21-52.
7. Ayala FJ. Science, evolution, and creationism. Proc Natl Acad Sci USA. 2008;105:3-4.
8. Kurjak A, Carrera JM. The beginning of human life—scientific and religious controversies. In: Kurjak A, Chervenak FA (Eds). Textbook of Perinatal Medicine. New Delhi: Jaypee Brothers Medical Publishers (P) Ltd; 2015. pp. 163-76.
9. Kurjak A, Spalldi Barišić L, Delic T, et al. Facts and Doubts about the Beginning of the Human Life and Personality. Donald School J Ultrasound Obstet Gynecol. 2016;10: 205-13.
10. Einstein A. Personal God Concept Causes Science-Religion Conflict. Sci News Lett. 1940;38:181-2.
11. Barbour I. Issues in Science and Religion. New York: Vantage; 1966.
12. Torrance TF. Theological Science. London: Oxford University Press; 1969.
13. Clark KJ. Religion and the Science Origins: Historical and Contemporary Perspectives. New York: Palgrave MacMillan; 2014.
14. Clark KJ, Barrett JL. Reidian Religious Epistemology and the Cognitive Science of Religion. J Am Acad Relig. 2011;79:639-75.
15. Barbour I. When Science Meets Religion: Enemies, Strangers, or Partners? New York: Harper Collins Publishers; 2000.
16. Gould SJ. Nonoverlapping magisteria. In: Pennock A (Ed). Intelligent Design Creationism and its Critics. Cambridge: MIT Press; 2001. pp. 737-49.
17. Dawes G. Galileo and the Conflict between Religion and Science. New York: Routledge; 2016.
18. Bowler P. Reconciling Science and Religion: The Debate in Early-Twentieth Century Chicago: University of Chicago Press; 2001.
19. Van Huyssteen, Wentzel J. Duet or Duel? Theology and Science in a Postmodern World. London: SCM Press; 1998.
20. Durkheim E. The Elementary Forms of the Religious Life: A Study in Religious Sociology. London: Allen & Unwin; 1915.
21. Freud S. Die Zukunft Einer Illusion. Leipzig, Wien and Zurich: Internationaler Psychoanalytischer Verlag-Gesammelte Werke.1927;14:325-80.
22. Collins F. The Language of God: A Scientists Presents Evidence for Belief. New York: Free Press; 2006.
23. Gervais WM, Norenzayan A. Analytic Thinking Promotes Religious Disbelief. Science. 2012;336:493-6.
24. Kurjak A. The beginning of human life and its modern scientific assessment. Clin Perinatol. 2003;30:27-44.
25. National Geographic. (2017). Origins of the Universe. [online] Available from www.nationalgeographic.com/science/space/universe/origins-of-the-universe/. [Accessed December, 2018].
26. Pitts JB. Why the Big Bang Singularity Does not help the Kalam Cosmological Argument for Theism. Br J Philosop Sci. 2008;59:675-708.
27. Godfrey J. The Pope and the Ontogeny of Person (commentary). Nature. 1995;273:100.
28. Rolston H. Science, religion, and the future. In: Richardson WM, Wildman WJ (Eds). Religion and Science History, Method, and Dialogue. New York: Routledge; 1996. pp. 21-82.
29. Mayr E. The growth of biological thought. Cambridge: Harvard University Press; 1982. p. 81.
30. Serra A, Colombo R. Identity and status of the human embryo: the contribution of biology. In: Correa DV, Sgreccia E (Eds). Identity and Statute of Human Embryo. New York: CRC Press; 1998. p. 128.
31. Beller FK, Zlatnik GP. The beginning of human life. J Assist Reprod Genet. 1995;12:477-83.
32. Kurjak A. When does human life begin? Encyclopedia Moderna. 1992;2:383-90.
33. Ventura-Junca P, Santos MJ. The beginning of life of a new human being from the scientific biological perspective and its bioethical implications. Biol Res. 2011;44:201-7.
34. Graham L. Foreword. In: Nathanielsz PW (Ed). Life before birth and the time to be born. New York: Promethean Press Ithaca; 1992.
35. Gilbert SF. Developmental biology. Sunderland: Sinauer Associates; 1991. p. 3.

36. Scarpelli EM. Postnatal through adult human life and the scientific deception. In: Atti del I (Ed). Congresso Nazionale della Societa Italiana di Medicina Materno Fetale. Italy: Medimond (International Proceedings); 2003. pp. 29-36.
37. Moore KL, Persaud TV. The developing human: Clinically oriented embryology, 7th edition. Philadelphia: Saunders; 2003.
38. Carlson BM. Human Embryology and Developmental Biology. Canada: Elsevier; 2004.
39. Moore KL. The Developing Human: Clinically Oriented Embryology. Philadelphia: Saunders; 1974. p. 1.
40. Moore KL. The Developing Human: Clinically Oriented Embryology, 10th edition. Philadelphia: Saunders; 2016. p. 11.
41. Schoenwolf GC. Larsen's Human Embryology, 5th edition. Philadelphia: Elsevier; 2015. pp. 2-14.
42. June PL, de Miranda F. When Human Life Begins. Am Coll Pediatr. 2017;2:23-41.
43. Vjugina U, Evans JP. New insights into the molecular basis of mammalian sperm-egg membrane interactions. Front Biosci. 2008;13:462-76.
44. Oren-Suissa O, Podbilewicz B. Cell fusion during development. Trends Biol. 2007;17:537-46.
45. Condic ML. When does human life begin? A scientific perspective. New York: Westchester Institute; 2008. p. 5.
46. Preembryo research: history, scientific background, and ethical considerations. ACOG Committee Opinion: Committee on Ethics. Number 136—April 1994. Int J Gynaecol Obstet. 1994;45:291-301.
47. Jirasek JE. An Atlas of the Human Embryo and Fetus. New York: Parthenon Publishing; 2001.
48. The Embryo as a Patient. Declaration of Professors from Five Faculties of Medicine and Surgery of the universities of Rome, organizers of the Conference. La Sapienza University Press; 2004.
49. Kurjak A, Stanojevic M, Azumendi G, et al. The potential of four-dimensional ultrasonography in the assessment of fetal awareness. J Perinat Med. 2005;33:46-53.
50. Watson JD, Crick F. Genetic implications of the structure of DNA. Nature. 1953;171:964-67.
51. Badregal P, Shand B, Santos MJ, et al. Contribution of epigenetics to understand human development. Rev Med Chile. 2010;138:366-72.
52. Santos MJ. Manipulacion genetica de seres humanos. Ars Medica. 1006;13:91-102.
53. Sass HM. Brain life and brain death: a proposal for normative agreement. J Med Philos. 1989;14:45-59.
54. Veatch RM. The beginning of full moral standing. In: Beller FK, Weir RF (Eds). The Beginning of Human Life. Dordrecht: Kluwer; 1994. p. 19.
55. Knutson AL. When does human life begin? Viewpoints of public health professionals. Am J Pub Health. 1967;57:21-67.
56. Bush GW. Inaugural speech. BBC News. 21 January, 2001. Online: http://news.bbc.co.uk/2/hi/americas.
57. Spalldi Barišić L, Kurjak A, Pooh KR, et al. Antenatal detection of fetal syndromes by ultrasound: From a single piece to a complete puzzle. Donald School J Ultrasound Obstet Gynaecol. 2016;10:63-77.
58. Spalldi Barišić L, Stanojević M, Kurjak A, et al. Diagnosis of fetal syndromes by three- and four-dimensional ultrasound: is there any improvement? J Perinat Med. 2017;45:651-65.
59. Engelhardt HT. The foundation of bioethics. New York: Oxford University Press; 1986.
60. Dunstan GR. The moral status of the human embryo. A tradition recalled. J Med Ethics. 1984;10:38-44.
61. Chervenak FA, McCullough LB, Kurjak A. Ethical implications of the embryo as a patient. In: Kurjak A, Chervenak FA, Carrera JM (Eds). The embryo as a patient. New York: Parthenon Publishing Group; 2001. pp. 226-30.
62. Curran CE. Abortion: Contemporary debate in philosophical and religious ethics. In: Reich WT (Ed). Encyclopedia of Bioethics. New York: Macmillan; 1978. pp. 17-26.
63. Ruddick W, Wilcox W. Operating on the fetus. Hastings Cen Report. 1982;12:10-4.
64. McCullough LB, Chervenak FA. Ethics in Obstetrics and Gynecology. New York. Oxford University Press; 1994.
65. Connery JR. The ancients and medievals on abortion. In: Horan DJ, Grant ER, Cunningham PC (Eds). Abortion and Constitution. Washington DC: Georgetown University Press; 1987. p. 124.
66. Pierre F, Soutoul JH. Medical and legal complications. J Gynecol Obstet Biol Reprod (Paris). 1994;23:516-9.
67. Scarpelli EM. Personhood: A biological phenomenon. J Perinat Med. 2001;29:417-26.
68. Ford NM. When did I Begin? Conception of the Human Individual in History, Philosophy and Science. Cambridge: Cambridge University Press; 1991. pp. 137-46.
69. McLaren A. Prelude to Embryogenesis in the Ciba Foundation, Human Embryo Research, Yes or No? New York: Tavistock; 1986. pp. 5-23.
70. Jacobs PA, Hassold T. Chromosome abnormalities: origin and etiology in abortions and livebirths. In: Vogel F, Sperling K (Eds). Human Genetics. Berlin; Springer-Verlag, 1987. pp. 233-44.
71. McCormick KA. Who or what is the preembryo? Kennedy Institute of Ethics J. 1991;1:24.
72. Mahoney SJ. Bioethics and belief. London: Sheed and Ward; 1984. p. 80.
73. Johnson M. Delayed hominization. Reflections on some recent Catholic claims for delayed hominization. Theological Stud. 1995;56:743-63.
74. Congregation for the Doctrine of the Faith, Instruction on respect for human life in its origin and on the dignity of procreation "Donum Vitae" (February 12, 1987). Acta Apostolicae Sedis. 1988;80:70-102.
75. Beazley JM. Fetal assessment from conception to birth. In: Kurjak A (Ed). Recent Advances in Ultrasound Diagnosis. Amsterdam: Excerpta Medica; 1980. p. 128.
76. Kurjak A. Kada pocinje zivot. In: Kurjak A (Ed). Ocekujuci novorodjence. Zagreb: Naprijed; 1987. pp. 18-28.
77. Mastroianni L. Ethical aspects of fetal therapy and experimentation. In: Schenker JG, Weinstein D (Eds). The

Intrauterine Life: Management and Therapy. Amsterdam: Excerpta Medica; 1986. pp. 3-10.
78. Beller FK, Reeve J. Brain life and brain death: The anencephalic as an explanatory example. J Med Philos. 1989;14:5-20.
79. Brody B. Abortion and the sanctity of human life: A philosophical view. Cambridge, MIT Press; 1975. p. 109.
80. Kupesic S. The first three weeks assessed by transvaginal color Doppler. J Perinat Med. 1996;24:310-7.
81. Sass HM. The moral significance of brain-life-criteria. In: Beller FK, Weir RF (Eds). The Beginning of Human Life. Dordrecht: Kluwer; 1994. pp. 57-70.
82. Kupesic S, Kurjak A, Ivancic-Kosuta M. Volume and vascularity of the yolk sac. J Perinat Med. 1999;27:91-6.
83. Kurjak A, Predanic M, Kupesic S. Transvaginal color Doppler study of middle cerebral artery blood flow in early normal and abnormal pregnancy. Ultrasound Obstet Gynecol. 1992;2:424-8.
84. Kurjak A, Kupesic S. Doppler assessment of the intervillous blood flow in normal and abnormal early pregnancy. Obstet Gynecol. 1997;89:252-6.
85. Kurjak A, Kupesic S, Hafner T. Intervillous blood flow in normal and abnormal early pregnancy. Croatian Med J. 1998;39:10.
86. Kurjak A, Kupesic S. Three-dimensional transvaginal ultrasound improves measurement of nuchal translucency. J Perinat Med. 1999;27:97-102.
87. Kurjak A, Kupesic S, Banovic I, et al. The study of morphology and circulation of early embryo by three-dimensional ultrasound and power Doppler. J Perinat Med. 1999;27:145-57.
88. Lee A. Four-dimensional ultrasound in prenatal diagnosis: Leading edge in imaging technology. Ultrasound Rev Obstet Gynecol. 2001;1:144-8.
89. Campbell S. 4D, or not 4D: That is the question. Ultrasound Obstet Gynecol. 2002;19:1-4.
90. de Vries JI, Visser GH, Prechtl HF. The emergence of fetal behaviour. I. Qualitative aspects. Early Hum Dev. 1982;7:301-22.
91. de Vries JI, Visser GH, Prechtl HF. The emergence of fetal behaviour. II. Quantitative aspects. Early Hum Dev. 1985;12:99-120.
92. Kurjak A, Vecek N, Hafner T, et al. Prenatal diagnosis: what does four-dimensional ultrasound add? J Perinat Med. 2002;30:57-62.
93. Kurjak A, Azumendi G, Vecek N, et al. Fetal hand movements and facial expression in normal pregnancy studied by four-dimensional sonography. J Perinat Med. 2003;31:496-508.
94. Okado N, Kojima T. Ontogenity of the central nervous system: Neurogenesis, fiber connection, synaptogenesis and myelinization in the spinal cord. In: Prechtl HF (Ed). Continuity of Neural Functions from Prenatal to Postnatal Life. Oxford: Blackwell Scientific Publishing; 1984. pp. 46-64.
95. Kurjak A, Azumendi G, Andonotopo W, et al. Three- and four-dimensional ultrasonography for the structural and functional evaluation of the fetal face. Am J Obstet Gynecol. 2007;196:16-28.
96. Kurjak A, Miskovic B, Andonotopo W, et al. How useful is 3D and 4D ultrasound in perinatal medicine? J Perinat Med. 2007;35:10-27.
97. Kurjak A, Miskovic B, Stanojevic M, et al. New scoring system for fetal neurobehavior assessed by three- and four-dimensional sonography. J Perinat Med. 2008;36:73-81.
98. Pooh RK, Kurjak A. Recent advances in 3D assessment of various fetal anomalies. Donald School J Ultrasound Obstet Gynecol. 2009;3:1-25.
99. Pooh RK, Shiota K, Kurjak A. Imaging of the human embryo with magnetic resonance imaging microscopy and high-resolution transvaginal 3-dimensional sonography: human embryology in the 21st century. Am J Obstet Gynecol. 2011;204:77.e1-16.
100. Pooh RK, Kurjak A. Three-dimensional/Four-dimensional Sonography moved Prenatal Diagnosis of Fetal Anomalies from the Second to the First Trimester of Pregnancy. Donald School J Ultrasound Obstet Gynecol. 2012;6:376-90.
101. Pooh RK, Kurjak A. Novel application of three-dimensional HDlive imaging in prenatal diagnosis from the first trimester. J Perinat Med. 2014;43:147-58.
102. Kurjak A, Spalldi Barišić L, Stanojevic M, et al. Are We Ready to investigate Cognitive Function of Fetal Brain? The Role of Advanced Four-dimensional Sonography. Donald School J Ultrasound Obstet Gynecol. 2016;10:116-24.
103. Pooh RK, Maeda K, Kurjak A, et al. 3D/4D sonography—any safety problem. J Perinat Med. 2016;44:125-9.
104. Pooh RK, Kurjak A. Donald School Atlas of Advanced Ultrasound in Obstetrics and Gynecology. New Delhi: Jaypee Brothers Medical Publishers (P) Ltd; 2015.
105. Salihagic-Kadic A, Kurjak A, Medić M, et al. New data about embryonic and fetal neurodevelopment and behavior obtained by 3D and 4D sonography. J Perinat Med. 2005;33:478-90.
106. Kurjak A, Antsaklis P, Stanojević M, et al. Multicentric studies of the fetal neurobehavior by KANET test. J Perinat Med. 2017;45:717-27.
107. Salihagić Kadić A, Kurjak A. Cognitive functions of the fetus. Ultraschall Med. 2018;39:181-9.
108. Pooh RK. A New Field of 'Fetal Sono-ophthalmology' by 3D HDlive Silhouette and Flow. Donald School J Ultrasound Obstet Gynecol. 2015;9:221-2.
109. Pooh RK. Neuroanatomy visualization by 2D and 3D. In: Pooh RK, Kurjak A (Eds). Fetal Neurology. New Delhi: Jaypee Brothers Medical Publishers (P) Ltd; 2009. pp. 15-38.
110. Zindani A-MA, Johnson EM, Ahmed MA, Goeringer GC, Simpson JL, Keith Moore K, et al. Human Development as Described in the Qur'an and Sunnah: Correlation with Modern Embryology. Islamic Academy for Scientific Research; 1994.

CHAPTER 5

Embryonic and Early Fetal Abnormalities Diagnosed with three-dimensional Ultrasound in the 1st Trimester

Eberhard Merz, Sonila Pashaj

INTRODUCTION

Three-dimensional (3D) ultrasound with its various display options[1-3] does not only allow to observe the normal embryonic and fetal anatomy in the 1st trimester but also to detect early malformations. Particularly, the transvaginal application of 3D ultrasound using the HDlive mode enables a near photographic demonstration of the surface of the embryo and fetus like in living embryology.[4] Nevertheless, the operator should know the normal embryonic/fetal development and the correct gestational age to avoid misdiagnoses.

EMBRYONIC PERIOD

The embryonic period begins at fertilization and ends after 8 weeks. This time span is divided into 23 Carnegie stages. The embryonic age (= conceptual age) measures the actual age of the embryo. In obstetrics, instead of the conceptual age, the gestational age is used which begins 2 weeks before conception with the 1st day of the last menstrual period.[5,6] Thus, the sonographically embryonic period lasts from gestational weeks 2–10.

NORMAL SONOGRAPHIC DEVELOPMENT OF THE EMBRYO

The earliest structure to be visualized in the chorionic sac is the yolk sac.[7] It is always seen in a mean sac diameter (MSD) of 8 mm using transvaginal approach.[8] The embryo is first visible at approximately 6 weeks of gestational age as a 1-2 mm hyperechoic structure at the periphery of the yolk sac[9] and should be definitely visualised at 25 mm MSD.[10] The thin amniotic membrane surrounding the embryo can be seen as early as 6.5 weeks of gestation.[11] With the production of the fetal urine at about 10 weeks of gestation, the amniotic cavity is enlarging and as a result, a fusion between the amnion and the chorion is seen at 14–16 weeks of gestation.[12]

Cardiac activity should be present at a crown-rump length of 7 mm.[10] The lower limit of the fetal heart rate at 6.2 weeks of gestation is 100 beats/min and at 6.3–7 weeks of gestation 120 beats/min.[13] A rapid heart rate of more than 135 beats/min or 155 beats/min, respectively before 6.3 weeks or after 6.3–7 weeks of gestation has a good prognosis, with a high likelihood of normal outcome.[14]

At 6 weeks of gestation, the brain is divided into three parts: (1) prosencephalon, (2) mesencephalon, and (3) rhombencephalon.[15] The rhombencephalon is the largest cavity with a pyramid-like shape.[16]

At 7 weeks of gestation, the yolk sac within the chorionic cavity can be clearly seen separately from the embryo in the amniotic cavity.[6]

At 8 weeks of gestation, the brain shows five brain vesicles: (1) telencephalon (the smallest brain structure), (2) diencephalon, (3) mesencephalon, (4) metencephalon (future cerebellum), and (5) myelencephalon (future medulla oblongata). The heart occupies 50% of the thoracic area.[17] The limb buds can be demonstrated in the surface mode. The spine is seen as two echogenic parallel lines.[18] Midgut herniation is also visible with the thick umbilical cord at the fetal side.[17]

At 9 weeks of gestation, the brain vesicles continues to develop and the choroid plexuses are visible on the lateral ventricles. The telencephalon will become larger in comparison to the rhombencephalon.[16] The upper extremities develop earlier than the lower ones. At this stage, we can recognize the upper arm, forearm and hand, thigh, lower leg, and foot. The limbs do not cross each other at the midline.[17]

At 10 weeks of gestation, the telencephalon structures are filled with the plexus chorioideus. The forebrain develops rapidly, while the hindbrain becomes smaller.[15] Using the 3D surface mode, the face can be demonstrated with eyes, nose, and mouth. The four-chamber view of the heart can be observed with high-resolution transvaginal probes.[17] HDlive allows the demonstration of the bowel

Table 5.1: Defects detectable and not detectable with three-dimensional (3D) ultrasound in the 1st trimester.

Defects detectable with 3D ultrasound in the 1st trimester	Defects not detectable with 3D ultrasound in the 1st trimester
Yolk sac abnormalities	Microcephaly
Umbilical cysts	Macrocephaly
Exencephaly/anencephaly	Ventriculomegaly
Encephalocele	Agenesis of corpus callosum
Holoprosencephaly	Subtle cardiac defects
Facial clefts/absent nasal bone/retrognathia	Lung abnormalities
Low-set ears	Bowel obstruction
Spina bifida	Hydronephrosis
Severe cardiac defects	Bladder exstrophy
Abdominal wall defects	Achondroplasia
Hydrops	Pena-Shokeir syndrome
Megacystis	
Achondrogenesis	
Limb defects/polydactyly	
Body stalk anomaly	
Kartagener syndrome	
Severe amniotic band syndrome	
Conjoined twins	
Single umbilical artery	

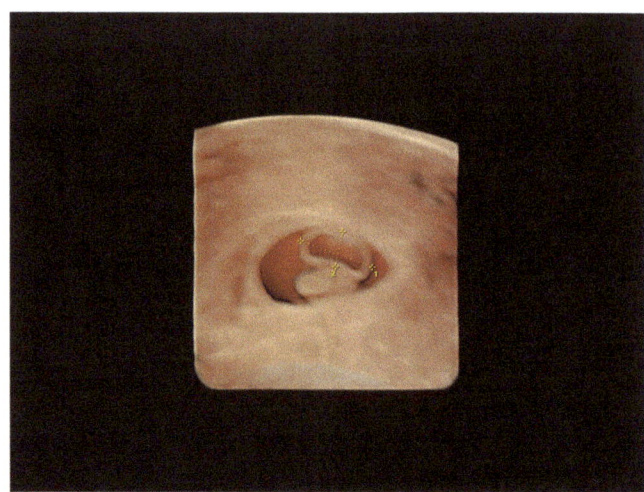

Fig. 5.1: Early pregnancy (7 + 3 weeks of gestation) showing deformed and enlarged yolk sac (9 × 4 mm), HDlive surface view of the cut plane.

loops inside the umbilical cord.[19] The upper and the lower extremities cross each other at the midline.[20]

FETAL PERIOD

After 10 weeks of gestation (respectively eight conceptual weeks), the fetal development starts.

EMBRYONIC/FETAL MALFORMATIONS

Using high-resolution transvaginal 3D probes, gross embryonic and early fetal abnormalities can be detected in a targeted examination. Table 5.1 gives an overview of defects which are detectable, respectively and not detectable during the 1st trimester.

YOLK SAC ABNORMALITY

Different authors have shown that abnormal yolk sac characteristics are associated with spontaneous abortion (Fig. 5.1).[21,22] In particular, an enlarged yolk sac more than 5 mm visualized before the 7th week is strongly associated with a significantly increased risk for spontaneous miscarriage.[22] In the study of Gersak et al.[23] none of the patients with a yolk size diameter more than 8 mm and viable pregnancy had a normal karyotype.

UMBILICAL CORD CYST

The prevalence of an umbilical cord cyst during the 1st trimester (Figs. 5.2A and B) varies from 0.4 to 3.4%, while in the 2nd and 3rd trimesters, the prevalence is unknown.[24,25] Umbilical cord cysts are classified as true cysts or pseudocysts.[26] *True cysts* are covered with epithelium and embryologically come from the allantois or the omphalomesenteric duct. They are generally located near the fetal cord insertion.[27] They can be associated with omphalocele, persistent urachus, and obstructive uropathy.[28,29] Omphalomesenteric duct cysts can be found in association with abdominal wall defects and with Meckel's diverticulum. *Pseudocysts* derived from local degeneration within Wharton's jelly and do not have an epithelium covering.

In prenatal diagnosis, umbilical cord cysts are reported in association with chromosomal defects such as trisomy 21, 18, and 13, as well as with structural malformations such as patient urachus, omphalocele, VACTERL association, vascular anomalies, and hypospadias.[24,30,31]

ACRANIA, ANENCEPHALY AND EXENCEPHALY

The ossification of the cranial bones starts from 10 weeks,[32] whether the skeletogenous layer surrounding the brain is present at 9 weeks.[33] Anencephaly develops from a failure of the anterior neuropore to close around the 26th

Chapter 5: Embryonic and Early Fetal Abnormalities Diagnosed with three-dimensional Ultrasound in the 1st Trimester

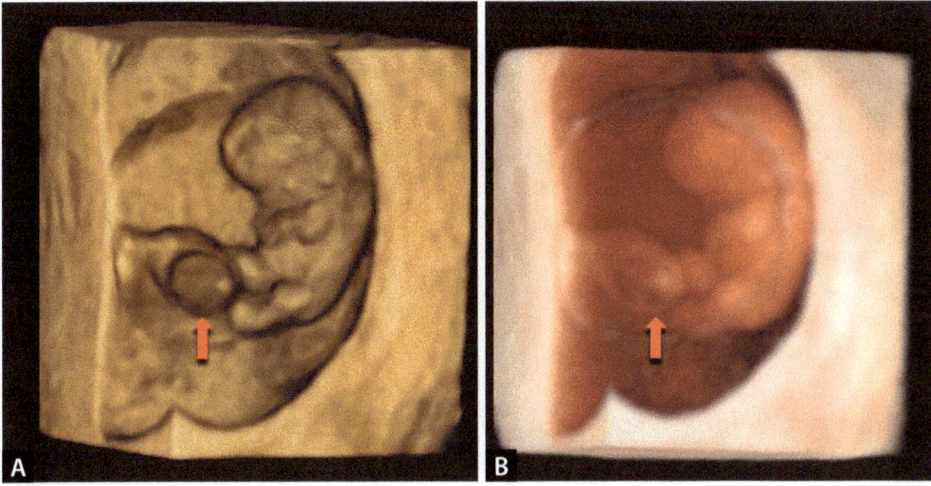

Figs. 5.2A and B: Embryo at 8 weeks of gestation, showing a cyst in the middle of the umbilical cord. (A) Surface mode; and (B) HDlive studio mode.

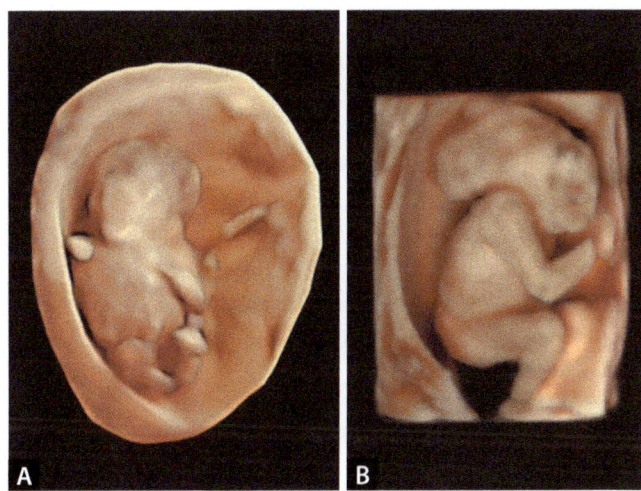

Figs. 5.3A and B: Surface demonstration (HDlive studio mode) of first trimester fetuses with head malformations at 13 weeks of gestation. (A) Anencephalus; and (B) Exencephaly.

postovulatory day of the embryonic period.[34] It is not clear whether exencephaly is a precursor of anencephaly (Fig. 5.3A) or exencephaly is a separated anomaly (Fig. 5.3B).[35] The exposure of brain tissue to amniotic fluid as well as repeated mechanical and chemical trauma in utero, due to the absence of calvarium, may be a theory to explain anencephaly.[22]

Exencephaly is reported as early as 9 weeks of gestation.[36] Anencephaly can be reliably diagnosed at the routine first trimester ultrasound scan (Fig. 5.3A).[37] A Mickey Mouse face is reported by different investigators.[3,38] Sepulveda[39] reported a progressive decrease in the ratio of crown-chin length to crown-rump length.

ENCEPHALOCELE

The ossification center in the occipital bone can be seen with transvaginal ultrasound in the 9th week of gestation.[40] An encephalocele may develop both from insufficient closure of the neural tube and the amniotic rupture sequence.

In ultrasound, at 11 weeks of gestation, it is described as a translucent area in the occipital region, which then changes to a more echogenic appearance with brain tissue protruding from the skull around 13 weeks of gestation.[40] During embryonic period, an enlarged rhombencephalon cavity is reported.[41]

Encephalocele is a part of syndrome such as Meckel-Gruber syndrome, Joubert syndrome, Walker–Warburg syndrome (Fig. 5.4), or cerebro-ocular-muscular syndrome.[42,43] Associated malformations to an enlarged rhombencephalon in Meckel-Gruber syndrome are polydactyly and renal abnormalities.

HOLOPROSENCEPHALY

Holoprosencephaly results from the failure of telencephalon to divide during the 7th week. As a result, a single cavity or a holosphere can be seen in ultrasound pictures.[44]

In embryos obtained through induced abortion in the 1st trimester, the incidence of holoprosencephaly was 1:250.[45] Histologically, the diagnosis can be performed as early as in Carnegie stage 13 weeks or 6 weeks of gestation, but most of the cases were reported in Carnegie stage 16 or 17 or 7 weeks of gestation.[45]

Using transvaginal sonography, it is possible to detect the malformation starting from 8 weeks of gestation.[42] Ultrasound markers are the large[46] or the small[44] monoventricular cavity at the endbrain. From 10–14 weeks of gestation, the lack of the typical, "butterfly" sign of normal choroid plexus suggest alobar holoprosencephaly (Figs. 5.5A to D).[47] Using 3D ultrasound with the inversion mode, it was possible to demonstrate holoprosencephaly as early as 9 weeks of gestation.[48]

Associated anomalies are facial malformations such as cyclopia, agnathia, otocephaly, and proboscis.[42]

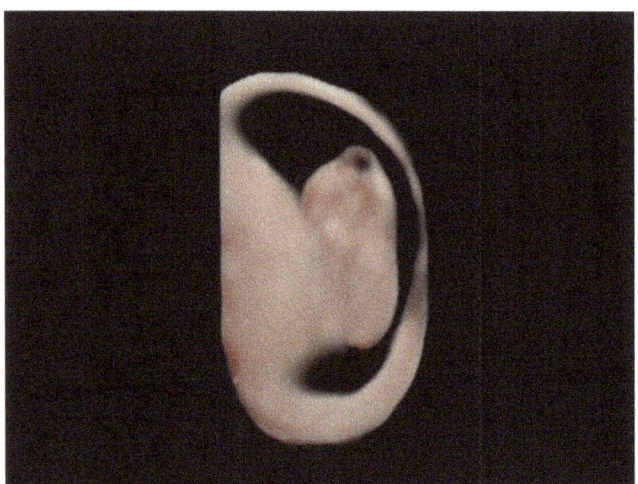

Fig. 5.4: Surface demonstration of a small encephalocele at 11 weeks of gestation (HDlive studio mode).

DANDY–WALKER MALFORMATION

Dandy-Walker malformation was first described by Dandy and Blackfan in 1914.[49] An obstruction of the foramina of Luschka and Magendie during embryological development is the main theory.[49,50]

A cystic structure in the fossa posterior can be seen as early as 11 weeks of gestation.[51] Sonographic findings in the 1st trimester include beside a cystic structure in the posterior portion of the brain also an increased intracranial translucency and an increased brain stem-to-occipital bone diameter.[52] Isolated enlarged fourth ventricle may be a transient finding during 11–14 weeks of gestation.[53]

CLEFT LIP/PALATE

Clefts of the upper lip and palate are present in 13% of all infants with congenital anomalies.[54] The etiology of cleft lip/palate is mostly unknown, but genetic and environmental factors play a role.[55] Both typical and atypical clefts can occur as an isolated anomaly, as part of a sequence of the primary defect, or as a multiple congenital anomaly.[56] In multiple congenital anomaly, the cleft anomaly could be part of a known monogenic syndrome, part of a chromosomal aberration, part of an association, or part of a complex of multiple congenital anomalies of unknown etiology.[57] The most common chromosomal abnormalities are trisomy 13, trisomy 18, and trisomy 21 (Fig. 5.6A).[57,58]

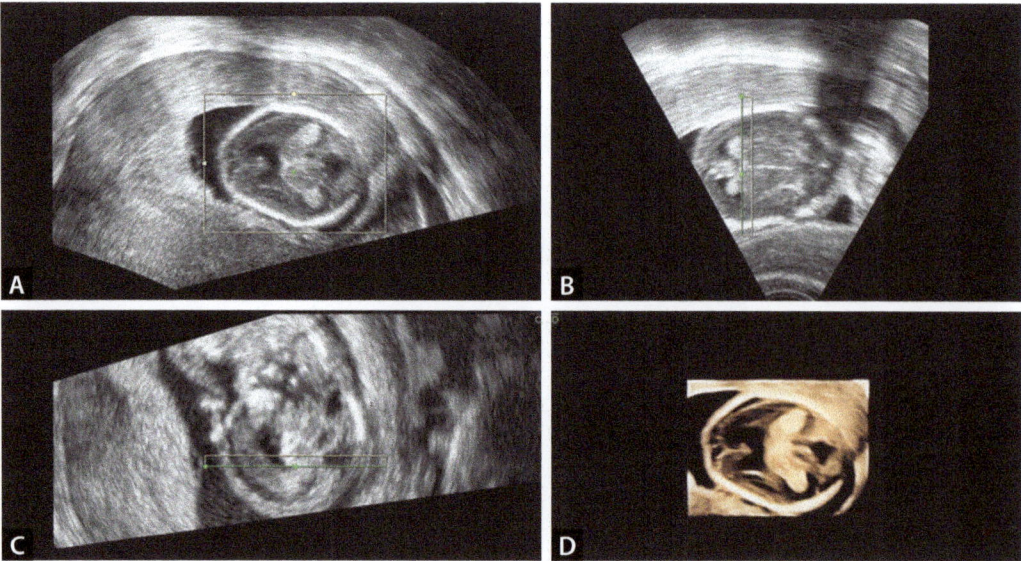

Figs. 5.5A to D: Alobar holoprosencephaly with a single brain ventricle at the anterior brain (13 weeks of gestation). (A to C) Multiplanar mode (A = axial view, B = coronal view, and C = sagittal view); and (D) Surface demonstration of the axial cut plane, showing the communicating hyperechoic choroid plexus.

RETRO-/MICROGNATHIA

Mandible anomalies are part of more than 100 genetic syndromes.[59] Micrognathia is a typical sign in Pierre-Robin syndrome, Franceschetti syndrome, Smith-Lemli-Opitz syndrome II, and Nager syndrome.[60] About 38% of fetuses with micrognathia show an abnormal karyotype.[61] The most common chromosomal abnormality is trisomy 18.[62] The sonographic profile view shows a small, receding chin (Fig. 5.6B).

LOW SET EARS

Low set ears can be found in different syndromes, such as Treacher-Collins syndrome, Kousseff syndrome, or Smith-Lemli-Opitz syndrome.[60] Looking at the fetal head from a side view, the low distance between the lower pole of the ear and the shoulder can be easily recognized (Figs. 5.7A and B). Malformations of the auricle are also found in various syndromes (Fig. 5.6B). However, in the 1st trimester, the pinna is yet not fully expressed and the C-shaped pattern of the auricle might feign a malformation.

ENLARGED NUCHAL TRANSLUCENCY

Nuchal translucency measurement is part of the noninvasive screening test that has gained worldwide importance.[63-65] A thickness above the 95th percentile is considered abnormal.[65,66] Some fetuses between 11 + 0 and 13 + 6 weeks' gestation show an unusual increased nuchal translucency (Fig. 5.8). This is not only a sign for chromosomal anomalies like trisomy 21, 18, and 13, but also provides evidence of fetal cardiac anomalies, genetic syndromes, or other fetal diseases.[65-68] The risk of a chromosomal defect or a cardiac malformation increases markedly with nuchal translucency thickness.[69,70]

The standard risk calculation using a certified computer program is performed on the basis of crown-rump length and nuchal translucency measurement, the maternal blood parameters like *pregnancy-associated plasma protein*-A (PAPP-A) and free beta-human chorionic gonadotropin (b-HCG), and the maternal age. The extended risk calculation includes the sonographic parameters like nasal bone, ductus venosus, and tricuspid flow in addition.[71-75] Absent nasal bone (Fig. 5.9), absent or reverse A-wave in ductus venosus Doppler, and tricuspid regurgitation increase the risk for a chromosomal defect.[76,77]

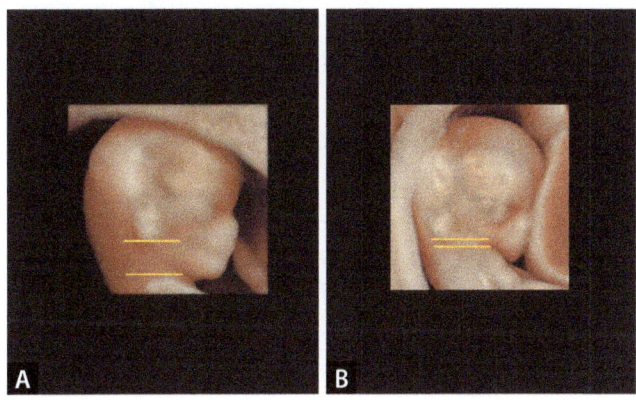

Figs. 5.7A and B: Surface side view of two fetal heads at 12 weeks of gestation (HDlive studio mode). (A) Normal shape and onset of the fetal ear (normal ear-shoulder distance); and (B) Low set ear with reduced ear-shoulder distance.

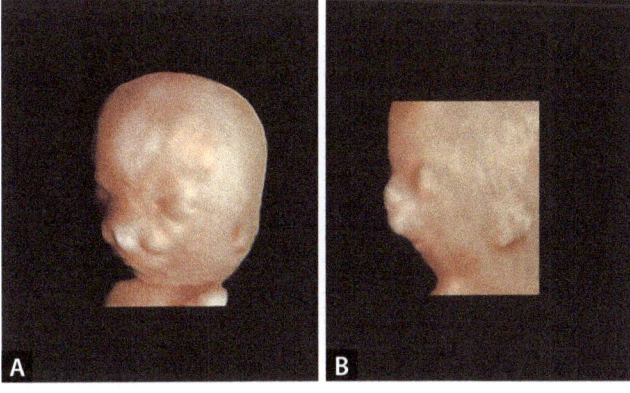

Figs. 5.6A and B: Surface demonstration of 1st trimester fetuses with face abnormalities (HDlive studio mode). (A) Fetus with trisomy 13, demonstrating bilateral cleft lip (13 weeks of gestation); and (B) Fetus with Franceschetti syndrome, showing severe retrognathia, microtia, and low set ear (13 weeks of gestation).

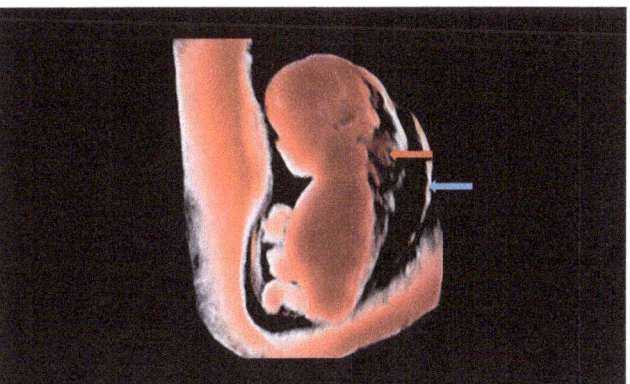

Fig. 5.8: Enlarged nuchal translucency (6.4 mm) (red arrow) in a fetus with trisomy 21 (11 + 5 weeks gestation) and amnion (blue arrow). HDlive surface demonstration, in which the fetus is illuminated by a virtual light source that is positioned behind the fetus.

CYSTIC HYGROMA

Cystic hygroma is a lymphatic malformation mainly located at the neck (Figs. 5.10A to D).[78] Hygromas can be uni- or multiloculated, lateral or posterior in the cervical region. They appear as thin-walled cystic structures, devoid of internal echos. There is an approximately 75% chance that the fetus has Turner syndrome (45,X0).[79] Differentiation includes meningocele, myelomeningocele, and hemangiomas. Color Doppler enables the differentiation from hemangiomas.

FETAL HYDROPS

Hydrops in the 1st trimester is a nonimmune one. The fetus has an appearance like a space suit (Fig. 5.11).[80] About 50% of cases have aneuploidy,[81] but also parvovirus infection[78] has been reported.

SPINA BIFIDA

Primary ossification of the vertebra starts in the cervical part of the spine at 10–11 weeks and is completed between 12 weeks and 14 weeks of gestation.[18]

The spine in the 1st trimester can be demonstrated as two parallel lines, representing the nonossified vertebra (Fig. 5.12A). Abnormalities of the spine are suspected in cases of widening of the two parallel lines or divergences from the parallel configuration.[18]

Diagnosis of neural tube defect are mainly performed in the postembryonic period, after 10 weeks of gestation with sacral irregularity or myelomeningocele.[29]

A retraction of the frontal bones resulting in an acorn-shaped head and the cerebral peduncles appearing parallel to each other are reported in 12 weeks fetuses.[38] However, with high-resolution transvaginal 3D ultrasound, a defect of the spine may be detected with the surface mode as early as 8 weeks of gestation (Fig. 5.12B), definitely with 13 weeks of gestation (Fig. 5.13).

Measurements of the fourth ventricle (=intracranial translucency) are performed during 11–13 weeks for the indirect detection of open spina bifida.[82] 3D ultrasound helps to obtain the mid-sagittal plane of the fetal brain.[83]

HEART DEFECTS

Transvaginal 1st trimester echocardiography has been performed since the beginning of the 1990.[84-86] A systematic approach should be used which includes assessment

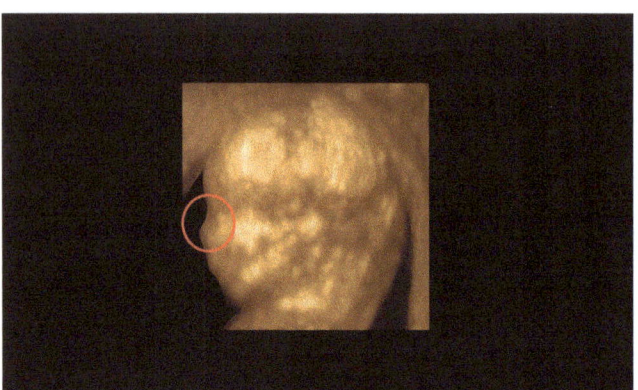

Fig. 5.9: Side view of a fetus with trisomy 21 at 12 weeks of gestation. The maximum mode shows the hyperechoic ossification centers in the head and absent nasal bone (O).

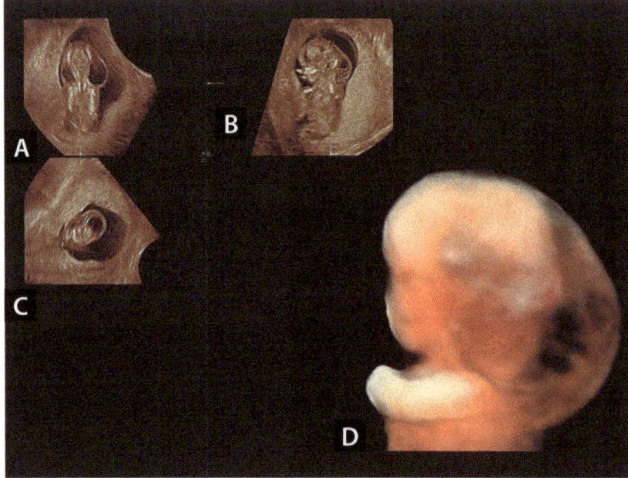

Figs. 5.10A to D: Fetus with hygroma colli at 13 weeks of gestation. (A to C) Multiplanar mode (A = coronal view, B = sagittal view, and C = axial view); and (D) Surface demonstration of the hygroma from a side view (HDlive studio mode).

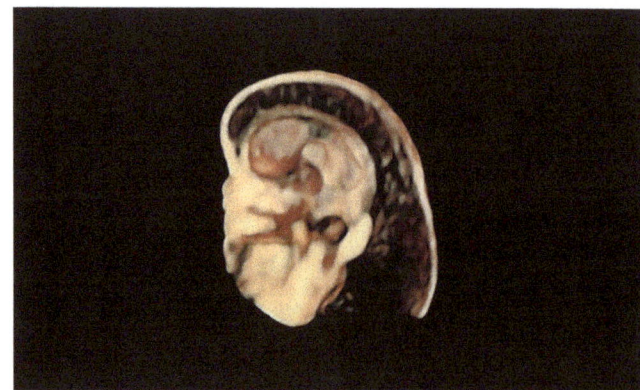

Fig. 5.11: Side view of a fetus with nonimmunologic hydrops at 11 + 5 weeks of gestation. After removing the left side of the fetal head with the electronic scalpel, the HDlive surface demonstration of the cut plane reveals massive edema from scalp to neck.

Chapter 5: Embryonic and Early Fetal Abnormalities Diagnosed with three-dimensional Ultrasound in the 1st Trimester 57

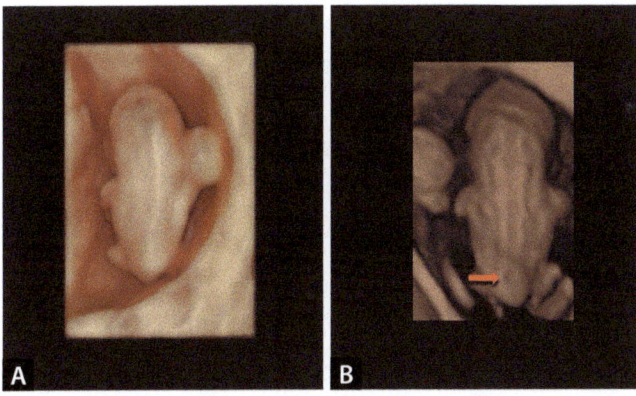

Figs. 5.12A and B: Surface demonstration of the back of two fetuses at 8 + 2 weeks. (A) Normal spine without any defect (HDlive studio surface mode); and (B) Small spina bifida at the lower part of the spine (red arrow) (surface mode).

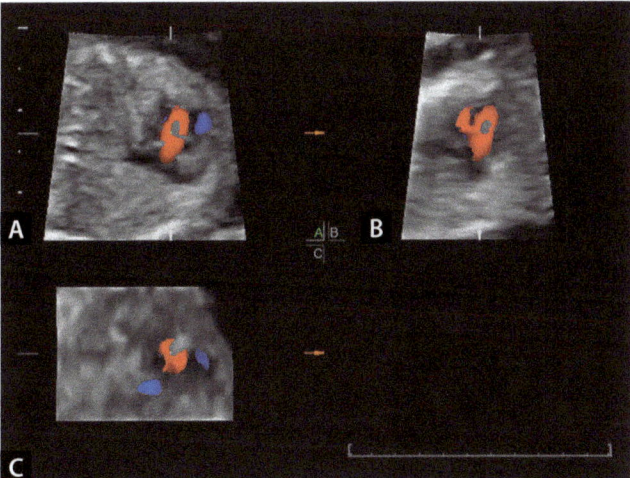

Figs. 5.14A to C: Fetal heart with single ventricle at 13 weeks of gestation. The color STIC mode (spatiotemporal image correlation) shows only a single flow from atrium to chamber in all three perpendicular planes (A = tilted axial plane; B = sagittal plane; and C = coronal plane).

Pentalogy of Cantrell

The Pentalogy of Cantrell was first described in 1958.[55] This includes ectopia cordis, anterior diaphragmatic defect, omphalocele, defect in the lower sternum, and congenital heart defect.[89] It is thought to result from a failure during migration of the paired mesoderm folds of the upper abdomen toward the midline between the 14th days and 18th days of intrauterine life.[90] The most common type of ectopia cordis is the thoracic or thoracoabdominal type.[91]

Toyama[89] proposed a classification for the Pentalogy of Cantrell: Class 1: all five defects are present; Class 2: four defects including intracardiac and ventral abdominal wall malformation; and Class 3: incomplete expression with various combinations of defects present, but always a sternal abnormality present.

Three-dimensional ultrasound helps us to demonstrate the different organs and the anatomical position of the heart. Using this technique, the diagnosis can be performed as early as 1 weeks of gestation (Fig. 5.15).

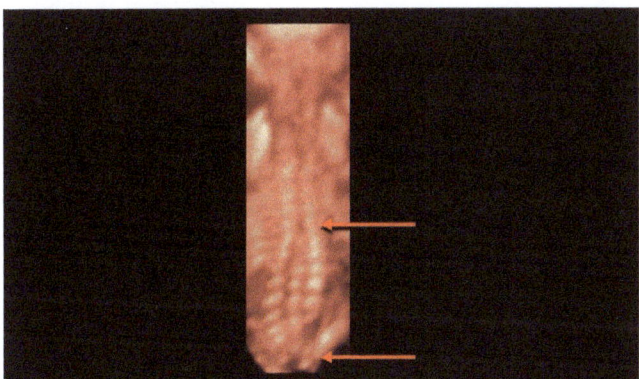

Fig. 5.13: Partial rachischisis with widening of the lower spinal canal (between red arrows). Surface mode, 13 + 6 weeks of gestation.

of the fetal position and orientation, examination of the four-chamber view to assess heart size, position, chamber sizes and the crux, assessment of the tricuspid valve, and the great arteries.[87] Color flow Doppler helps in the demonstration of the great vessels. Sonographic markers that have been studied in relation to congenital heart anomalies are nuchal translucency, abnormal flow in the ductus venosus, and tricuspid regurgitation.[88]

Recent development in 3D/4D ultrasound enables a better anatomical orientation in the fetal heart, facilitating the diagnosis of congenital heart anomalies.

Single Ventricle

A single ventricle refers to a group of heart defects (hypoplastic left heart syndrome, pulmonary atresia or tricuspid atresia) in which the heart functionally has only one pumping chamber which can be demonstrated with STIC technology (Figs. 5.14A to C).

ABDOMINAL WALL DEFECTS

Abdominal wall defects include gastroschisis, omphalocele, eventration, body stalk anomaly, and bladder exstrophy.

Gastroschisis

There are many theories attempting to explain gastroschisis. Some authors propose the premature regression of one or two omphalomesenteric arteries connecting the yolk sac with the dorsal aorta between the 5th weeks and 8th weeks of gestation.[92] Another theory explains gastroschisis as an abnormal development of the umbilical vein.[93] The right location of gastroschisis is explained by persistence or atrophy of the right umbilical vein.[9] Rupture of the amniotic membrane at the base of the umbilical cord is also proposed.[94,95]

Ultrasound features include the absence of a herniated sac, the bowel loops are extruded from the paraumbilical defect on the right side of the abdomen, and float freely in the amniotic fluid (Fig. 5.16A).[96]

Reports on gastroschisis in the 1st trimester are rare because the wall defect is small and bowel peristaltic does begin after 14 weeks of gestation.[97,98]

Omphalocele

An omphalocele is a ventral abdominal wall defect that occurs during the 3rd week of embryonic development. It results from primary deficient closure of the ventral abdominal wall, marked by failure of formation of the umbilical ring.[99] The herniated sac may contain different abdominal viscera (bowel, liver, and stomach) (Fig. 5.16B).[96] Sometimes, ascites can be seen within the sac.

The differential diagnosis between an omphalocele and a physiological midgut herniation in the 1st trimester[100] is performed based on its sonographic appearance and time of appearance. Physiological umbilical herniation is a temporary change at the embryonic umbilical cord insertion that can typically be observed during prenatal ultrasound examination between 9 and 10 gestational weeks.[19] During that time, the intestine herniates into the umbilicus, twists 90°, and concludes with a 180° counterclockwise rotation after descending back into the abdominal cavity.[19] If the rotation is incomplete, an *umbilical hernia* is formed.[101] Such a defect is smaller than an omphalocele and contains only bowel.

Eventration

Eventration is an extensive abdominal wall defect with protrusion of abdominal viscera (Fig. 5.16C). The defect is

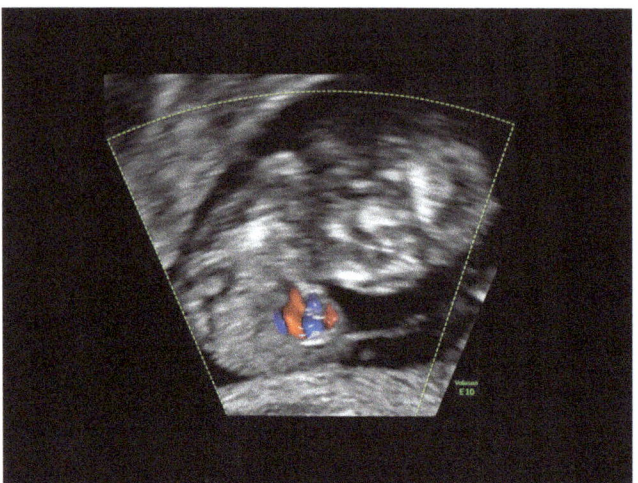

Fig. 5.15: Pentalogy of Cantrell at 11 weeks of gestation. The fetal heart is located outside of the thorax (radiant flow).

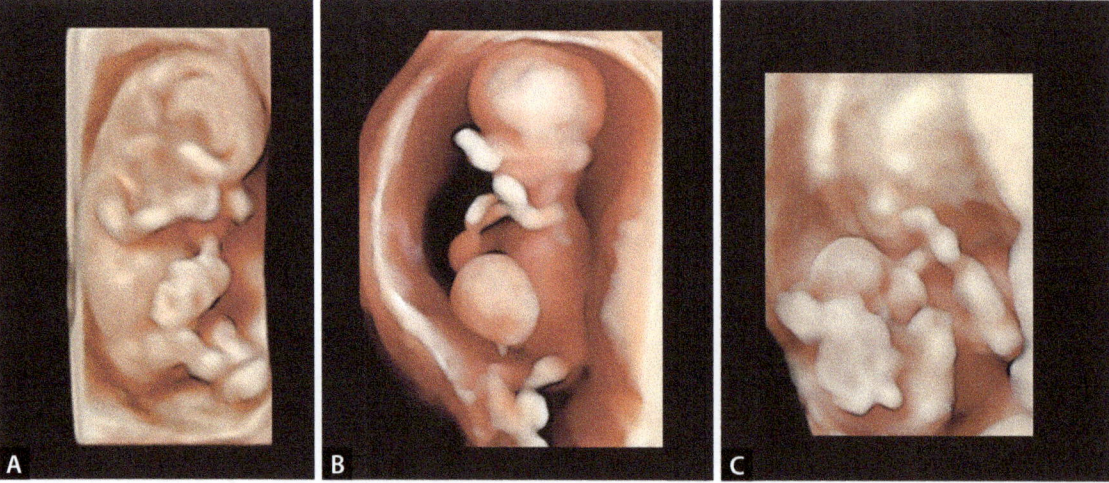

Figs. 5.16A to C: Surface demonstration of 1st trimester fetuses with abdominal wall defects (HDlive studio mode). (A) Fetus with gastroschisis (11 + 4 weeks of gestation); (B) Fetus with omphalocele (13 + 2 weeks of gestation); and (C) Fetus with eventration, showing liver and bowel surrounded by amniotic fluid (13 + 2 weeks of gestation).

found in connection with an absent umbilical cord (body stalk anomaly) or amniotic band sequence.[96]

Body Stalk Anomaly

Body stalk anomaly is the rarest and the most severe abdominal wall malformation. Due to an absence of the umbilical cord, the abdominal organs lie outside the abdominal cavity in a sac of amnion mesoderm which is limited by the placenta at one side and amnion on the other side. The umbilical vessels cross the amniotic portion of the amniotic sac usually with a single umbilical artery (SUA).[102] While the upper part of the fetus may look normal, the lower part is missing (Fig. 5.17).

Hyperechogenic Bowel

Hyperechogenic bowel is an observation during prenatal ultrasound examination, in which the fetal bowel appears with similar or greater echogenicity than surrounding bone (Figs. 5.18A to D).[103,104] A grading scale was proposed by Slotnick et al.[105]: Grade 0 = normal, Grade 1 = increased echogenicity, but less echogenic than bone, Grade 3 = echogenicity equal to bone, and Grade 4 = echogenicity greater than bone. The sign of hyperechogenic bowel belongs to the soft markers that can be associated with different pathologic conditions, especially fetal aneuploidy (trisomy 21, less frequently trisomy 13, 18, and X0).[104]

URINARY TRACT ANOMALIES

Using transvaginal ultrasound the kidneys can be visualized as hypoechoic oval structures on both sides of the embryonic spine as early as 9 weeks of gestation. Transabdominally, they can be visualized in all fetuses after 12 weeks of gestation.[106,107] Nomograms of the kidneys are published by Rosati and Guariglia.[108] Bilateral renal

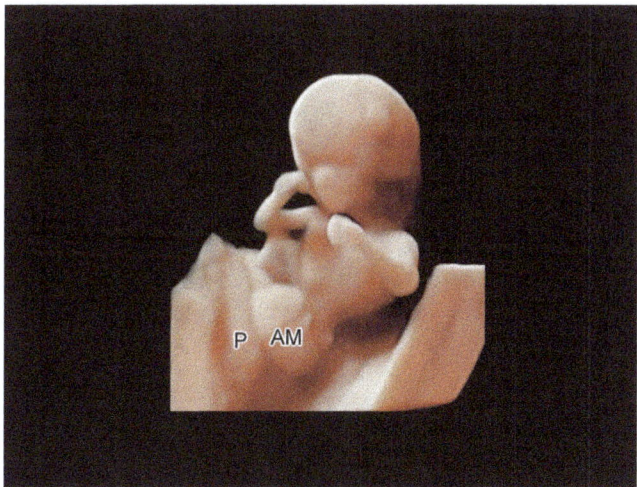

Fig. 5.17: Surface demonstration of a fetus with body stalk anomaly (HDlive studio mode) at 12 + 2 weeks of gestation. The abdominal organs lie in a sac of amnion mesoderm (AM) between abdominal wall and placenta (P).

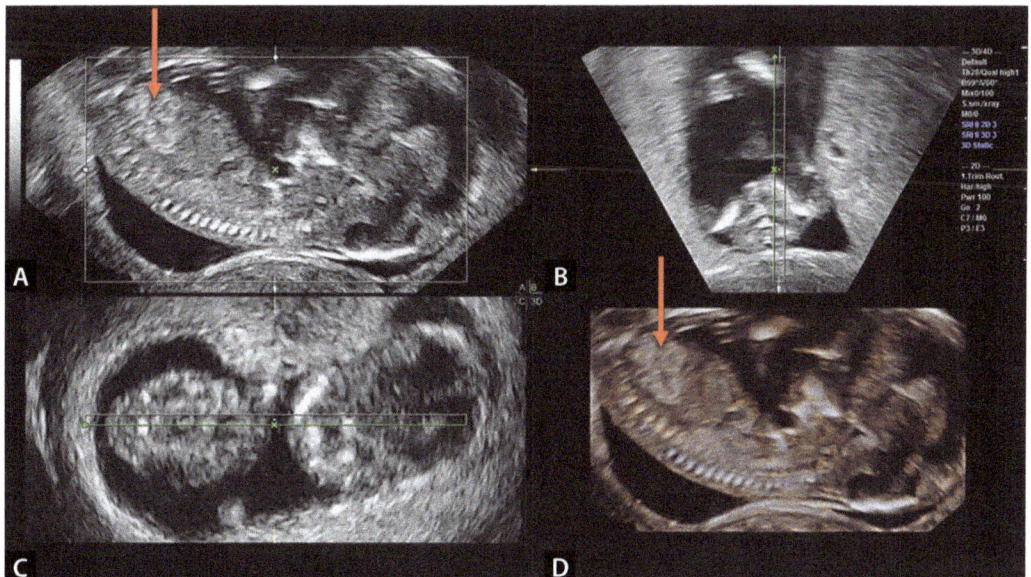

Figs. 5.18A to D: Hyperechogenic bowel (arrows) in a fetus with triploidy (69, XXX) at 13 weeks of gestation. (A to C) Multiplanar mode (A = sagittal view, B = axial view, and C = coronal view); and (D) Surface demonstration of the sagittal cut plane.

agenesis after 12 weeks of pregnancy is reported, while a polycystic kidney disease was possible to be diagnosed after 14 weeks of gestation.[109,110]

The enlargement of the bladder more than 6 mm between 11 weeks and 14 weeks of gestation is defined as megacystis.[111] In the majority of chromosomally normal fetuses with mild or moderate enlargement of the bladder (8–12 mm), there was spontaneous resolution of the megacystis by 20 weeks of gestation without any obvious adverse effects on renal development and function. However, in some cases megacystis is associated with progressive obstructive uropathy, chromosomal defects or extrarenal malformations.[111,112] In *prune belly syndrome*, not only megacystis but also several other defects can be observed—absence of the abdominal wall muscles, renal dysplasia, and in males absence of the prostate and cryptorchidism.[113]

Using HDlive or HDlive Silhouette mode, we can see the fluid-filled structures in the urinary tract allowing a better diagnosis (Figs. 5.19A and B).

LIMB ANOMALIES

Limb anomalies are published in the literature as early as 9 weeks of gestation.[114] In the 1st trimester, a number of malformations are reported, including amelia,[115] radial aplasia,[116] clubfoot,[117] and sirenomelia.[118,119]

Three-dimensional ultrasound with its different display modes does not only offer a precise demonstration of limb defects but also reveals an extra digit (Fig. 5.20A) or a deviation of the limb axis (Fig. 5.20B).

CONJOINED TWINS

In monochorionic, monoamniotic twin pregnancy, there is always a risk of conjoined twins. The 3D ultrasound enables the operator to demonstrate such an abnormality already in the 1st trimester very convincingly (Fig. 5.21).

SINGLE UMBILICAL ARTERY

Several studies have shown that there is an association between a SUA and an increased incidence of structural and chromosomal anomalies and growth restriction.[120-125] In 1st trimester, prevalence of SUA was 1.1% in single pregnancies and 3.3% in twin pregnancies. 17.6% of cases had associated malformations.[126]

In the 1st trimester, a SUA can be identified at the level of the bladder using color Doppler.[127] The cross-section

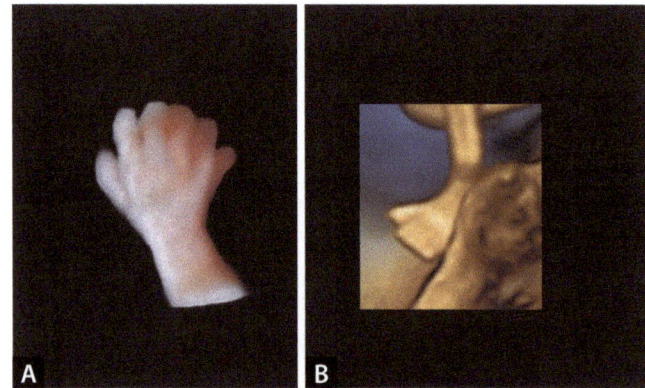

Figs. 5.20A and B: Surface demonstration of limb anomalies. (A) Hexadactyly at 13 weeks of gestation (HDlive studio mode); and (B) Clubfoot left at 13 weeks of gestation (soft surface mode).

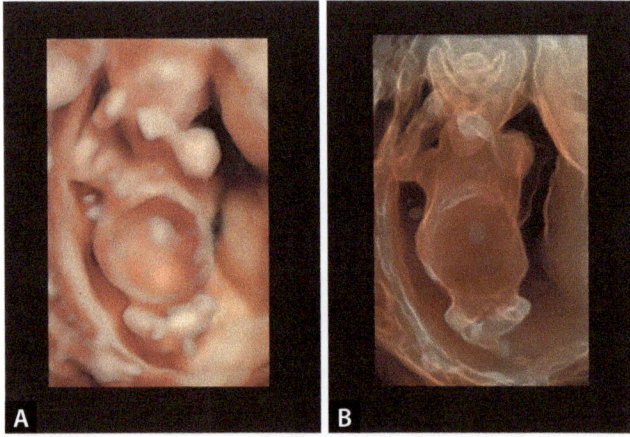

Figs. 5.19A and B: Surface view of a fetus with prune belly syndrome at 11 weeks of gestation. (A) HDlive studio mode; and (B) Silhouette mode, demonstrating the enlarged bladder.

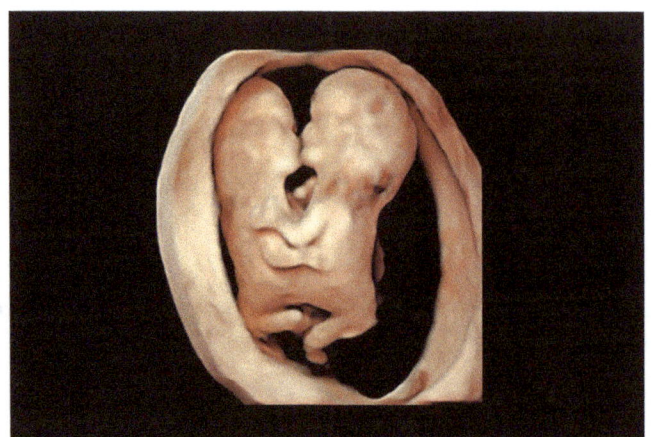

Fig. 5.21: Surface demonstration of conjoined twins (thoracopagus) at 12 weeks of gestation (HDlive studio mode).

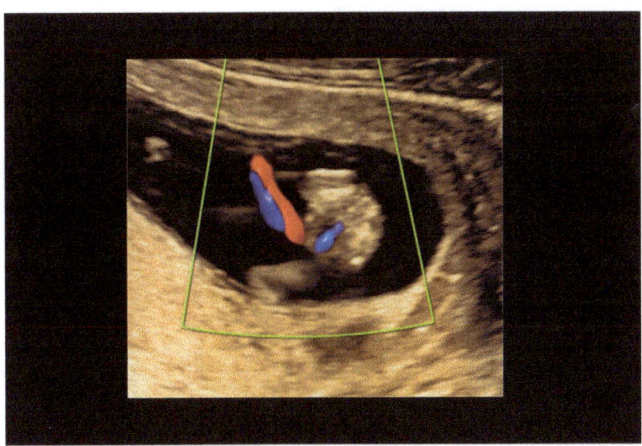

Fig. 5.22: Single umbilical artery at 13 weeks of gestation. The radiant flow reveals only the right umbilical artery next to the urinary bladder (breech presentation) and in the umbilical cord only two vessels can be seen.

of the fetal pelvis reveals only one artery next to the fetal bladder (Fig. 5.22).

CONCLUSION

In comparison to two-dimensional (2D) ultrasound, 3D sonography offers, particularly the experienced operator, several advantages in the demonstration of fetal malformations in the 1st trimester: several display modes, no limitation of scan planes, standardization of planes, virtual scanning facilities, long-term storage of volumes, and the possibility to demonstrate normal and abnormal anatomy of the embryo/fetus to the parents like on a photograph.

REFERENCES

1. Merz E, Weber G, Bahlmann F, et al. Application of transvaginal and abdominal three-dimensional ultrasound for the detection or exclusion of malformations of the fetal face. Ultrasound Obstet Gynecol. 1997;9:237-43.
2. Merz E, Abramowicz JS. 3D/4D ultrasound in prenatal diagnosis: is it time for routine use? Clin Obstet Gynecol. 2012;55:336-51.
3. Merz E, Pashaj S. Advantages of 3D ultrasound in the assessment of fetal abnormalities. J Perinat Med. 2017;45:643-50.
4. Pooh RK, Kurjak A. Novel application of three-dimensional HDlive imaging in prenatal diagnosis from the first trimester. J Perinat Med. 2014;43:147-58.
5. Merz E. Normal early pregnancy (first trimester). In: Merz E (Ed). Ultrasound in Obstetrics and Gynecology, 1st edition. Philadelphia: Williams and Wilkins; 2005. pp. 17-25.
6. Callen PW. Ultrasonography in Obstetrics and Gynecology. New York: Elsevier; 2000. pp. 105-45.
7. Lindsay DJ, Lovett IS, Lyons EA, et al. Yolk sac diameter and shape at endovaginal US: predictors of pregnancy outcome in the first trimester. Radiology. 1992;183:115-8.
8. Levi CS, Lyons EA, Lindsay DJ. Early diagnosis of nonviable pregnany with transvaginal US. Radiology. 1988:167;383-5.
9. Bree RL, Edwards M, Böhm-Vélez M, et al. Transvaginal sonography in the evaluation of normal early pregnancy: correlation with hCG level. Am J Roentgenol. 1989;153:75-9.
10. Doubilet PM, Benson CB, Bourne T, et al. Diagnostic criteria for nonviable pregnancy early in the first trimester. N Engl J Med. 2013;369:1443-51.
11. Yegul NT, Filly RA. The expanded amnion sign: evidence of early embryonic death. J Ultrasound Med. 2009;28:1331-5.
12. Yeh HC, Rabinowitz JG. Amniotic sac development: ultrasound features of early pregnancy—the double bleb sign. Radiology. 1988;166:97-103.
13. Doubilet PM, Benson CB. Embryonic heart rate in the early first trimester: what rate is normal? J Ultrasound Med. 1995;14:431-4.
14. Doubilet PM, Benson CB, Chow JS. Outcome of pregnancies with rapid embryonic heart rates in the early first trimester. AJR Am J Roentgenol. 2000;175:67-9.
15. Bayer AS, Altman J. The Human Brain during the Late First Trimester. New York: CRC Press; 2006.
16. Timor-Tritsch I. A close look at early embryonic development with high-frequency transvaginal transducer. Am J Obstet Gynecol. 1988;159:676-81.
17. Blaas HG, Eik-Nes SH, Kiserud T, et al. Early development of the abdominal wall, stomach and heart from 7 to 12 weeks of gestation: a longitudinal ultrasound study. Ultrasound Obstet Gynecol. 1995;6:240-9.
18. van Zalen-Sprock MM, van Vugt JM, van Geijn HP. First and early second trimester diagnosis of anomalies of the central nervous system. J Ultrasound Med. 1995;14:603-10.
19. Merz E. Physiological umbilical herniation—a distinctive sonographic feature in the embryonic stage. Ultraschall Med. 2017;38:123-4.
20. Yamada SH, Takakuwa T. Introduction—Developmental Overview of the Human Embryo. Hum Embr. 2012;2:1-20.
21. Moradan S, Forouzeshfar M. Are abnormal yolk sac characteristics important factors in abortion rates? Int J Fertil Steril. 2012;6:127-30.
22. Tan S, Gülden-Tangal N, Kanat-Pektas M, et al. Abnormal sonographic appearances of the yolk sac: which can be associated with adverse perinatal outcome? Med Ultrasound. 2014;16:15-20.
23. Gersak K, Veble A, Mulla ZD, et al. Association between increased yolk sac diameter and abnormal karyotypes. J Perinat Med. 2012;40:251-4.
24. Sepulveda W, Leibe S, Ulloa A, et al. Clinical significance of the first trimester umbilical cord cysts. J Ultrasound Med. 1999;18:95-9.
25. Ghezzi F, Raio L, DI Naro E, et al. Single and multiple umbilical cord cysts in early gestation: two different entities. Ultrasound Obstet Gynecol. 2003;21:215-9.
26. Benirschke J, Kaufmann P. Anatomy and pathology of the umbilical cord and major fetal vessels. In: Benirschke J,

Kaufmann P (Eds). Pathology of the Human Placenta. New York: Springer; 2000. pp. 355-98.
27. Frazier HA, Guerrieri JP, Thomas RI, et al. The detection of a patent urachus and allantoic cyst of the umbilical cord on prenatal ultrasonography. J Ultrasound Med. 1992;11:117-20.
28. Sepulveda W, Bower S, Dhillon HK, et al. Prenatal diagnosis of congenital patent urachus and allantoic cyst: the value of the color flow imaging. J Ultrasound Med. 1995;14:47-51.
29. Weissman A, Jakobi P, Bornstein M, et al. Sonographic measurements of the umbilical cord and vessels during normal pregnancies. J Ultrasound Med. 1994;13:11-4.
30. Shipp TD, Bromley B, Benacerraf BR. Sonographically detected abnormalites of the umbilical cord. Int J Gynaecol Obstet. 1995;48:179-85.
31. Smith GN, Walker M, Johnston S, et al. The sonographic finding persistent umbilical cord cystic masses are associated with lethal aneuploidy and/or congenital anomalies. Prenat Diagn. 1996;16:1141-7.
32. Cullen MT, Green J, Whetham J, et al. Transvaginal ultrasonographic detection of congenital anomalies in the first trimester. Am J Obstet Gynecol. 1990;163:466-76.
33. O´Rahilly R, Müller F. Developmental Stages in Human Embryos. Washington: Carnegie Institution Publications; 1987.
34. Moore KL, Persaud TV. Embryologie 4. AuflageVelrag: Schattauer; 1996. p. 485.
35. Hardt W, Entezami M, Vogel M, et al. Die fetale Exenzephalie—Vorstadium der Anenzephalie? Ein kasuistischer Beitrag. Geburtsh Frauenheilk. 1999;59:135-8.
36. Becker R, Mende B, Stiemer B, et al. Sonographic markers of exencephaly at 9 + 3 weeks of gestation. Ultrasound Obstet Gynecol. 2000;16:582-4.
37. Johnson SP, Sebire NJ, Snijders RJ, et al. Ultrasound screening for anencephaly at 10–14 weeks of gestation. Ultrasound Obstet Gynecol. 1997;9:14-6.
38. Chatzipapas IK, Whitlow BJ, Economides DL. The "Mickey Mouse" sign and diagnosis of anencephaly in early pregnancy. Ultrasound Obstet Gynecol. 1999;13:196-9.
39. Sepulveda W, Sebire NJ, Fung TY, et al. Crown-chin length in normal and anencephalic fetuses at 10-14 weeks gestations. Am J Obstet Gynecol. 1997;176:852-5.
40. van Zalen-Sprock MM, van Vugt JM, van dHarten HJ, et al. Cephalocele and cystic hygroma: diagnosis and differentiation in the first trimester of pregnancy with transvaginal sonography. Report of two cases. Ultrasound Obstet Gynecol. 1992;2:289-92.
41. van Zalen-Sprock MM, van Vugt JM, van Geijn HP. First trimester sonographic detection of neurodevelopment abnormalities in some single gene disorders. Prenat Diagn. 1996;16:199-202.
42. Blaas HG, Eik-Nes HS. Sonoembryology and early prenatal diagnosis of neural anomalies. Prenat Diagn. 2009;29:312-25.
43. Nishi T, Nakano R. First trimester diagnosis of exencephaly by transvaginal ultrasonography. J Ultrasound Med. 1994;13:149-51.
44. Blaas H. Picture of the month. Holoprosencephaly at 10 weeks 2 days (CRL 33 mm). Ultrasound Gynecol Obstet. 2000;15:86-7.
45. Matsunaga E, Shiota K. Holoprosencephaly in human embryos: Epidemiologic studies of 150 cases. Teratology. 1977;16:226-32.
46. Sepulveda W, Lutz I, Be C. Holoprosencephaly at 9 weeks 6 days in a triploid fetus. J Ultrasound Med. 2007;26:411-4.
47. Sepulveda W, Dezerega V, Be C. First-trimester sonographic diagnosis of holoprosencephaly: value of the "butterfly" sign. J Ultrasound Med. 2004;23:761-5.
48. Timor-Tritsch IE, Monteagudo A, Santos R. Three-dimensional inversion rendering in the first- and the early second-trimester fetal brain: its use in holoprosencephaly. Ultrasound Obstet Gynecol. 2008;32;744-50.
49. Dandy WE, Blackfan KD. Internal hydrocephalus and experimental, clinical and pathological study. Am J Dis Child. 1914;8:406-82.
50. Taggart JK, Walker AE. Congenital atresia of the foramens of Luschka and Magendie. Arch Neurol Psychiatr. 1942;48:583-612.
51. Achiron R, Achiron A, Yagel S. First trimester transvaginal sonographic diagnosis of Dandy-Walker malformation. J Clin Ultrasound. 1993;21:62-4.
52. Bornstein E, Goncalves Rodriguez JL, Alvares Pavon EC, et al. First trimester sonographic findings associated with a Dandy-Walker Malformation and inferior vermian hypoplasia. J Ultrasound Med. 2013;32:1863-998.
53. Bornstein M, Zimmer EZ, Blazer S. Isolated large fourth ventricle in the early pregnancy—a possible benign transient phenomenon. Prenat Diagn. 1998;18:997-1000.
54. Gorlin RJ, Cervenka J, Pruzansky S. Facial clefting and its syndromes. Birth Defects Orig Artic Ser. 1971;7:3-49.
55. Lidral AC, Moreno LM, Bullard SA. Genetic factors and orofacial clefting. Semin Orthod. 2008;14:103-14.
56. Merz E, Pashaj S. Prenatal detection of orofacial clefts. Ultraschall Med. 2016;37:133-5.
57. Tolarová MM, Cervenka J. Classification and birth prevalence of orofacial clefts. Am J Med Genet. 1998;75:126-37.
58. Doray B, Badila-Timbolschi D, Schaefer E, et al. Epidemiology of orofacial clefts (1995-2006) in France (Congenital Malformations of Alsace Registry). Arch Pediatr. 2012;19:1021-9.
59. Jones KL. Smith's Recognizable Patterns of Human Malformation, 5th edition. London: WB Saunders; 1997.
60. Merz E. Anomalies of the head. In: Merz E (Ed). Ultrasound in Obstetrics and Gynecology. New York: Elsevier; 2005. pp. 212-45.
61. Turner GM, Twining P. The facial profile in the diagnosis of fetal abnormalities. Clin Radiol. 1993;47:389-95.
62. Nicolaides KH, Salvesen DR, Snijders RJ, et al. Fetal facial defects: associated malformations and chromosomal abnormalities. Fetal Diagn Ther. 1993;8:1-9.
63. Nicolaides KH, Spencer K, Avgidou K, et al. Multicenter study of first-trimester screening for trisomy 21 in 75,821 pregnancies: results and estimation of the potential impact of

individual risk-orientated two stage first-trimester screening. Ultrasound Obstet Gynecol. 2005;25:221-6.
64. Merz E, Thode C, Alkier A, et al. A new approach to calculating the risk of chromosomal abnormalities with first-trimester screening data. Ultraschall Med. 2008;29:639-45.
65. Kagan KO, Wright D, Baker A, et al. Screening for trisomy 21 by maternal age, fetal nuchal translucency thickness, free beta-human chorionic gonadotropin, and pregnancy-associated plasma protein-A. Ultrasound Obstet Gynecol. 2008;31:618-24.
66. Merz E, Thode C, Eiben B, et al. Prenatal Risk Calculation (PRC) 3.0: An extended DoE based first-trimester screening algorithm allowing for early blood sampling. Ultrasound Int Open. 2016;2:E19-26.
67. Hyett JA, Perdu M, Sharland GK, et al. Using fetal nuchal translucency to screen for congenital cardiac defects at 10–14 weeks of gestation: population-based cohort study. Br Med J. 1999;318:81-5.
68. Souka AP, Krampl E, Bakalis S, et al. Outcome of pregnancy in chromosomally normal fetuses with increased nuchal translucency in the first trimester. Ultrasound Obstet Gynecol. 2001;18:9-17.
69. Snijders RJ, Pandya P, Brizot ML, et al. First trimester fetal nuchal translucency. In: Snijders RJ, Nicolaides KH (Eds). Ultrasound Markers for Fetal Chromosomal Defects. Carnforth: Parthenon Publishing; 1996. pp. 121-56.
70. Ghi T, Huggon IC, Zosmer N, et al. Incidence of major structural cardiac defects associated with increased nuchal translucency but normal karyotype. Ultrasound Obstet Gynecol. 2001;18:610-4.
71. Cicero S, Avgidou K, Rembouskos G, et al. Nasal bone in first-trimester screening for trisomy 21. Am J Obstet Gynecol. 2006;195:109-14.
72. Borrell A, Gonce A, Martinez JM, et al. First-trimester screening for Down syndrome with ductus venosus Doppler studies in addition to nuchal translucency and serum markers. Prenat Diagn. 2005;25:901-5.
73. Maiz N, Plasencia W, Dagklis T, et al. Ductus venosus Doppler in fetuses with cardiac defects and increased nuchal translucency thickness. Ultrasound Obstet Gynecol. 2008;31:256-60.
74. Faiola S, Tsoi E, Huggon IC, et al. Likelihood ratio for trisomy 21 in fetuses with tricuspid regurgitation at the 11 to 13 + 6-week scan. Ultrasound Obstet Gynecol. 2005;26:22-7.
75. Scala C, Morlando M, Familiari A, et al. Fetal Tricuspid Regurgitation in the First Trimester as a Screening Marker for Congenital Heart Defects: Systematic Review and Meta-Analysis. Fetal Diagn Ther. 2017;42:1-8.
76. Ghaffari SR, Tahmasebpour AR, Jamal A, et al. First-trimester screening for chromosomal abnormalities by integrated application of nuchal translucency, nasal bone, tricuspid regurgitation, and ductus venosus flow combined with maternal serum free β-hCG and PAPP-A: a 5-year prospective study. Ultrasound Obstet Gynecol. 2012;39:528-34.
77. Wassef M, Blei F, Adams D, et al. Vascular anomalies classfication: recommendations from the International Society for the Study of vascular anomalies. Pediatrics. 2015;136: e203-14.
78. Sohan K, Carrol S, Byrne D, et al. Parvovirus as a differential diagnosis of hydrops fetalis in the first trimester. Fetal Diagn Ther. 2000;15:234-6.
79. Merz E. Transvaginal detection of fetal anomalies. In: Merz E (Ed). Ultrasound in Obstetrics and Gynecology. New York: Elsevier; 2005. pp. 45-8.
80. Shulman LP, Phillips OP, Emerson DS, et al. Fetal "space-suit" hydrops in the first trimester: differentiating risk for chromosomal abnormalities by delineating characteristics of nuchal translucency. Prenat Diagn. 2000;20: 30-2.
81. Has R, Recep H. Non-immune hydrops fetalis in the first trimester: a review of of 30 cases. Clin Exp Obstet Gynecol. 2000;28:187-90.
82. Chaoui R, Benoit B, Mitkowska-Wozniak H, et al. Assessment of intracranial translucency (IT) in the detection of spina bifida at the 11-13 week scan. Ultrasound Obstet Gynecol. 2009;34:249-52.
83. Chaoui R, Nicolaides KH. From nuchal translucency to intracranial translucency: toward the early detection of spina bifida. Ultrasound Obstet Gynecol. 2010;35:133-8.
84. Gembruch U, Knopfle G, Chatterjee M, et al. First-trimester diagnosis of fetal congenital heart disease by transvaginal two-dimensional and Doppler echocardiography. Obstet Gynecol. 1990;75:496-8.
85. Dolkart LA, Reimers FT. Transvaginal fetal echocardiography in early pregnancy: normative date. Am J Obstet Gynecol. 1991;165:688-91.
86. Johnson P, Sharland G, Maxwell D, et al. The role of transvaginal sonography in the early detection of congenital heart disease. Ultrasound Obstet Gynecol. 1992; 2:248-51.
87. Allan L, Cook A, Huggon I. First trimester fetal heart scanning. In: Allan L, Cook A, Huggon I (Eds). Fetal Echocadrdiography—A Practical Guideline. Cambridge: Cambridge University Press; 2009. pp. 190-202.
88. Khalil A, Nicoloaides KH. Fetal heart defects: Potential pitfalls of first trimester detections. Semin Fetal Neonat Med. 2013;18:251-60.
89. Toyama WM. Combined congenital defects of the anterior abdominal wall, sternum, diaphragm, pericardium, and heart: a case report and review of the syndrome. Pediatrics. 1972;50:778-9.
90. Cantrell JR, Heller RJ, Ravitch MM. A syndrome of congenital defects involving the abdominal wall, sternum, diaphragm, pericardium, and heart. Surg Gynecol Obstet. 1958;107: 602-14.
91. Dobell AR, William HB, Long RW. Staged repair of ectopia cordis. J Pediatr Surg. 1982;17:353-8.
92. Hoyme HE, Higginbottom MC, Jones KL. The vascular pathogenesis of gastroschisis: intrauterine interruption of the omphalomesenteric artery. J Pediatr. 1981;98:228-31.
93. de Vries PA. The pathogenesis of gastroschisis and omphalocele. J Pediatr Surg. 1980;15:245-51.

94. Perrella RR, Ragavendra N, Tessler FN, et al. Fetal abdominal wall mass detected on prenatal sonography: gastrischisis vs. omphalocele. Am J Roentgenol. 1991;157:1065-8.
95. Shaw A. The myth of gastroschisis. J Pediatr Surg. 1975;10:235-44.
96. Merz E. Anomalies of the gastrointestinal tract and anterior abdominal wall. In: Merz E (Ed). Ultrasound in Obstetrics and Gynecology. New York: Elsevier; 2005. pp. 297-311.
97. Guzman ER. Early prenatal diagnosis of gastroschisis with transvaginal ultrasonography. Am J Obstet Gynecol. 1990;162:1253-4.
98. Whitlow BJ, Chatzipapas IK, Lazanakis ML, et al. The value of sonography in early pregnancy for the detection of fetal abnormalities in an an unselected population. Br J Obstet Gynecol. 1999;106:929-36.
99. Duhamel D. Embryology of exomphalos and allied malformations. Arch Dis Child. 1963;38:142-7.
100. Howell H, Fox BT. First trimester diagnosis of omphalocele. Differentiating between the omphalocele and normal physiologic gut herniation. J Diagn Med Sono. 2015;31:261-4.
101. Klein MD, Kosloske AM, Hertzler JH. Congenital defects of the abdominal wall: a review of the experience in New Mexico. J Am Med Assoc. 1981;245:1643-6.
102. Ginsberg NE, Cadkin A, Strom C. Prenatal diagnosis of body stalk anomaly in the first trimester of pregnancy. Ultrasound Obstet Gynecol. 1997;10:419-21.
103. Lince DM, Pretorius DH, Manco-Johnson ML, et al. The clinical significance of increased echogenicity in the fetal abdomen. AJR Am J Roentgenol. 1985;145:683-6.
104. De Oronzo MA. Hyperechogenic fetal bowel: an ultrasonographic marker for adverse fetal and neonatal outcome. J Prenat Med. 2011;5:9-13.
105. Slotnick RN, Abuhamad AZ. Prognostic implications of fetal echogenic bowel. Lancet. 1996;13:85-7.
106. Green JJ, Hobins JC. Abdominal ultrasound examination of the first trimester fetus. Am J Obstet Gynecol. 1988;159:165-75.
107. Braithwaite JM, Armstrong MA, Economides DL. Assessment of fetal anatomy at 12-13 weeks of gestation by transabdominal and transvaginal sonography. Br J Obstet Gynecol. 1996;103:82-5.
108. Rosati P, Guariglia L. Transvaginal sonographic assesment of the fetal urinary tract in early pregnancy. Ultrasound Obstet Gynecol. 1996;7:95-100.
109. Bornstein M, Amit A, Achiron R, et al. The early prenatal diagnosis of renal agenesis: techniques and possible pitfalls. Prenat Diagn. 1994;14:291-7.
110. Bornstein M, Bar-Hava I, Blumenfeld Z. Clues and pitfalls in the early prenatal diagnosis of "late onset" infantile polycystic kidney. Prenat Diagn. 1992;12:293-8.
111. Sebire NJ, von Kaisenberg C, Rubio C, et al. Fetal megacystis at 10-14 weeks of gestation. Ultrasound Obstet Gynecol. 1996;8:387-90.
112. Jouannic JM, Hyett JA, Pandya PP, et al. Perinatal outcome in fetuses with megacystis in the first half of the pregnancy. Prenat Diagn. 2003;23:340-4.
113. Moerman P, Fryns JP, Goddeeris P, et al. Pathogenesis of the prune belly syndrome: a functional urethral obstruction caused by prostatic hypoplasia. Pediatrics. 1984;73:470-5.
114. Timor-Tritsch IE, Monteagudo A, Peisner DB. High-frequency transvaginal sonographic examination for the potential malformation assessment of the 9-week fetus. J Clin Ultrasound. 1992;20:231-8.
115. Bianca S, Bartoloni G, Libertini C, et al. Fetal upper limb amelia with increased nuchal translucency. Congenit Anom (Kyoto). 2009;49:121-2.
116. Rice KJ, Ballas J, Lai E, et al. Diagnosis of fetal limb abnormalities before 15 weeks: cause for concern. J Ultrasound Med. 2011;30:1009-19.
117. Bornshtein M, Keret D, Deutsch M, et al. Transvaginal sonographic detection of skeletal anomalies in the first trimester and early second trimester. Prenat Diagn. 1993;13:597-601.
118. Van Keirsbilck J, Cannie M, Robrechts C, et al. First trimester diagnosis of sirenomelia. Prenat Diagn. 2006;26:684-8.
119. Singh C, Lodha P, Arora D, et al. Diagnosis of sirenomielia in the first trimester. J Clin Ultrasound. 2014;6:335-9.
120. Thummala MR, Raju TN, Langenberg P. Isolated single umbilical artery anomaly and the risk for congenital malformations—a meta-analysis. J Pediatr Surg. 1998;33:580-5.
121. Chow JS, Benson CB, Doubilet PM. Frequency and nature of structural anomalies in fetuses with single umbilical arteries. J Ultrasound Med. 1998;17:765-8.
122. Rinehart BK, Terrone DA, Taylor CW, et al. Single umbilical artery is associated with an increased incidence of structural and chromosomal anomalies and growth restriction. Am J Perinatol. 2000;17:229-32.
123. Rembouskos G, Cicero S, Longo D, et al. Single umbilical artery at 11–14 weeks' gestation: relation to chromosomal defects. Ultrasound Obstet Gynecol. 2003;22:567-70.
124. Dagklis T, Defigueiredo D, Staboulidou I, et al. Isolated single umbilical artery and fetal karyotype. Ultrasound Obstet Gynecol. 2010;36:291-5.
125. Voskamp BJ, Fleurke-Rozema H, Oude-Rengerink K, et al. Relationship of isolated single umbilical artery to fetal growth, aneuploidy and perinatal mortality: systematic review and meta-analysis. Ultrasound Obstet Gynecol. 2013;42:622-8.
126. Martínez-Payo C, Cabezas E, Nieto Y, et al. Detection of single umbilical artery in the first trimester ultrasound: its value as a marker of fetal malformation. Biomed Res Int. 2014;2014:548729.
127. Blazer S, Sujov P, Escholi Z, et al. Single umbilical artery right or left? Does it matter? Prenat Diagn. 1997;17:5-8.

CHAPTER 6

Behavior of the Embryo

Toshiyuki Hata, Uiko Hanaoka, Mohamed Ahmed Mostafa AboEllail, Nobuhiro Mori, Kenji Kanenishi, Megumi Ito

INTRODUCTION

The brain develops from the neural tube that is cranial to the fourth to sixth somite pairs. The development of three primary brain vesicles (forebrain or prosencephalon, midbrain or mesencephalon, and hindbrain or rhombencephalon) occurs at 6 weeks of gestation. Two vesicles, the telen- and diencephalon, are formed by partial division of the forebrain at 7 weeks of gestation, and meten- and myelencephalon are formed by partial division of the hindbrain. Consequently, there are five secondary brain vesicles.[1] Using intrauterine ultrasonography with a 20-MHz flexible catheter-based, high-resolution, real-time miniature transducer, the parallel lines of the neural tube can be noted at 6 weeks of gestation.[2] At 7 weeks of gestation, one-half of embryos still had primary brain vesicles, but the other half had secondary brain vesicles.[3] At 8 weeks of gestation, all embryos had secondary brain vesicles.[3] Using transvaginal three-dimensional (3D) ultrasound with the inversion mode, the brain vesicles were the most prominent, multilobular consecutive structures, and all embryos had secondary brain vesicles at 7 weeks and 8 weeks of gestation.[4,5]

Fetal movement reflects the activity of the fetal central nervous system (CNS).[6] At 6 weeks of gestation, embryo immobility is characteristic.[7] After 7 weeks of gestation, embryonic movements are identifiable.[8,9] However, little is known regarding the behavior of the embryo early in the first trimester of pregnancy. This chapter describes the neurological development of the embryo, reviews the literature on conventional two-dimensional (2D) sonographic and four-dimensional (4D) ultrasound assessments of embryonic behavior, and makes recommendations regarding future research on embryonic behavior using the latest advances in 4D ultrasound in this field, such as HDlive.

NEUROLOGICAL DEVELOPMENT OF THE EMBRYO

At 6 weeks of gestation, the embryo is devoid of synapses. The motor neuropil of the cervical cord shows the development of a few axodendritic synapses, and the motor neuropil exhibits the first axosomatic synapses at 7 gestational weeks. Synapse formation outside the motor neuropil of the cervical cord can be noted at 8 gestational weeks, during the onset period of the precocious reflex.[10]

At 6-7 gestational weeks, the human embryonic brainstem develops and then undergoes a caudal to rostral arc, consequently leading to the medulla, pons, and midbrain. The state of arousal, breathing, pulse, and gross body and head movements are mediated by the medulla, and these medullary functions precede those of the pons, which in turn precede those of the midbrain. Therefore, spontaneous movements can be noted by 7-9 gestational weeks.[8]

Local reflexes (spontaneous vermicular movements) consistent with the "total pattern" type of movements arise at 7.5 gestational weeks, marking the development of the first afferent-efferent circuits within the spinal cord.[11] From 8 to 9 gestational weeks, general body movements involving head, trunk, and limb movements are observable.[7,12]

TWO-DIMENSIONAL SONOGRAPHIC STUDY ON EMBRYONIC BEHAVIOR

In the first-generation 2D sonographic studies, only heart activity was evident at 7 weeks of gestation, embryonic trunk movement could be noted from 8 weeks of gestation, and isolated limb movement could be identified from 9 weeks of gestation.[13-16] In the second-generation 2D sonographic investigations, sideways bending of the embryo was noted at 7 weeks of gestation, general and startle movements

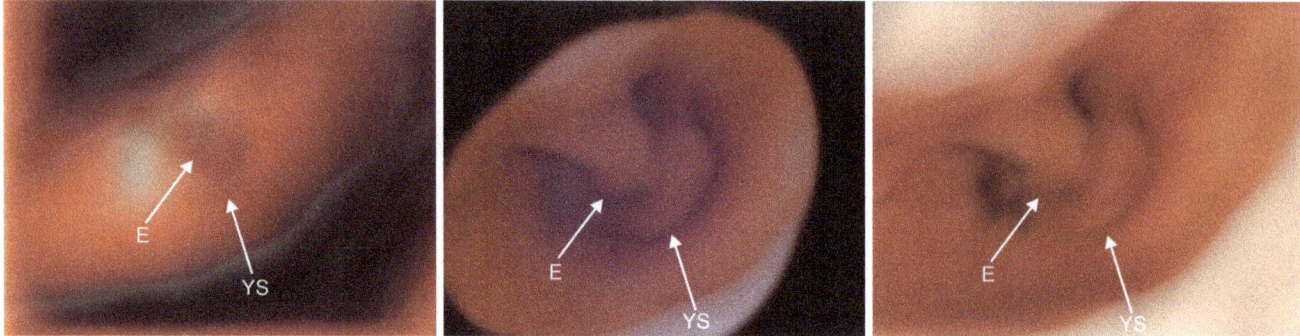

Fig. 6.1: The embryo (E) and yolk sac (YS) at 5 weeks and 3 days of gestation.

were recognized at 8 weeks of gestation, and fetal hiccups, isolated arm and leg movements, and sucking and swallowing appeared at 9 weeks of gestation.[12,17-19]

In the latest 2D sonographic study,[20] the earliest form of motility was noted at 7 gestational weeks and comprised small and simple sideways bending of the head and/or rump, with an approximately 1-second duration. Between 7 weeks and 8.5 weeks, this progresses to movements involving one or two arms or legs; although such movements are still slow and unidirectional, their duration is prolonged to a few seconds. At 9–10 weeks, there is a progression to general movements, which is characterized by changes in the participating body parts and amplitude, speed, and direction over longer time.

In pregnant women with type 1 diabetes, a delay of 1–2 weeks was noted in the initial appearance of all patterns of movement that can typically be observed during the first 12 weeks of pregnancy.[21] This delay in embryonic/fetal motor development in diabetic women may be due to hyperglycemia because the periconceptional quality of glucose control is poor.

FOUR-DIMENSIONAL ULTRASOUND STUDY ON EMBRYONIC BEHAVIOR

At 5 weeks of gestation, a small dot-like embryo adjacent to the yolk sac was noted as a round to oval structure (Fig. 6.1). Heart activity could be sometimes recognized, but embryonic movement could not be depicted.

At 6 weeks of gestation, the embryo is a solid, comma-shaped structure adjacent to the yolk sac (Fig. 6.2), but embryonic movements cannot be identified during this

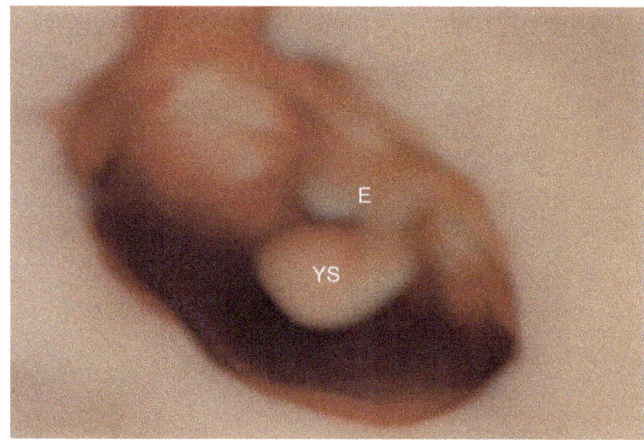

Fig. 6.2: The embryo (E) and yolk sac (YS) at 6 weeks and 6 days of gestation.

stage. Using the latest 4D ultrasound apparatus with high-frame rates (19 Hz/second), embryonic heart activity could be clearly identified (Figs. 6.3A to D).

At 7 weeks of gestation, embryonic limb movements (Figs. 6.4A to D) and a changing body direction (Figs. 6.5A to D) were noted.

At 8 weeks of gestation, various types of movements such as bending of the wrist (Figs. 6.6A and B), upper and/or lower limb (Figs. 6.7 to 6.12), twisting (Figs. 6.13 and 6.14), startle (Figs. 6.15A and B), and general movements (Figs. 6.16 and 6.17) could be clearly identified.

Kurjak et al.[22] reported the first study on 4D-ultrasound assessment of embryonic and fetal behaviors before 12 weeks of gestation. General body movements were noted at 7–8 weeks of gestation, limb body movements

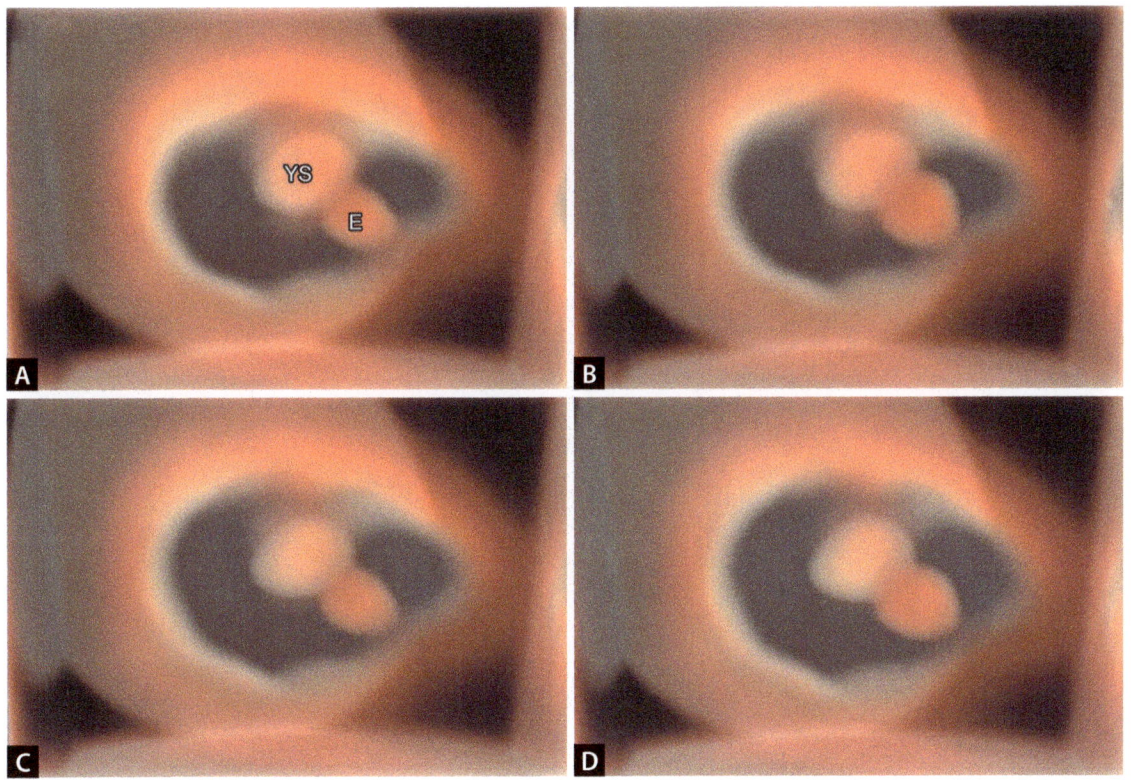

Figs. 6.3A to D: The embryo (E) and yolk sac (YS) at 6 weeks and 2 days of gestation. The crown-rump length is 2.8 mm. Embryonic heart activity can be clearly identified (A to D).
Note: The frame rate is 19 Hz.

were recognized at 9–10 weeks, and complex limb movements appeared at 11–12 weeks.

Kurjak et al.[23] counted the frequencies of seven parameters—general movements, startle, stretching, isolated arm movements, isolated leg movements, head retroflexion, head rotation, and head anteflexion in the first trimester of pregnancy. Head retroflexion and head rotation could not be detected at 7–8 weeks of gestation, but the other five movements were noted.

Andonotopo et al.[24] attempted to determine the accuracy of 4D ultrasound in the assessment of embryonic and early fetal behaviors in the first trimester of pregnancy, in comparison with 2D sonography. General body, head and limb movements recorded by 2D sonography were also depicted by 4D ultrasound. Some movement patterns such as sideways bending, hiccups, breathing movements, mouth opening, and facial movements could be observed only with 2D sonography.

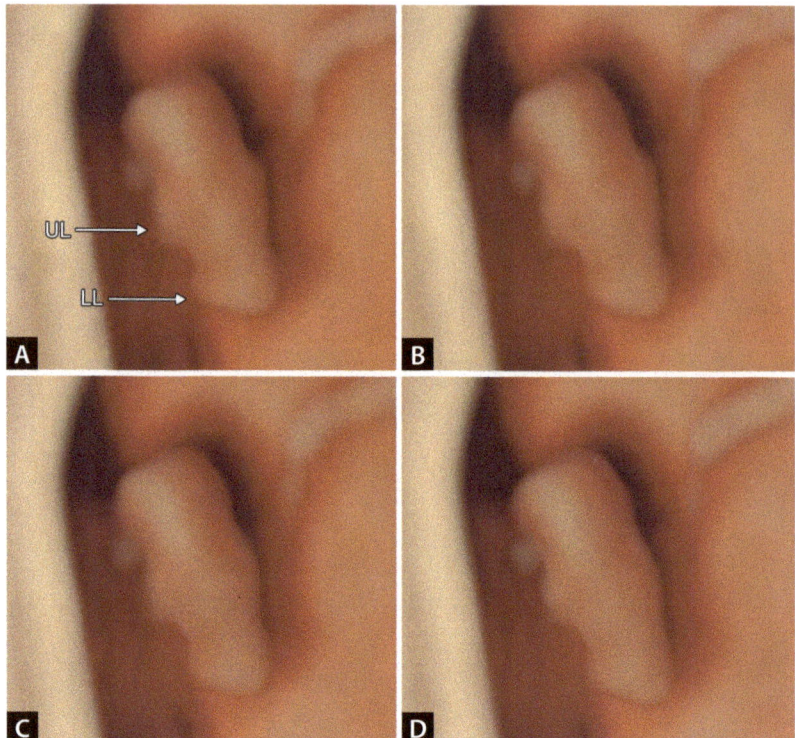

Figs. 6.4A to D: Embryonic upper limb (UL) and lower limb (LL) movements at 7 weeks and 5 days of gestation (A to D).
Note: The frame rate is 7 Hz.

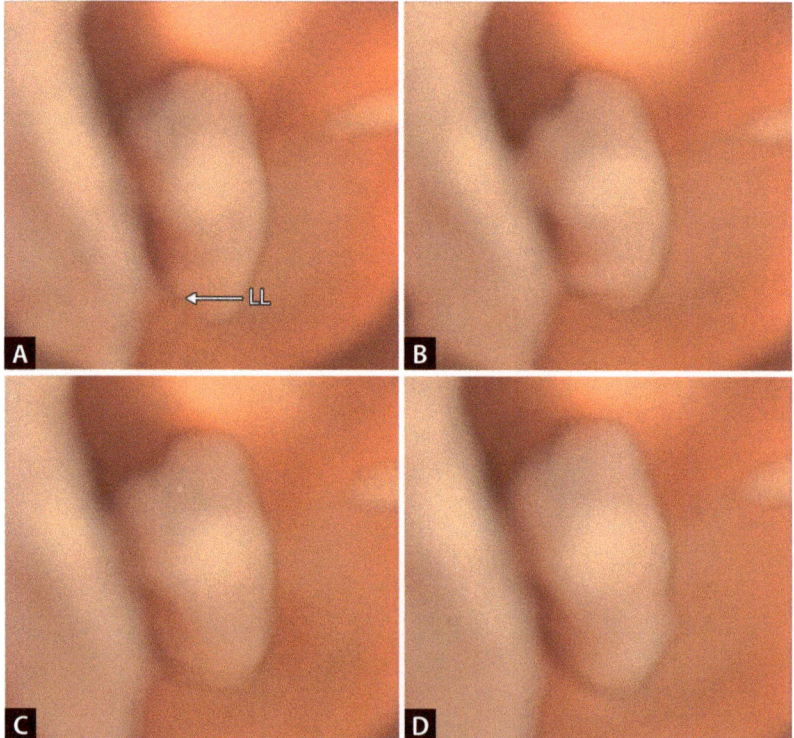

Figs. 6.5A to D: Changing the body direction (right-angled turn) at 7 weeks and 5 days of gestation (A to D). (LL: lower limb)
Note: The frame rate is 7 Hz.

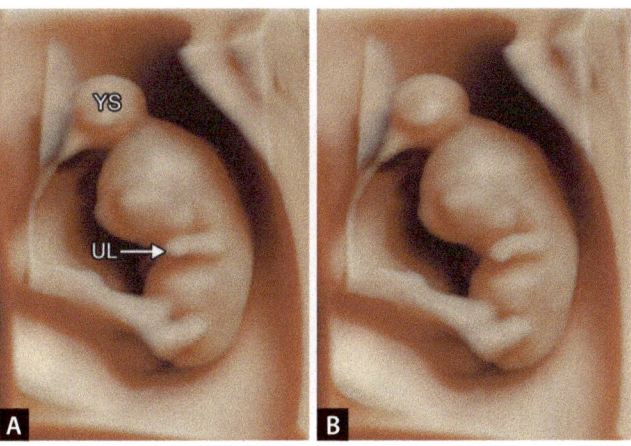

Figs. 6.6A and B: Left upper limb (UL) wrist movement at 8 weeks and 6 days of gestation (A and B). (YS: yolk sac)
Note: The frame rate is 11 Hz.

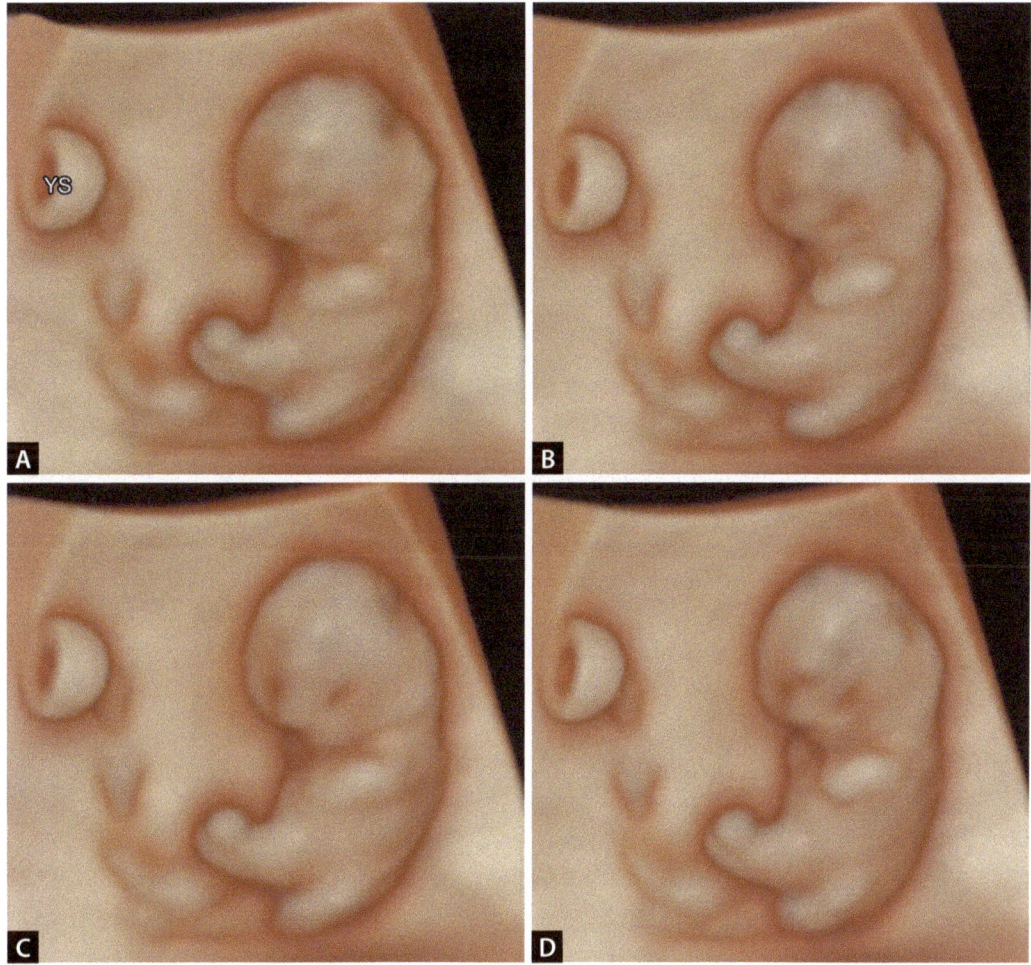

Figs. 6.7A to D: Upper and lower limb movements at 8 weeks and 3 days of gestation (A to D). (YS: yolk sac)
Note: The frame rate is 8 Hz.

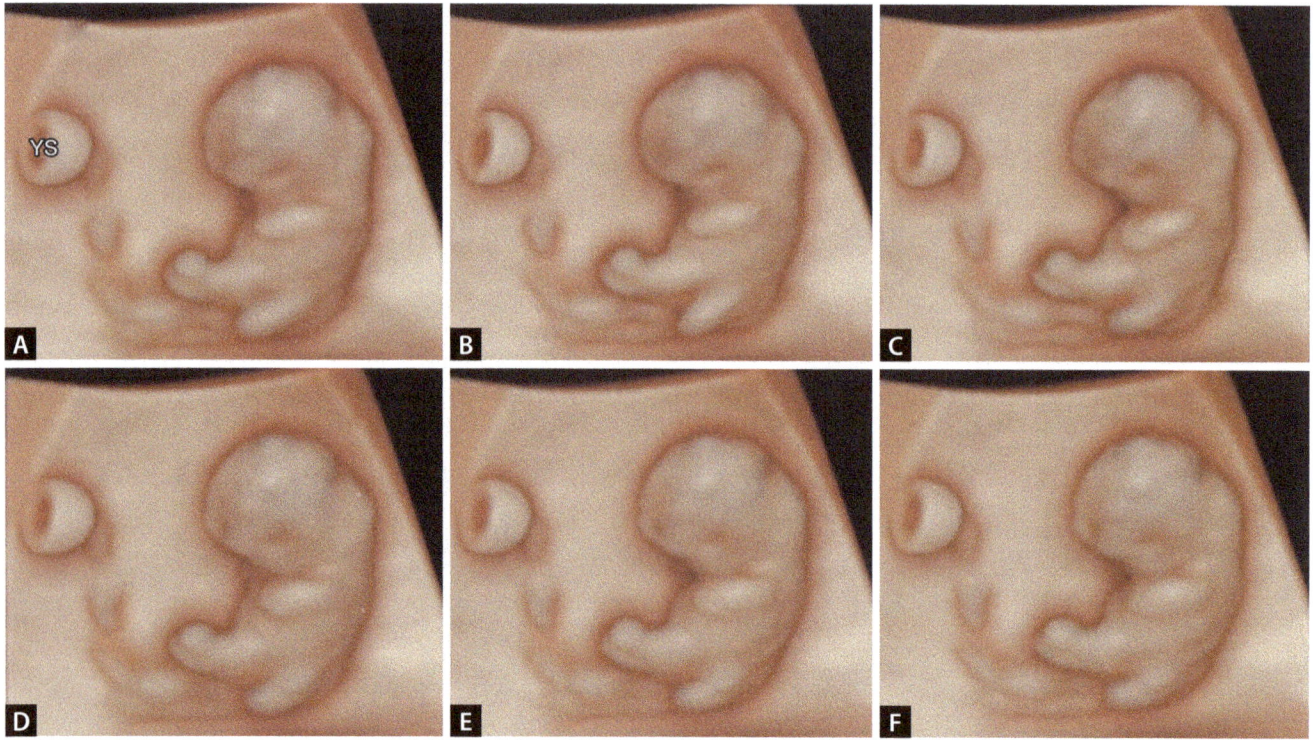

Figs. 6.8A to F: Upper and lower limb movements at 8 weeks and 3 days of gestation (A to F). (YS: yolk sac)
Note: The frame rate is 8 Hz.

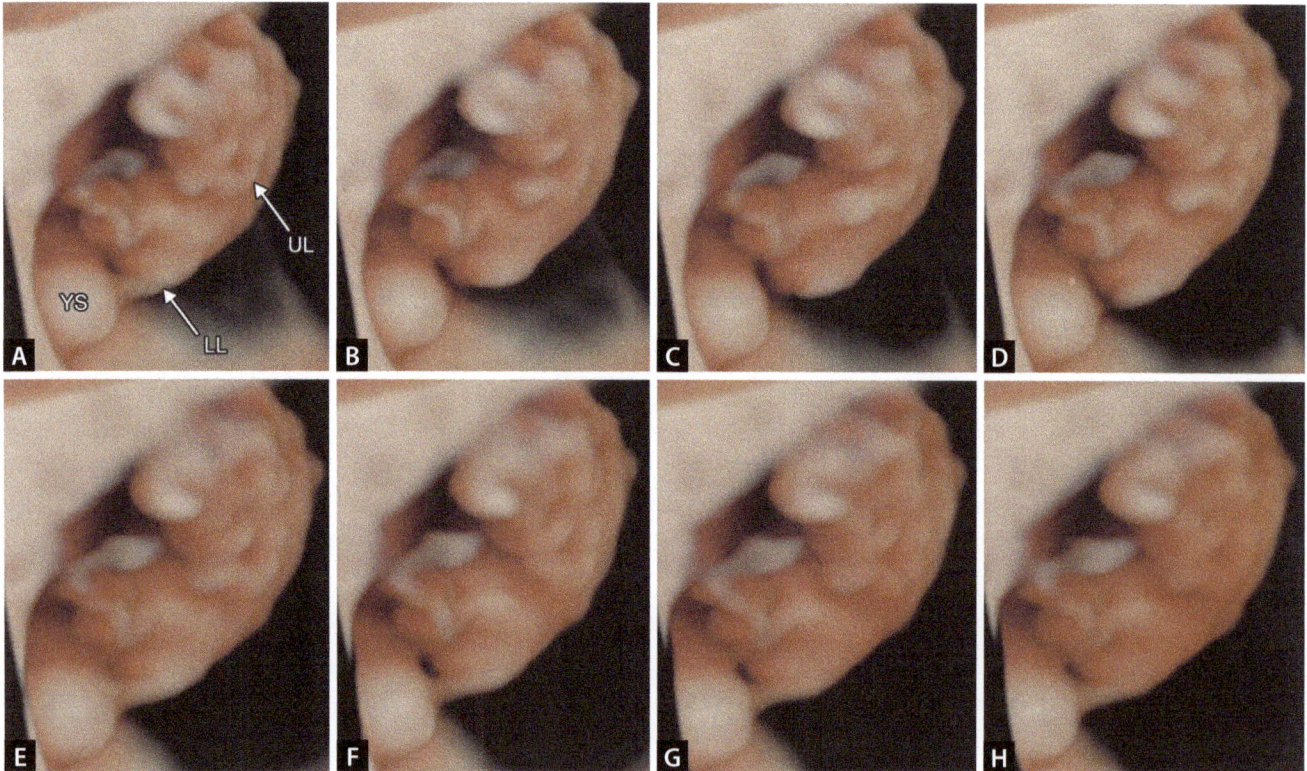

Figs. 6.9A to H: Upper (UL) and lower limb (LL) movements at 8 weeks and 5 days of gestation (A to H). (YS: yolk sac)
Note: The frame rate is 11 Hz.

Chapter 6: Behavior of the Embryo 71

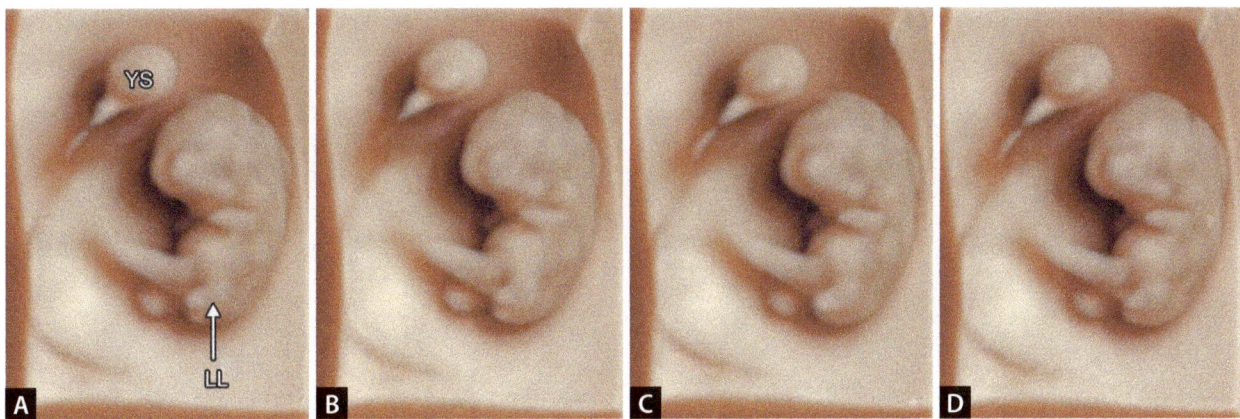

Figs. 6.10A to D: Lower limb (LL) movements at 8 weeks and 6 days of gestation (A to D). (YS: yolk sac)
Note: The frame rate is 11 Hz.

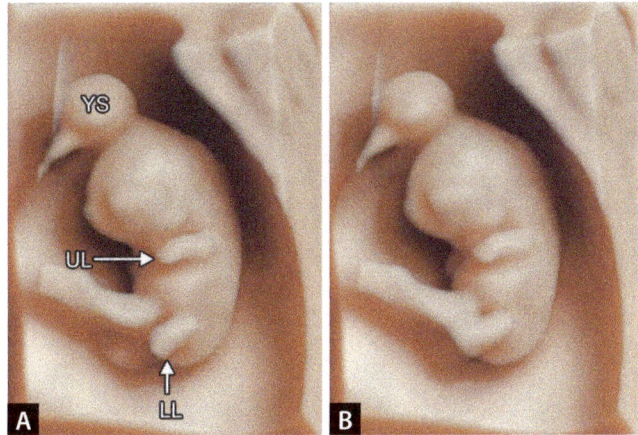

Figs. 6.11A and B: Upper limb (UL) wrist and lower limb (LL) movements at 8 weeks and 6 days of gestation (A and B). (YS: yolk sac)
Note: The frame rate is 11 Hz.

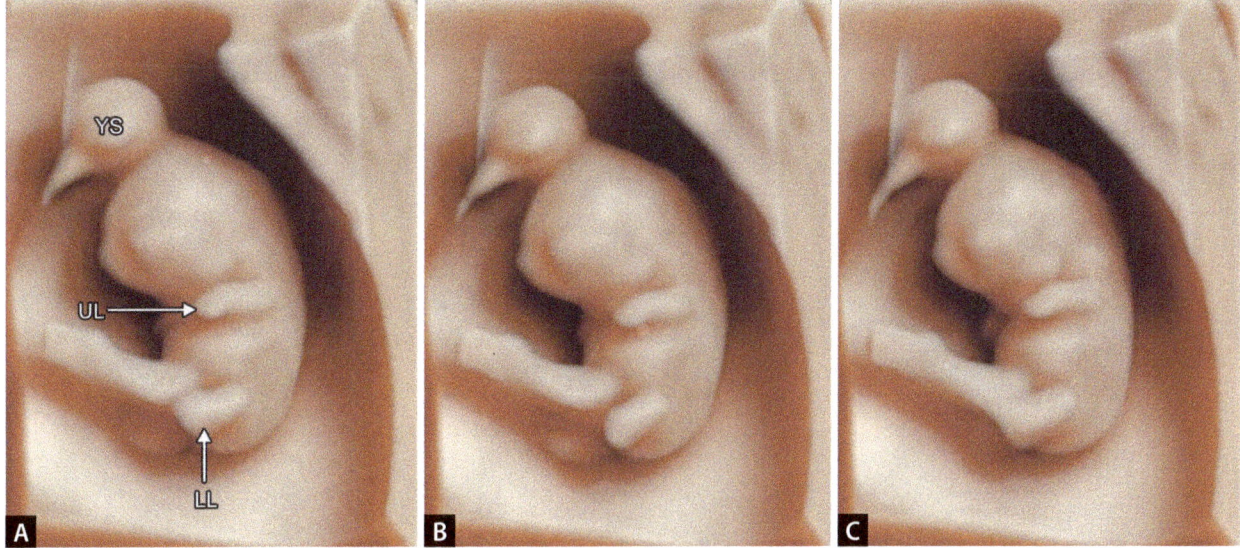

Figs. 6.12A to C: Upper (UL) and lower (LL) limb movements at 8 weeks and 6 days of gestation (A to C). (YS: yolk sac)
Note: The frame rate is 11 Hz.

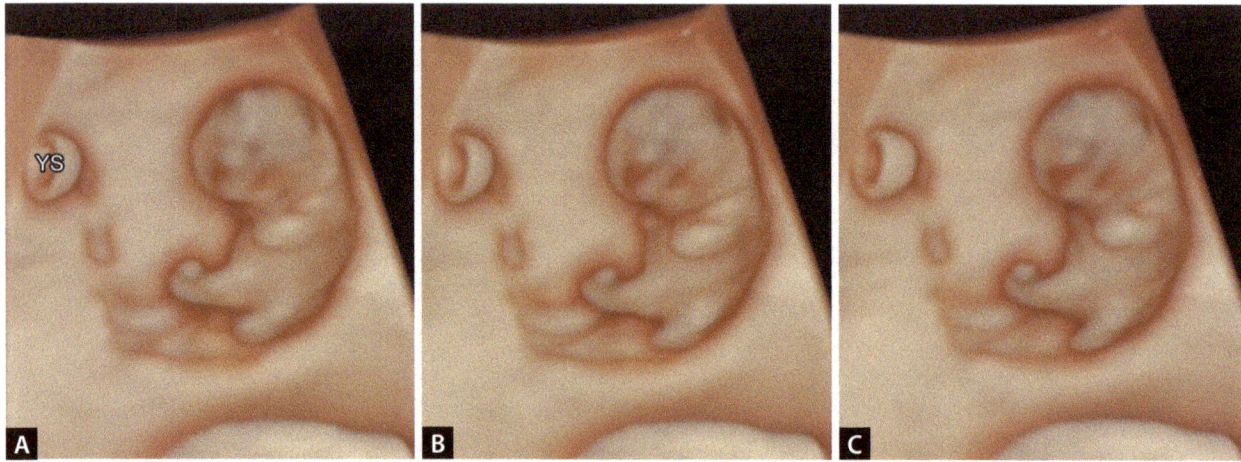

Figs. 6.13A to C: Twisting movement at 8 weeks and 3 days of gestation (A to C). (YS: yolk sac)
Note: The frame rate is 8 Hz.

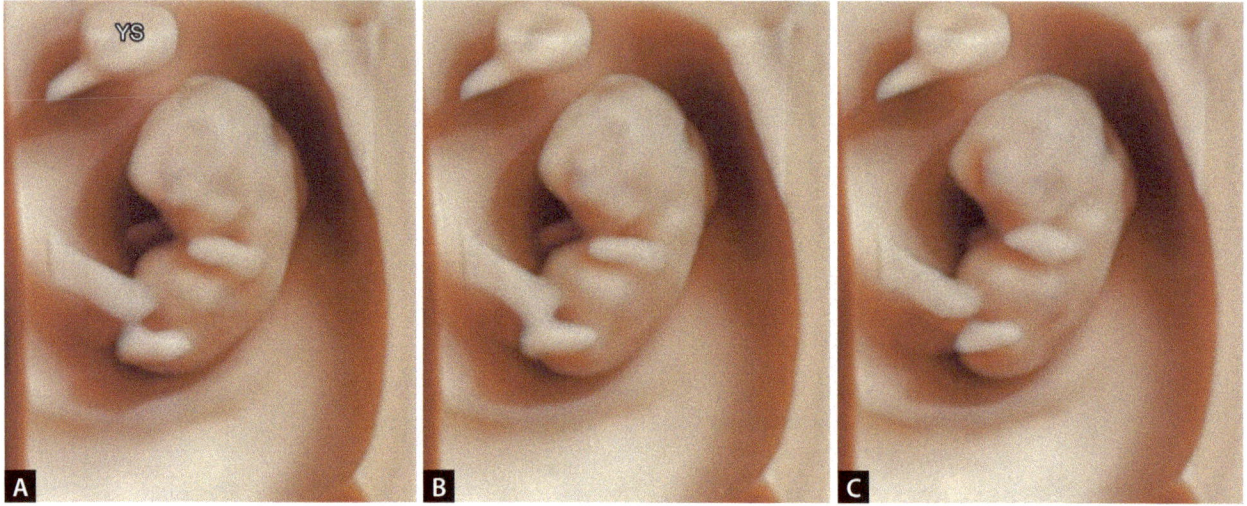

Figs. 6.14A to C: Twisting movement at 8 weeks and 6 days of gestation (A to C). (YS: yolk sac)
Note: The frame rate is 11 Hz.

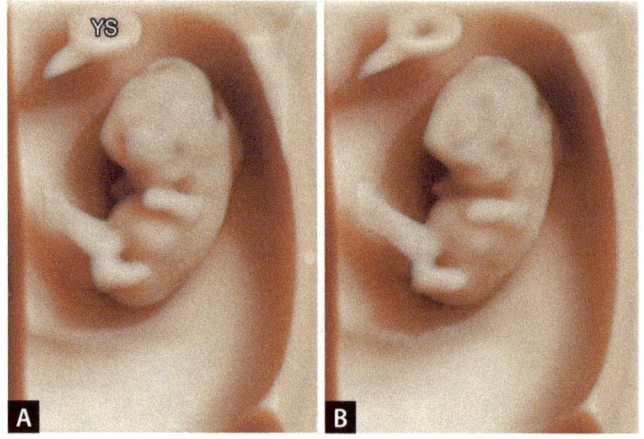

Figs. 6.15A and B: Startle movement at 8 weeks and 6 days of gestation (A and B). (YS: yolk sac)
Note: The frame rate is 11 Hz.

Chapter 6: Behavior of the Embryo 73

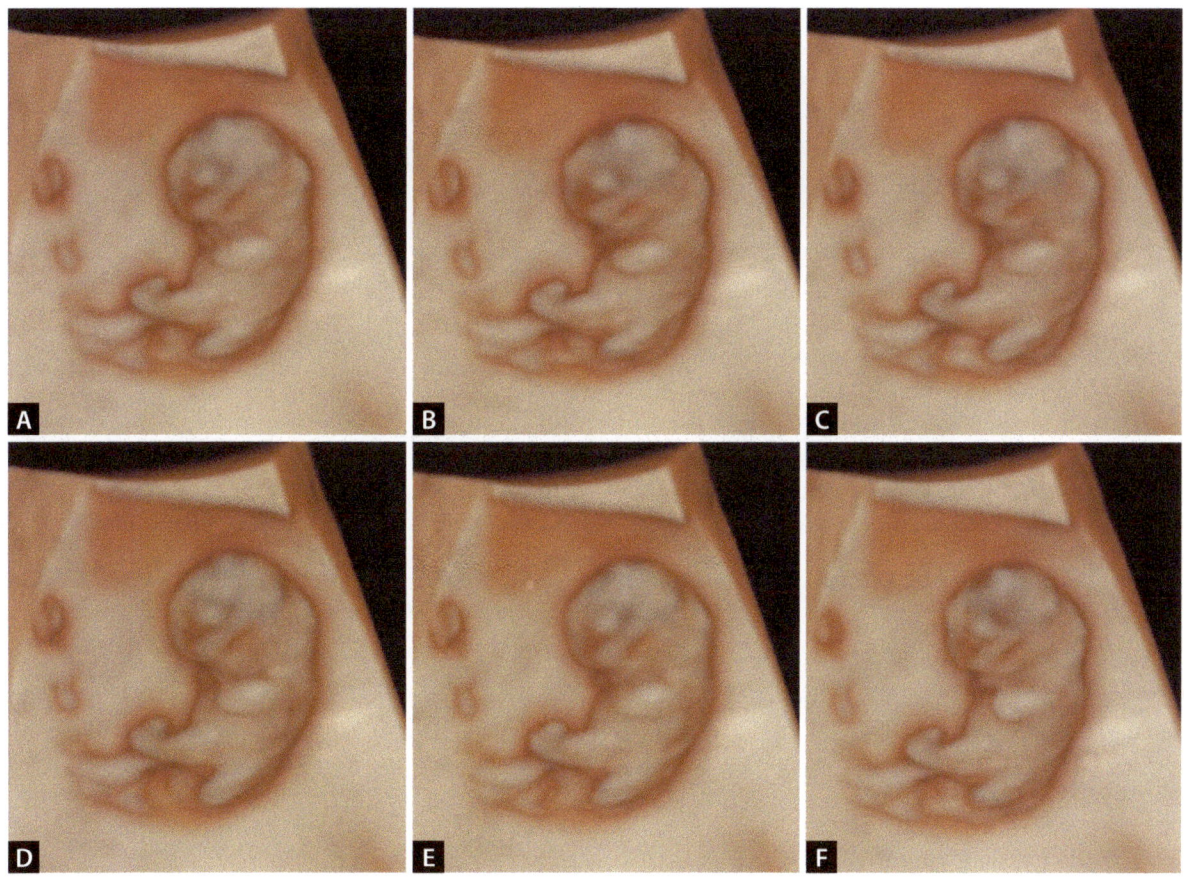

Figs. 6.16A to F: General movement at 8 weeks and 3 days of gestation (A to F).
Note: The frame rate is 8 Hz.

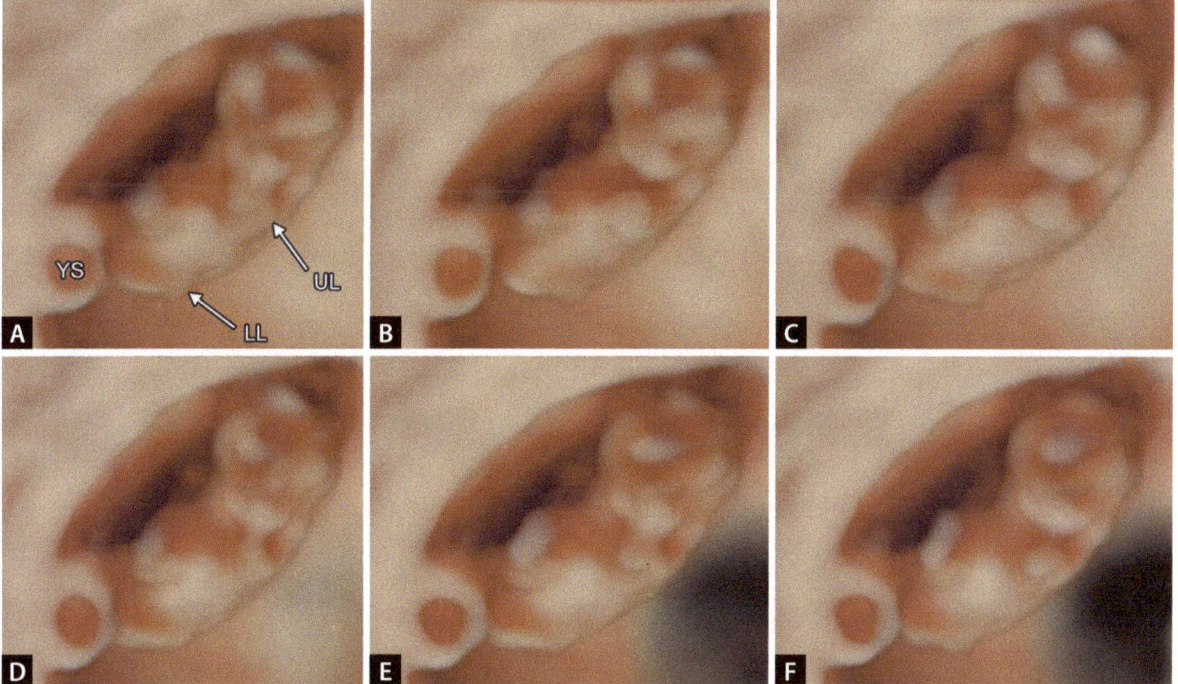

Figs. 6.17A to F: General movement at 8 weeks and 5 days of gestation (A to F). (YS: yolk sac; LL: lower limb; UL: upper limb)
Note: The frame rate is 12 Hz.

CONCLUSION

With the latest 4D ultrasound, the frame rates of the transvaginal probe on clinical application were around 7-20 frames per second before 8 weeks of gestation. Because of 3D-imaging capabilities, 4D ultrasound should be superior to 2D sonography to assess embryonic behaviors early in the first trimester of pregnancy. Therefore, 4D ultrasound will help to discover novel embryonic behavioral functions early in the first trimester of pregnancy. Studies on embryonic behavior will help to elucidate the functioning of the embryonic central nervous system, and to shed light on new areas of embryonic development. Further studies involving larger sample sizes are needed to assess the detailed behavior of the embryo early in the first trimester of pregnancy.

Conflict of interest: The authors have no conflict of interest.

REFERENCES

1. Moore KL, Persaud TVN, Torchia MG. The Developing Human: Clinically Oriented Embryology, 10th edition. Philadelphia: Elsevier Inc.; 2015.
2. Hata T. Intrauterine ultrasonography for the assessment of embryonic development. Med Imag Int. 1996;6:11-6.
3. Fujiwaki R, Hata T, Hata K, et al. Intrauterine ultrasonographic assessments of embryonic development. Am J Obstet Gynecol. 1995;173:1770-4.
4. Kim MS, Jeanty P, Turner C, et al. Three-dimensional sonographic evaluations of embryonic brain development. J Ultrasound Med. 2008;27:119-24.
5. Hata T, Dai SY, Kanenishi K, et al. Three-dimensional volume-rendered imaging of embryonic brain vesicles using inversion mode. J Obstet Gynaecol Res. 2009;35:258-61.
6. Nijhuis JG. Fetal behavior. Neurobiol Aging. 2003;24:S41-S46.
7. Salihagic-Kadic A, Predojevic M. What we have learned from fetal neurophysiology? Donald School J Ultrasound Obstet Gynecol. 2012;6:179-88.
8. Joseph R. Fetal brain behavior and congnitive development. Dev Rev. 2000;20:81-98.
9. Andonotopo W, Stanojevic M, Kurjak A, et al. Assessment of fetal behavior and general movements by four-dimensional sonography. Ultrasound Rev Obstet Gynecol. 2004;4:103-14.
10. Okado N, Kakimi S, Kojima T. Synaptogenesis in the cervical cord of the human embryo: Sequence of synapse formation in a spinal reflex pathway. J Comp Neurol. 1979;184:491-518.
11. Okado N. Onset of synapse formation in the human spinal cord. J Comp Neurol. 1981;201:211-9.
12. de Vries JIP, Visser GHA, Prechtl HFR. The emergence of fetal behaviour. I. Qualitative aspects. Early Hum Dev. 1982;7:301-22.
13. Van Dongen LGR, Goudie EG. Fetal movement patterns in the first trimester of pregnancy. Br J Obstet Gynaecol. 1980;87:191-3.
14. Shawker TH, Schuette WH, Whitehouse W, et al. Early fetal movement: A real-time ultrasound study. Obstet Gynecol. 1980;55:194-8.
15. Ianniruberto A, Tajani E. Ultrasonographic study of fetal movements. Sem Perinatol. 1981;5:175-81.
16. Tuck SM. Ultrasound monitoring of fetal behaviour. Ultrasound Med Biol 1986;12:307-17.
17. de Vries JIP, Visser GHA, Prechtl HFR. The emergence of fetal behaviour. II. Quantitative aspects. Early Hum Dev. 1985;12:99-120.
18. Goto S, Kato T. Spontaneous movements of embryos and fetuses in the early stage of life. Gin Pol. 1987;58:61-75.
19. de Vries JIP, Fong BF. Normal fetal motility: an overview. Ultrasound Obstet Gynecol. 2006;27:701-11.
20. Luchinger AB, Hadders-Algra M, van Kan CM, et al. Fetal onset of general movements. Pediatr Res. 2008;63:191-5.
21. Mulder EJH, Visser GHA. Growth and motor development in fetuses of women with type-1 diabetes. II. Emergence of specific movement patterns. Early Hum Dev. 1991;25:107-15.
22. Kurjak A, Vecek N, Hafner T, et al. Prenatal diagnosis: what does four-dimensional ultrasound add? J Perinat Med. 2002;30:57-62.
23. Kurjak A, Andonotopo W, Hafner T, et al. Normal standards for fetal neurobehavioral developments—longitudinal quantification by four-dimensional sonography. J Perinat Med. 2006;34:56-65.
24. Andonotopo W, Medic M, Salihagic-Kadic A, et al. The assessment of fetal behavior in early pregnancy: comparison between 2D and 4D sonographic scanning. J Perinat Med. 2005;33:406-14.

CHAPTER 7

Pre-embryo: Medical, Moral and Legal Aspects

Joseph G Schenker

INTRODUCTION

Pre-embryo is defined as the period from fertilization in vivo and in vitro until implantation. Fertilization is not a single event but it is an event that includes several steps.

EVENTS OF FERTILIZATION

Following sperm entry into the oocyte, the male chromatin decondenses rapidly while the oocyte resumes meiosis and extrudes the second polar body. Male and female pronuclei become visible and migrate until they are in close apposition. At that stage, the membranes of the pronuclei disappear, the male and female chromosomes intermingle and syngamy is achieved.

Fertilization Steps

- Sperm capacitation
- Sperm-zona pellucida binding
- The acrosome reaction
- Penetration of the zona pellucida
- Sperm-oocyte binding
- Egg activation and the cortical reaction
- The zona reaction
- Postfertilization events.

Recently a new biomarker "zinc sparks" was introduced to determine the moment when the process of fertilization is completed, transition of an oocyte to pre-embryo.[1]

A stunning explosion of zinc fireworks occurs when a human egg is activated by a sperm enzyme, and the size of these "sparks" is a direct measure of the quality of the egg and its ability to develop into an embryo.

PRE-EMBRYO DEVELOPMENT IN VITRO

- Mean time for the first (2-cell) and second (4-cell) cleavages: 35 h and 45 h postinsemination (day 2)
- Mean time for the third cleavage (8-cell): 54 hours postinsemination (day 3)
- Activation of the embryonic genome: utilization of embryonic mRNA for protein synthesis.

Morula: Compacted embryo, 16–32-cell
- External cells will give rise to the trophoblast cells
- Internal cells will become the inner cell mass (ICM)

Blastocyst: Day 5–6
- Cavitation: The trophoblast cells secrete a fluid to create a blastocoel cavity
- The ICM, which will give rise to the embryo, is clearly distinct from the trophoblast cells which are required for implantation
- The percentage of 2-cell embryos reaching the blastocyst stage is usually (25%).

Fast cleaving pre-embryos, with good morphology (no fragments, regular blastomeres) able to reach the blastocysts stage is considered as good quality pre-embryos with a high implantation potential. This quality depends on intrinsic characteristics of the pre-embryos but also on the cultures conditions.

PRE-EMBRYO CULTURE CONDITIONS

Pre-embryo culture conditions are important for the assisted reproductive technology (ART) outcome its pre- and postimplantation development. The pioneer units of in vitro fertilization (IVF) were making their own culture media.

The culture medium supports the pre-embryo from the very beginning until the transfer. After the first mitotic divisions, zygotic genome activation, compaction, morula formation, cavitation and blastocyst formation.[2]

The development of ART over the past 35 years has led to a huge commercial activity of cultural media.

Over the years, basic research on the metabolism of preimplantation embryos revealed that there are specific needs depending on the developmental stage of the embryo.

Gardner et al.[3] showed significant differences in the concentrations of various metabolites between the fallopian tube and the uterus. Cleaving embryos use pyruvate and lactate as energy sources and nonessential amino acids for protein metabolism. From the 8-cell stage, the major energy source is glucose and for protein metabolism the embryos use essential amino acids.

Based on their studies they formulate the composition of two culture media G1 and G2.

G1 supports the in vitro development of the zygote, 8-cell stage, and G2 development from 8-cells to blastocyst.[4]

Sequential media are now being used successfully in IVF treatment all over the world.

These laboratory-controlled environmental variables can effect media efficacy and embryo development, resulting in significantly different outcomes among facilities. Specifically, conditions within the laboratory incubator, such as oxygen tension, pH, and temperature stability, can all significantly impact embryo development.

COMPOSITION OF THE EMBRYO CULTURE MEDIUM[5]

Culture media containing a phosphate buffer or HEPES organic buffer is used for procedures that involve handling of gametes outside of the incubator, flushing of follicles and micromanipulation.

Most culture media utilize a bicarbonate/CO_2 buffer system to keep pH in the range of 7.2–7.4.

A humidified incubator with a temperature setting of 37.0–37.5°C should be used for oocyte fertilization and pre-embryo culture.

Pre-embryos should be cultured under paraffin oil, which prevents evaporation of the medium preserving a constant osmolarity.

The medium is composed of 99% water. Purity of the water is crucial,[5] and is achieved by ultrafiltration.

The medium contains recombinant albumin or synthetic serum.

Salt solution of NaCl, KCl, CaCl, Mg, and $NaHCO_3$.

Carbohydrates together with the amino acids are the main energy source for the pre-embryo.

Media that support the development of 8-cell embryos up to the blastocyst stage contain pyruvate and lactate in low concentrations and a higher concentration of glucose. Supplement of the culture medium with amino acids is necessary for pre-embryo development.

Media that support the development of zygotes up to 8-cells are supplemented with no essential amino acids while supporting the development of 8-cell pre-embryos up to the blastocyst stage is supplemented with essential amino acids. Most media contain vitamins and antibiotics to minimize the risks of microbial growth. Ethylenediaminetetraacetic acid (EDTA) is used as a chelator in medium that supports the embryo from the zygote stage to 8-cells and prevents abnormal glycolysis.

PRE-EMBRYO CRYOPRESERVATION

Since the first pregnancy and delivery with cryopreserved pre-embryo was reported [Trounson and Mohr, (1983)].[6] Cryopreservation of pre-embryos is a routine and essential aspect of ART.

Cryopreservation of pre-embryos decreased the number of fresh embryo transfers, reduced multiple pregnancies and maximized the effectiveness of the IVF. Cryopreservation of pre-embryos is a crucial approach in cases of cancelled embryo transfer due to OHSS risk, uterine bleeding and unsuspected medical conditions of the woman.[7,8]

The proportion of cryopreserved embryo transfer cycles compared with fresh cycles is growing worldwide.

Two freezing technologies are applied worldwide to cryopreserve human pre-embryo in cleavage stage, zygote to blastocyst, slow freezing and vitrification.

Slow freezing involves the addition of a cryoprotective agent to prevent the formation of ice crystals in the cells, after the cells are cooled gradually under computer control to –196°C.

Vitrification method is rapid cooling of pre-embryo so fast that ice crystals never form. It has been shown to be superior to slow freezing especially freezing of blastocyst. In the early days of freezing, approximately 20% of embryos did not survive the freezing or thawing process, thought to be due to subtle damage suffered by the embryo during the cooling and/or warming transition.

Several factors influence the success rate of freeze–thaw cycles, including the age of the patient at the time of cryopreservation, cause of infertility, grade of the embryos being transferred and the extent of embryo damage after thawing cryopreservation techniques. Present data can ensure maximal frozen embryo viability and minimal risk of cryodamage.

Recent studies have found that children born after transfer of frozen-thawed embryos have better perinatal outcomes than those born after transfer of fresh embryos: lower rate of preterm birth, low birth weight, growth restriction, perinatal mortality, and malformation rates.[8]

In blastocyst stage, vitrification is more efficient than slow freezing for, in terms of postwarming survival rate.

Pre-embryo cryopreservation generated ethical, moral, and legal issues. Some countries have enacted specific laws that restrict pre-embryo freezing.

PRE-EMBRYO ASSESSMENT—NONINVASIVE METHODS

Morphological scoring of pre-embryos has been used since the introduction of IVF[9] to define embryo development. An urgent need for a simple and practical method for embryo selection is required in order to maximize the chances of success and minimize the problems of multiple pregnancies in couples treated with assisted reproduction.

Assessment of morphological feathers as a reliable noninvasive method that provides valuable information in prediction of IVF outcome has been practiced for 40 years.

Pre-embryo assessment has many potential benefits such as:
- Accurate selection of embryos prior to transfer
- Reduction of the risk of multiple pregnancies
- Assessment of different culture media.

Morphological noninvasive quality assessments are performed at different stages of pre-embryo development:
- Cleavage stage embryos (day 3 after insemination)
- Blastocyst stage embryos (day 5 after fertilization).

At cleavage stage the different morphological parameters that are evaluated:
- Pronuclear scoring systems
- Cleavage-stage scoring systems
- Cell number
- Fragmentation
- Symmetry
- Multinucleation.

At blastocyst stage: The degree of blastocyst expansion as well as the morphological appearance of the ICM and the trophectoderm cells are assessed.[10]

Four decades of ART practice have shown that none of the morphological assessments have a high accuracy to identify the embryos that have good implantation potential.

In recent years,[11] it has been shown that pre-embryos can be selected on the basis of their morphokinetic changes from the time of fertilization until blastocyst formation using time-lapse photography. An automatic system is introduced into the incubator.

GENETIC TESTING OF PRE-EMBRYO

Preimplantation genetic diagnosis (PGD) application has become possible through the development of artificial reproductive technology and sensitive molecular methods allowing genetic analysis at the single-cell level.

The first clinical application of PGD was described by Handyside et al. (1990).[12]

The goal of preimplantation testing (PGS/PGD) is to reduce the likelihood of conceiving a child with severe disease or to reduce miscarriages. It may also increase the chance of pregnancy in the case of couples with advanced maternal age, recurrent pregnancy loss, or repeated IVF failures.[13]

Preimplantation genetic diagnosis followed by implantation of unaffected embryos offers high-risk couples the option to decrease the risk of genetic disease in their offspring without the dilemma of a prenatal diagnosis that may be followed by a termination of pregnancy.

There are several techniques to sample DNA at this early stage without having an impact on the viability of the conceptus. These include biopsy of the first and second polar bodies when a mutation is maternally inherited, aspiration of one or two cells from a 6–8-cell embryo at 2–3 days postconception (blastomere biopsy), and, although rarely performed, biopsy of the trophectoderm taken from an embryo at the blastocyst stage.

Genetic analysis involves DNA amplification using a variety of strategies [whole-genome amplification, polymerase chain reaction (PCR) amplification], followed by use of one of several available platforms for analysis of the amplified DNA.[14]

At present a new terminology of genetic evaluation of pre-embryo was introduced: Preimplantation Genetic Testing (PGT) which includes following categories:[15]

Preimplantation Genetic Testing for Aneuploidy

This is to identify embryos with de novo aneuploidy, including sib-chromosomal deletion and additions in pre-embryos of couple presumed to be chromosomally normal.

Preimplantation genetic testing for aneuploidy also known as PGS (preimplantation genetic screening) is a genetic test that allows the determination of the chromosomal status of IVF embryos by screening all 23 pairs of human chromosomes. Only embryos with the correct number of chromosomes will be able to develop into a healthy baby.

The PGT-A test is able to identify those embryos free from chromosome abnormalities (euploid embryos) that are more likely to implant and result in a healthy live birth. By selecting healthy embryos with the right number of chromosomes to be transferred to the uterus.

The PGT-A is genetic testing for aneuploidy: Improves IVF success, increasing the likelihood of pregnancy per transfer.
- Reduces the risk of miscarriage
- Allows for confident single embryo transfer, reducing the risks and complications associated to multiple pregnancies
- Reduces time to pregnancy by allowing the identification of a normal embryo as soon as possible
- Avoids the live birth of a baby with genetic disorders.

Preimplantation Genetic Testing for Monogenic (Single-gene) Disorders

Preimplantation genetic testing for monogenic (single-gene) disorders (PGT-M) testing is to establish a pregnancy that is unaffected by specific genetic characteristics, such as a known heritable genetic mutation carried by one or both biological parents. It is also used to select embryos for transfer that has specific characteristics, such as a particular gender or compatible human leukocyte antigen complex type.

Preimplantation genetic testing for monogenic diseases for adult-onset conditions is ethically permissible for a range of conditions including when the condition is serious and not safe, effective interventions are available.

Preimplantation Genetic Testing for Structural Rearrangements

Preimplantation genetic testing for structural rearrangements (PGT-SR) is to establish a pregnancy that is unaffected by a structural chromosomal abnormality (translocation) in a couple with a balanced translocation or deletion or duplication. New technology may actually distinguish normal noncarrier embryos from balanced carriers.

In PGT, a biopsy is necessary for obtaining embryonic material for genetic analysis. PGT requires an invasive biopsy to obtain embryonic material for genetic analysis. PGT may result in damage to the pre-embryo or may lower the implantation potential of the pre-embryo. This is less likely if the pre-embryo biopsied is at the blastocyst stage. Recent studies demonstrated that aspiration of blastocyst fluid is a promising alternative source of DNA for PGT.

LEGAL STATUS OF THE PREIMPLANTED PRE-EMBRYO[16-18]

The legal status of the pre-embryo is difficult to establish.

If it is regarded as a person, or even a potential person. It has no legal status according to the law in most countries. There is a suggestion that the pre-embryo is property. However, this definition offends ethical principles. The above suggestions leave a open the legal question of the right to use, to dispose, to sell and to purchase a pre-embryo. A pre-embryo seems not to be a human being for the purposes of criminal law. Deliberate destruction of a pre-embryo is not a criminal "Abortion" Act. The legislation regarding storage of pre-embryos in the UK, Australia, and regulations in other countries give the gamete donors the right to decide its fate. According to the wishes and consent of the gamete donors it can be disposed of, donated to other couples or given for research (this differs from country to country).

Present consensus on the status of the pre-embryo has been documented by several ethical committees. USA Advisory Board states: The pre-embryo is entitled to profound respect, but this does not necessarily give him the full legal and moral rights attributed to persons.

The Warnock committee: The human embryo is not, under the present to the law of the United Kingdom, accorded the same status as the living child or an adult.

The proposed Federal Human Life Bill in the USA would not give all the legal rights of personhood to the pre-embryo from the moment of conception. This is not similar in all states. The legislation in Illinois (USA), applied to the pre-embryo's legal status in vitro, is that of the 1877 Child Abuse Act. The physician is criminally liable if he endangers the life or health of the pre-embryo. This may lead to the situation whereby physicians can be prosecuted when the in vitro fertilized pre-embryo is damaged during its growth in vitro by changing the growth medium, temperature or following use of manipulation techniques.

A further question arises as to whether the physician commits a crime if he discards a pre-embryo that is not dividing properly or is damaged by the procedure of in vitro fertilization or its storage.

There is a general consensus that the pre-implanted pre-embryo is not a person but should have its own legal rights, and should be treated with special respect since it may become a person. Therefore, any intervention with the pre-embryo that is subsequently transferred to the uterus, creates obligations not only to avoid hurting or injuring it, but even to apply therapeutic measures since, following transfer, it may be born. This view point imposes the traditional duty of reasonable prenatal care and raises the question that if therapy is not undertaken, can the physicians and the parents, the donors of the gametes, be sued for wrongful life? The basis for this assumption may be a decision by the Supreme Court of the State of Israel on the issue of wrongful life. The Israeli Supreme Court of Appeals decided that it has the power to deal with the matter of the right not to be born, and decided that the minor has a valid claim against the physician. Therefore, the physician has a duty to care for the unborn. Damages were assessed against the physician for wrongful life so, according to this decision, it seems that the minor has the right to sue his negligent parents if antenatal care, even at the pre-embryo stage, is not undertaken.

MORAL STATUS OF PRE-EMBRYO[19-21]

The central question regarding therapeutic approaches to the preimplantation pre-embryo is its moral status. There are three options for the definition of the moral status of the pre-embryo:

- *The pre-embryo has no moral status*: It is a collection of undifferentiated cells lacking individuality, and therefore has a status which is no different from that of any other human tissue. The consequences of this assumption are that we have no obligation to treat the pre-embryo
- The pre-embryo has the full status of a human being. The bases for this assumption are:
  – A new genotype is established during fertilization
  – Some of the pre-embryos have the potential to become full-term fetuses, children, and adults. The consequences of this assumption are that the pre-embryo has its own rights, the gamete donors are the guardians of the pre-embryo and the interests of the mother are irrelevant to the future of the pre-embryo. Therefore, society has an obligation to apply therapeutic measures to the pre-embryo
- The pre-embryo is a potential human being. This definition is a new philosophical entity, representing a compromise between the other two, and is the one accepted today by most of the scientists, physicians, and ethicists. Even though the pre-embryo is a potential human being, it should be handled with dignity and its rights should be respected as long as they do not harm major social, maternal or other interests.

Life has been defined as ending when brain activity ceases.

Therefore, some consider that life begins when brain activity starts.

The beginning of life is 8 weeks after conception at the point when the embryo is responsive to stimuli. Human life begins when the human conceptus becomes a person, has some degree of sentience or even an active volition.

According to the above statements, apart from the one supported by the Catholic Church that human life begins at conception, human life cannot be attributed to the pre-embryo in the in vitro status.

Therefore, the question arises whether the gamete donors and the medical staff have an obligation to apply medical measures.

HUMAN GENOME EDITING

Genome editing is a technology able to change the DNA of a cell or organism by adding or removing DNA in the genome. The technology uses specific enzyme nucleases which cuts the genome in a specific place. The specific nucleases are made up of two parts:

- Nuclease part that cuts the DNA
- DNA-targeting part that is designed to guide the nuclease to a specific sequence of DNA

After cutting the DNA in a specific place, the cell will naturally repair the cut DNA. It is possible to manipulate the repair process, to make changes to the DNA in that location in the genome.[22]

There are two different categories of gene therapies:
1. Germline gene therapy
2. Somatic therapy.

Genome editing of human somatic cells aims to repair or eliminate a mutation that could cause disease like cancer patients.

Clinical experiments demonstrated positive results. It was approved to modify human blood cells to treat conditions including patients with malignancy and acquired immunodeficiency syndrome (AIDS). Changes to DNA of somatic cells affect only the person who receives the gene therapy.

Germline gene therapies change DNA in reproductive cells (sperm, oocyte, pre-embryo) are passed down from generation-to-generation.

Genome editing of pre-embryo has the potential to cure and eradicate genetic diseases. On the other hand, deliberately changing the genes passed on to children and future generations creating genetically modified people.

Chinese scientists led by Junjiu Huang[23] have reported editing the genomes of human embryos. The team was using "nonviable" embryos, which cannot result in a live birth, because were obtained from local fertility clinics.

The team attempted to modify the gene responsible for β-thalassemia, a potentially fatal blood disorder, using a gene-editing technique known as clustered regularly interspaced palindromic repeats (CRISPR/Cas9).

Huang and his colleagues set out to see if the procedure could replace a gene in a single-cell fertilized human embryo; in principle, all cells produced as the embryo developed would then have the repaired gene.

The results revealed that only part of the cells were successfully spliced, and that only a fraction of those contained the replacement genetic material. His team also found a high rate mutations assumed to be introduced by the CRISPR/Cas9 complex acting on other parts of the genome. Unintended mutations observed with gene editing could be harmful. It prevents its introduction into practice.

Genome editing of pre-embryos at present was not proved to be save. Questions are raised by society regarding—social, legal, ethical, religious, and economic implications of the technique.

At present ethical committees[24] support research aimed at making gene editing safe in order to medically treat existing people, but urge a prohibition on its use to create genetically modified humans.

MITOCHONDRIA MANIPULATION: A THREE-PARENT BABIES

Mitochondria are located in the cytoplasm of cells along with other organelles of the cell. Pre-embryo possesses a nucleus that contains a genome comprising nuclear DNA from both the father and the mother and mitochondria that house a distinct genome, which is solely composed of mitochondrial DNA.

Maternally inherited mitochondrial DNA (mtDNA) accounts for only a very small percentage of the total DNA in cells and less than 1%. Mutations in mtDNA are a cause of mitochondrial disease. Correlations have been identified between reduced mtDNA quantity and infertility, as well as between mtDNA mutations and fertilization rates.

Mitochondrial genetic disorders can be caused by the mtDNA or nuclear DNA that lead to dysfunction of the mitochondria and inadequate production of energy. Those caused by mutations in mtDNA are transmitted by maternal inheritance.

There are a few methods of transferring mitochondria:
- Pronuclear transfer
- Spindle transfer.

In pronuclear transfer, both the maternal oocytes and the donor one are fertilized via IVF. The fertilized pronucleus of the donor oocyte is destroyed and replaced with the fertilized nucleus of the maternal oocyte which has the DNA of the mother and the father.

In spindle transfer, the nuclear DNA from the mother (known as a spindle) is transplanted into the donor's oocyte replacing the donor's DNA. This new oocyte is fertilized by the father's sperm via intracytoplasmic sperm injection.

Defective mitochondria of the woman's oocyte are replaced with mitochondria from a donor who did not carry the mutation. IVF is performed, the resulting child carried DNA from three people: the female nuclear DNA donor (mother), the male nuclear DNA (father) or sperm donor, and the female mitochondria donor (additional mother).

The first baby born using mitochondrial replacement therapy was Jordanian couple by Dr Zhang and colleagues.[25] The mother of the baby boy is a carrier of Lehigh disease, a rare neurometabolic disorder that decimates a child's muscular system and often results in respiratory failure and death.

The three-parent babies will still resemble the men and women whose sperm and oocyte combined to produce the 23 chromosomes in the nucleus of that first cell. At present the technology of mitochondria manipulation is forbidden in USA but permitted in UK.[26]

REFERENCES

1. Kim AM, Bernhardt ML, Kong BY, et al. Zinc sparks are triggered by fertilization and facilitate cell cycle resumption in mammalian eggs. ACS Chem Biol. 2011;6(7):716-23.
2. Cockburn K, Rossant J. Making the blastocyst: lessons from the mouse. J Clin Invest. 2010;120(4):995-1003.
3. Karamalegos C, Bolton VN. A prospective comparison of 'in house' and commercially prepared Earle's balanced

salt solution in human in-vitro fertilization. Hum Reprod. 1999;14(7):1842-6.
4. Gardner DK, Schoolcraft WB, Wagley L, et al. A prospective randomized trial of blastocyst culture and transfer in in-vitro fertilization. Hum Reprod. 1998;13(12):3434-40.
5. Lopata A. Personal communication; 1981.
6. Trounson A, Mohr L. Human pregnancy following cryopreservation, thawing and transfer of an eight-cell embryo. Nature. 1983;305(5936):707-9.
7. Fasouliotis SJ, Schenker JG. Cryopreservation of embryos: Medical, ethical and legal issues. J Assist Reprod Genetics. 1996;13(10):763-8.
8. Shufaro Y, Schenker JG. Cryopreservation of human genetic material. Ann N Y Acad Sci. 2010;1205:220-4.
9. Edwards RG, Fishel SB, Cohen J, et al. Factors influencing the success of in vitro fertilization for alleviating human infertility. J In Vitro Fert Embryo Transf. 1984;1(1):3-23.
10. Gardner DK, Lane M, Stevens J, et al. Blastocyst score affects implantation and pregnancy outcome. Fertil Steril. 2000;73(6):1155-8.
11. Kirkegaard K, Agerholm IE, Ingerslev HJ. Time-lapse monitoring as a tool for clinical embryo assessment. Hum Reprod. 2012;27(5):1277-85.
12. Handyside AH, Kontogianni EH, Hardy K, et al. Pregnancies from biopsied human preimplantation embryos sexed by Y-specific DNA amplification. Nature. 1990;344(6268):768-70.
13. Harper JC, Wilton L, Traeger-Synodinos J, et al. The ESHRE PGD Consortium: 10 years of data collection. Hum Reprod Update. 2012;18(3):234-47.
14. Fasouliotis SJ, Schenker JG: Preimplantation genetic diagnosis, principles and ethics. Human Reprod. 1998;13(8):2238-045.
15. Glenn Schattman, Kangpu Xu. (2018). Preimplantation genetic testing. [online] Available from https://www.uptodate.com/contents/preimplantation-genetic-testing/print/. [Accessed December, 2018].
16. Eisenberg VH, Schenker JG. The ethical, legal and religious aspects of preembryo research. Eur J Obstet and Gynecol Reprod Biol. 1997;75(1):11-24.
17. Eisenberg VH, Schenker JG. Pre-embryo donation: ethical and legal aspects. Int J Gynecol and Obstet. 1998;60(1):51-7.
18. Schenker JG. Oocyte and embryo donation. In: Asch RH, Ballmaced JP, Johnston I (Eds). Gamete Physiology. Serono Symposia USA; 1990, pp. 319-29.
19. Schenker JG. The beginning of human life: Status of embryo. Perspectives in Halakha (Jewish Religious Law). J Assist Reprod Genet. 2008;25(6):271-6.
20. Schenker JG. Research on human embryos. Eur J Obstet Gynecol Reprod Biol. 1990;36(3):267-73.
21. Schenker JG (moderator). The ethical, legal and religious aspects of the modern diagnostic and therapeutic approach to the fetus. Round-table discussion. In: Schenker JG, Weinstein D, (Eds). The Intrauterine Life: Management and Therapy. Amsterdam: Elsevier; 1986. pp. 9-19.
22. Dance A. Core concept: CRISPR gene editing. Proc Natl Acad Sci USA. 2015;112(20):6245-6.
23. Huang J, Wang Y, Zhao J. CRISPR editing in biological and biomedical investigation. J Cell Physiol. 2018;233(5):3875-91.
24. Committee on Science, Technology, and Law; Policy and Global Affairs; National Academies of Sciences, Engineering, and Medicine, et al. International Summit on Human Gene Editing: A Global Discussion. Washington (DC): National Academies Press (US); 2016.
25. Zhang J, Liu H, Luo S, et al. Corrigendum to 'Live birth derived from oocyte spindle transfer to prevent mitochondrial disease.' Reprod Biomed Online. 2017;35(6):750.
26. Ravitsky V, Birko S, Dupras-Leduc R. The "Three-Parent Baby": A Case Study of How Language Frames the Ethical Debate Regarding an Emerging Technology. Am J Bioeth. 2015;15(12):57-60.

CHAPTER 8

The Moral Status of the Embryo in Professional Obstetric Ethics

Frank A Chervenak, Laurence B McCullough

INTRODUCTION

The ethical concept of the embryo as a patient is an essential component of assisted reproductive medicine and of obstetric management of early pregnancy as embryologic development transitions to fetal development and therefore in professional obstetric ethics.[1,2] In this chapter, we provide an account of this ethical concept and identify its implications in clinical practice. To accomplish this goal, we begin with accounts of ethics and professional medical ethics, including a brief overview of their historical development. There then follows a section on definitional issues, which includes an account of the ethical concept of moral status. The material presented in this chapter provides the basis for a practical examination of the clinical and research implications for the ethical concept of the embryo as a patient, a pragmatic, clinically applicable concept free of metaphysical baggage. These implications are separately identified for the in vitro embryo as a patient and for the in vivo embryo as a patient.

ETHICS

Ethics is the disciplined study of morality, our actual beliefs about right and wrong, and good and bad. Ethics assumes that these beliefs—as well as behavior and character traits based on these beliefs—can be improved. Ethics uses two tools to do so. The first tool is patient analysis of relevant ethical concepts with the goal of expressing them as clearly as possible. Unclear or confused concepts disable ethical reasoning from its very start, and therefore must be replaced with clear concepts. The second tool is identifying the implications of clearly expressed concepts for behavior and character. The goal of ethical reasoning is to reach well-reasoned ethical judgments that classify types of behavior and character traits as ethically permissible, ethically obligatory, or ethically impermissible. Ethics accepts only well-reasoned judgment, i.e. those that are established on the basis of ethical analysis and argument. Judgments made without this basis are to be considered "mere opinion," as Plato and Socrates teach in the *Dialogues* 2,500 years ago. "Mere opinion" therefore has no place in ethics and therefore no place in the professional ethics of obstetrics and gynecology.[3]

Beginning in the world of ancient Greece and China, two fundamental methods of ethical reasoning emerged. The first method can be described as a quest for certainty.[4] By grounding ethical reasoning in sources that are not of human making, one seeks to identify ethical judgments that are true and therefore transcultural, transnational, and transreligious. This philosophical tradition begins with Plato (427-347 BCE) and includes the most important philosopher of the German Enlightenment, Immanuel Kant (1724-1804 CE). One prominent example is the ethical concept of a natural right, a right that all human beings possess in virtue of shared human nature no matter their nationality, culture, or religion. The second method can be described as the quest for reliability.[4] This philosophical tradition begins with Confucius (551-479 BCE) and Aristotle (384-322 BCE). Ethical judgments evoke ethical concepts that human beings have invented in a specific cultural setting, but have become durable. This occurs when, over time, an ethical concept becomes transcultural, transnational, and transreligious. One prominent example is the ethical concept of a human right, which was invented shortly after World War II and has since then gathered persuasive power as it was repeatedly and successfully invoked utility to call governments to account for abuse of human beings. The discourse of human rights has been endorsed by the United Nations.[5]

Professional Ethics in Obstetrics and Gynecology

Professional medical ethics undertakes to improve clinical practice, research, and health policy. Professional medical ethics accomplishes this goal of constant improvement by deploying the tools of philosophical ethics to reach reasoned judgments about how physicians should act and what character traits or professional virtues they should cultivate in patient care, in scientific and clinical research, and in contributing to the formation and implementation of health policy.

Many physicians believe that professional medical ethics was introduced into the history of medical ethics in the ethical texts of the Hippocratic Corpus, including the Hippocratic Oath. This common belief, however, is mistaken. There is no concept of medicine as a profession in the Hippocratic Oath. Instead, medicine was understood by the authors of the Hippocratic Oath and other ethical writings in the Hippocratic Corpus to be entrepreneurial and self-interested, and thus dominated by the physician's concern for a good reputation (which was then in scarce supply). These texts are also shaped by the self-interests of physicians as a group to maintain market share in a highly competitive and unforgiving market to medical services. This group's self-interest is evidenced in the dismissal of surgeons in the Hippocratic Oath and the prohibition of surgery because its frightful mortality rates would bring disrepute on all physicians.[6]

Professional medical ethics, including professional ethics in obstetrics and gynecology, was invented in the late 18th century. The ethical concept of medicine as a profession was introduced into the history of medical ethics by two British physician-ethicists, John Gregory (1724–1773) of Scotland and Thomas Percival (1740–1804). This ethical concept calls for physicians to make three commitments: to become and remain scientifically and clinically competent; to protect and promote the patient's health-related interests as the physician's primary concern and motivation, keeping individual self-interest systematically secondary; and to protect and promote the patient's health-related interests as the physician's primary concern and motivation, keeping group self-interest systematically secondary.[3,6]

Gregory and Percival put forth this concept to correct three major problems. First, many practitioners were incompetent, given the absence of uniform training and state licensure. Second, many practitioners were "men of interest" who made money and fame their primary consideration, as one would expect of entrepreneurs (this was the true legacy of the Hippocratic texts). Third, many practitioners made the protection of the market share and power of medical guild, known as the Royal Colleges, their primary consideration. The result was rampant distrust of the sick in physicians, surgeons, apothecaries, and other medical practitioners.[6]

Making the three commitments of the ethical concept of medicine as a profession transformed the relationship between physicians and the sick. The historical legacy of the Hippocratic texts was that this relationship was contractual and nothing more. Physicians made no commitment other than to deliver promised services, just as in every other commercial enterprise. This had resulted in profound distrust of physicians. The relationship was a "the sick-the physician" (an admittedly awkward phrase) relationship of *caveat emptor* on the part of the sick individual contracting for medical services. The professional relationship is very different. In this relationship the sick individual is not on his/her own, always wary and distrustful, but protected by the physician's three commitments.[6]

Two ethical principles and one professional virtue are essential for undertaking professional medical ethics.[3] Ethical principles provide general guides to action. Professional virtues shape the professional character of the obstetrician-gynecologist.

Ethical Principle of Beneficence

This is the oldest ethical principle in the history of medical ethics. It creates the ethical obligation of the obstetrician-gynecologist to identify and provide forms of clinical management that are reliably predicted to result in net clinical benefit for the patient. Beneficence-based ethical judgments should be evidence-based. The reliability of beneficence-based ethical judgment varies directly with the level of evidence for the prediction of net clinical benefit.

The ethical principle of beneficence is essential for understanding the clinical ethical concept of a medically reasonable alternative.[3] A form of clinical management should be considered medically reasonable only when two conditions are met:
- The form of clinical management is technically feasible
- There is a sufficient evidence base for the prediction of net clinical benefit.

Ethical Principle of Respect for Autonomy

Gregory insisted that every patient has a "right to speak," one of the earliest expressions of respect for patient autonomy.[6] In contemporary professional ethics in obstetrics and gynecology, the ethical principle of respect for patient autonomy creates the ethical obligation to empower the pregnant patient with information about the progress and current state of her condition, including pregnancy, the medically reasonable alternatives for managing her pregnancy, and the clinical benefits and risks of each medically reasonable. The obstetrician should support the pregnant woman as she evaluates this information and expresses a decision based on such evaluation. The obstetrician should also be alert to potentially controlling influences on the woman's decision-making process and protect her from such influences. The goal is to enable the woman to make informed and take voluntary decisions.[3]

Professional Virtue of Integrity

Fulfilling the three commitments of the ethical concept of medicine as a profession sets the physician on the path of the pursuit of excellence in patient care, research, and health policy. The experience of such excellence integrates the physician's character in a life of service to patients. The professional virtue of integrity requires lifelong and rigorous adherence to the three commitments of the ethical concept of medicine as a profession.[3,6]

Definitional Issues

The Meaning of "Embryo" in Reproductive Medicine

The word "embryo" as two distinct meanings in reproductive medicine. The first meaning is: "the fertilized ovum after it has begun the process of cell division."[7] This is the meaning used in in vitro fertilization (IVF). This first meaning is the in vitro definition of "embryo." The second meaning is the biological entity that comes into existence when the blastocyst implants in the uterine wall until the 8th week of development, after which it becomes a fetus.[8] This is the meaning used in obstetrics and gynecology. This is the in vivo definition of "embryo."

The Ethical Concept of Moral Status

The attribution of moral status to an entity means that other have the ethical obligation to recognize the existence of that entity and to protect its interests or stakes that it has in the present and future. There are two kinds of moral status.

The Ethics Concept of a Person

In philosophy, the first kind of moral status is known as "independent" moral status; some property or properties constitutive of the entity that has independently of all other entities originate moral status.[3] In philosophical ethics, a paradigm of independent moral status is known as a "person." The word "person" thus has a distinctive meaning in philosophy. There are, to be sure, different meanings of the word, "person," with different implications for moral status. These concepts of being a person, especially in religion, are explored elsewhere in this volume.

The ethical concept of independent moral status and therefore the ethical concept of being a person apply only to individuals. In Western metaphysics, an entity becomes an individual if and only if satisfies two criteria (which can be thought of an inclusion criteria for being an individual). The first criterion is that the entity is distinct from other entities: we can pick it out separately from other entities. The in vitro embryo and the in vivo embryo are distinct, thus satisfying the first criterion for being an individual. The second criterion is indivisibility: the entity cannot divide into two entities of the same species. In embryological development this division is known as twinning. Twinning, a phenomenon with which obstetricians are already familiar, has important metaphysical implications, which we now, briefly, explore.

As long as the embryo retains the potential to twin, it is divisible, not indivisible, into two human beings. It follows necessarily that an embryo that can twin is not an individual and therefore cannot have independent moral status. It also follows necessarily that the ethical concept of being a person cannot apply to the embryo with the potential to twin. No in vitro embryo is a person.

The embryo that no longer has the potential to twin is indeed an individual, because it has become indivisible. However, while it is metaphysically necessary for being a person that one is an individual, it is metaphysical insufficient for being a person, by itself, that one is an in individual. One must also be an entity that self-generates the constitutive property that is the basis for independent moral status as an individual. In Western metaphysics, it is generally accepted an entity with the constitutive property of rational self-consciousness, which is a function of a highly developed sensory and nervous systems. Neither the in vitro embryo nor the in vivo embryo has such sensory and nervous systems. It necessarily follows that neither the in vitro embryo nor the in vivo embryo is a person.

Some Western philosophers hold that the capacity for awareness of pain establishes the basis for the independent moral status of an individual as a person. Awareness of pain is a function of highly developed sensory and nervous systems. Neither the in vitro embryo nor the in vivo embryo has such sensory and nervous systems. It necessarily follows that neither the in vitro embryo nor the in vivo embryo can be aware of pain. It also follows that neither has independent moral status nor can be a person.

The ethical concept of being a person provides no applicable ethical guidance for the professionally responsible management of clinical practice and research on in vitro embryos or the clinical management of in vivo embryos. The ethics of the clinical management and research on in vitro embryos or the clinical management of in vivo embryos is therefore free the metaphysics of being an individual and being a person. Finally, the metaphysics of being an individual and being a person is distinctively Western, calling into serious question whether the ethical concept of the embryo as a person is a transnational, transcultural, and transreligious concept. The ethical concept of the embryo as a person therefore has no place in the professional ethics of obstetrics and gynecology.

Ethical Concept of being a Patient

The second kind of moral status is known as "dependent" moral status; an entity occupies as social role that has been created to protect all entities in that role.[3] In philosophical ethics a paradigm of dependent moral status is a child; a human entity in social role that creates ethical obligations of parents to protect and promote the interests of their child. The concept of dependent moral status is pragmatic; it is a concept invented and sustained over time because of its utility, in this case, its utility for the professional ethics of obstetrics and gynecology. The concept is therefore not metaphysical, freeing it from the metaphysical baggage that burdens the ethical concept of being a person.

The Hippocratic texts and the later Latin texts in the Hippocratic tradition do not use the word "patient" but instead the word "the sick one" or "the sick individual." This discourse signals an ethics of the marketplace.

Gregory and Percival rejected the discourse of "the sick" with the ethical concept of being a patient. The professional relationship becomes the physician-patient relationship. The ethical concept of being a patient derives from their invention of the ethical concept of medicine as a profession. Being a patient means that one has been presented to a physician and their exist forms of clinical management that are reliably predicted to protect and promote the patient's health-related interests (in reducing the risk of mortality and morbidity).

The physician's three commitments to professionalism create the social role of being a patient. Being a patient therefore is a form of dependent moral status. This has a crucial clinical implication—having independent moral status, or being a person (in the philosophical meaning above) is not required in order to become a patient. This is why the embryo can sometimes be considered a patient.

The Ethical Concept of the Embryo as a Patient

An embryo becomes a patient when it is presented, in vitro or in vivo, to a physician and there exist forms of clinical management that are reliably expected to protect and promote the embryo's health-related interests. For the in vitro embryo this presentation occurs in the IVF laboratory, unmediated by any other human being. This is not the case for the in vivo embryo, the presentation of which is mediated by the pregnant woman. This means that whether the in vivo embryo becomes a patient, it is a function of the pregnant woman's autonomous decision to present for obstetric management and to continue her pregnancy to live birth. The dependent moral status of the in vivo embryo is therefore more complex ethically than the dependent moral status of the in vitro embryo. This difference requires that the clinical ethical implications of the embryo as a patient differ for the in vitro embryo and for the in vivo embryo.

Clinical and Research Implications: the Ethical Concept of the in vitro Embryo as a Patient

Transferring Embryos to Initiate a Pregnancy

The in vitro embryo can become an in vivo patient only with the informed consent of the woman into whose uterus it is to be transferred to confer this dependent moral status. The in vitro embryo can become a research subject that will not be transferred only with the informed consent of the couple from whom the in vitro embryo was derived. When the woman is initiating pregnancy with in vitro embryos, her gynecologist and the in vitro team have a beneficence-based ethical obligation to the future fetal patient(s) not to transfer a number that will result in high-order pregnancy that will increase in utero and perinatal risks to the fetal patient(s).[9] The gynecologist and in vitro team also have a beneficence-based obligation to the woman to prevent the biopsychosocial risks to her of a high-order pregnancy. Existing guidelines from such organizations as the American Society for Reproductive Medicine (ASRM),[10] the American College of Obstetricians and Gynecologists (ACOG),[11] or the European Society of Human Reproduction and Embryology[12] (ESHRE) should be followed. The informed consent process should include information about the IVF group's outcomes, including both percent of pregnancies initiated and percent of live births.

Preimplantation Diagnosis

If preimplantation genetic or genomic diagnosis is to be performed, the woman should be provided information about the categories of results. These include results pertaining to each embryo:
- A genetic or genomic diagnosis of an embryo
- Risk assessment, i.e. the increased likelihood of disease in a future child or in genetic kinfolk
- Pharmacogenomic information about medication of the future child
- Alleles of uncertain clinical significance, i.e. not previously reported alleles in genes known or suspected to be pathogenic
- Previously unreported alleles in healthy genes, the clinical significance of which is unknown.[13]

These also include results to the sources of gametes, either by implication or when they are also genomically assessed, (e.g. in "trio" testing). The results will fall into the same five categories.

Counseling the woman and her partner about the interpretation of results must recognize that reports from genome laboratories can be cognitively demanding for the physician and will be even more cognitively demanding for the woman and her partner. The results should be organized into the above five categories and presented in order clinical significance for which embryo(s) are considered appropriate for transfer. The likelihood of there being no results in any of the five categories is very low, given the inherent errors of human reproduction. This should be explained, so that the woman and her partner are disabused of the search for the "perfect baby."[14] It should be made very clear from the outset that the decision about which embryos she considers appropriate to transfer is the woman's decision and that the gynecologist's professional judgment may differ, in which case the differences will need to mediated. The IVF laboratory should have a policy to guide such mediation that expressly states the laboratory's exclusion criteria, which should be consistent with guidance from ASRM, ACOG, or ESHRE.

Responding to Requests for High Number of Embryos to be Transferred

A request from a woman to depart from these guidelines should be managed by informing her the risks of high-order pregnancy and recommending that these guidelines be followed for her benefits and for the benefit of future and neonatal patients. If this attempt to transform her request into the informed consent process fails to persuade to withdraw her request, then the gynecologist and in vitro team should, as a matter of professional integrity, refuse the request. The gynecologist should document this process in detail.

Seamless Transfer of Patient Care

The gynecologist has a strict professional obligation to ensure a seamless transfer of care to the woman's obstetrician after transfer. The referring obstetrician should receive a clinical report, especially detailing any complications or poor prognosis, so that her obstetrician has the clinical information that he or she needs to create an appropriate care plan with the pregnant woman.

Research with in vitro Embryos

In vitro embryos should be used for research (an experiment undertaken with a group of subjects in order to create generalizable knowledge) only under a protocol approved by the appropriate Institutional Review Board (IRB) or Research Ethics Committee (REC). Failure to obtain IRB or REC approval for research on human embryos constitutes an egregious failure of scientific and professional integrity and is therefore ethically impermissible. There are no exceptions.

Clinical Implications and the Ethical Concept of the in vivo Embryo as a Patient

The in vivo embryo can become a patient only with the informed consent of the pregnant woman to confer this dependent moral status. The pregnant woman is free to confer, withhold, or having once conferred, withdraw the moral status of being a patient from the in vivo embryo.[3]

Counseling about the Termination of Pregnancy

There are a number of clinical circumstances in which it is ethically obligatory to offer (but not recommend) termination of early first-trimester pregnancy.[15] The first occurs when a woman expresses ambivalence or uncertainty about remaining pregnant and raises the issue directly. The second occurs when her pregnancy has resulted from rape or incest. The second occurs when noninvasive risk assessment indicates an increased risk of a fetal anomaly, provided that the obstetrician explains that risk assessment is not diagnosis, which requires invasive assessment. For some women, the increased risk, by itself, will be unacceptable. The third occurs when invasive assessment results in the diagnosis of a fetal anomaly, in which circumstances it is exclusively the woman's decision about whether she wants to continue her pregnancy. The fourth occurs when a high-order pregnancy is diagnosed. Selective feticide is known to improve the perinatal outcomes for a twin or singleton pregnancy, information that a pregnant needs to make an informed decision about continuation of a high-order pregnancy. The fifth occurs when the pregnant woman has a serious medical condition (the mortality and morbidity risks) of which a coexisting pregnancy could increase. This is information that a pregnant needs to make an informed decision about continuation of her pregnancy. Termination of an early first-trimester pregnancy remains legally permissible in most legal jurisdictions.

This counseling should focus on assisting the woman to have the clinical information that is salient to her decision. This information should be presented free of bias. It is ethically impermissible to limit information based on the obstetrician's personal beliefs or statutory law. It is also ethically impermissible to make any recommendation of any kind, especially one based on the obstetrician's personal beliefs. Counseling therefore should be strictly nondirective. A shared decision-making process should be adopted and driven by the patient's informational needs, values, and beliefs. She should be encouraged to draw on her social supports as she deems valuable. She should be supported in her decision about whom to involve and she should be assured that the professional of confidentiality will be adhered to without exception and as required by law.

Counseling about Obstetric Management

Pregnant women should be routinely informed that 2–3% of pregnancies are affected by fetal anomalies. If one is diagnosed later in pregnancy, the pregnant woman may confront a decision about continuation of her pregnancy (subject to applicable legal restrictions).[15] Pregnant should also be informed that a normal, low-risk pregnancy can become high-risk quickly and without warning, especially during the intrapartum period. In this case, when evidence-based clinical judgment supports doing so, her obstetrician may recommend cesarean. To prevent the effects on decision-making in a high-stress and time-compressed environment, the obstetrician should take advantage of prenatal visits to discuss intrapartum management in such clinical circumstances and document the results in the patient's record, so that decision-making intrapartum can be guided by the patient's expressed values and beliefs.[16]

CONCLUSION

The ethical concept of the embryo as a patient plays a foundational role in professional obstetric ethics[3,17] and therefore in both IVF and in nondirective counseling about a newly initiated pregnancy. This concept is beneficence-based and autonomy-based. The purpose of the counseling process should be integrate beneficence with respect for autonomy to guide a professionally responsible counseling process that is designed to empower the woman to make informed decisions about initiating and continuing pregnancy and to implement the professional virtue of integrity.

REFERENCES

1. Kurjak A, Chervenak FA (Eds). Controversies on the Beginning of Human Life, 1st edition. New Delhi: Jaypee Brothers Medical Publishers; 2008.
2. Kurjak A, Chervenak FA, McCullough LB (Eds). Science and Religion: Synergy not Skepticism. New Delhi: Jaypee Brothers Medical Publishers; 2017.
3. Chervenak FA, McCullough LB. The Professional Responsibility Model of Perinatal Ethics. Berlin: Walter de Gruyter; 2014.
4. Gracia D. Philosophy: ancient and contemporary approaches. In: Sugarman J, Sulmasy DP (Eds). Methods in Medical

Ethics, 2nd edition. Washington: Georgetown University Press, 2010. pp. 55-72.
5. McKeon R. The philosophical basis and material circumstances of the rights of man. Ethics. 1948;58:180-7.
6. McCullough, Laurence B. John Gregory and the Invention of Professional Medical Ethics and the Profession of Medicine. Dordrecht: Springer; 1998.
7. Society for Assisted Reproductive Technology. (2018). Embryo. [online] Available from https://www.sart.org/topics/topics-index/embryo/ [Accessed November, 2018].
8. American College of Obstetrics and Gynecology. (2018). How your fetus grows during pregnancy. [online] Available from https://www.acog.org/-/media/For-Patients/faq156.pdf?dmc=1&ts=20180615T1523286650. [Accessed on November, 2018]
9. Chervenak FA, McCullough LB. Professional integrity, respect for autonomy, and the self-regulation of reproductive endocrinology. Am J Obstet Gynecol. 2009;201(1):3-4.
10. Practice Committee of the American Society for Reproductive Medicine. Performing the embryo transfer: a guideline. Fertil Steril. 2017;107(4):882-96.
11. American College of Obstetricians and Gynecologists, Society for Maternal-Fetal Medicine. ACOG Practice Bulletin No. 144: Multifetal gestation: twin, triplet, and higher-order multifetal pregnancies. Obstet Gynecol. 2014;123(5):1118-32.
12. Magli MC, Van den Abbeel E, Lundin k, et al. ESHRE Pages Revised guidelines for good practice in IVF laboratories. Hum Reprod. 2008;23(6):1253-62.
13. McCullough LB, Brothers KB, Chung WK, et al. Clinical Sequencing Exploratory Research (CSER) Consortium Pediatrics Working Group. Professionally responsible disclosure of genome sequencing results in pediatric practice. Pediatrics. 2015;136(4):e974-82.
14. Chervenak FA, McCullough LB, Brent RL. The perils of the imperfect expectation of the perfect baby. Am J Obstet Gynecol. 2010;203(2):101.e1-5.
15. Chervenak FA, McCullough LB. An ethically justified approach to offering, recommending, performing, and referring for induced abortion and feticide. Am J Obstet Gynecol. 2009;201(6):560.e1-6.
16. Chervenak FA, McCullough LB. Preventive ethics for cesarean delivery: the time has come. Am J Obstet Gynecol. 2013;209(3):166-7.
17. Chervenak FA, McCullough LB, Brent RL. The professional responsibility model of obstetric ethics: avoiding the perils of clashing rights. Am J Obstet Gynecol. 2011;205(4):315.e1-5.

CHAPTER 9

Invasive Diagnostic Procedures in Embryonic Period

Giovanni Monni, Ambra Iuculano, Cristina Peddes, Maria Carla Monni, Valentina Corda

INTRODUCTION

Invasive diagnostic sampling procedures are all techniques used for analyzing embryofetal and placental tissues, amniotic fluid or fetal blood to avoid birth defects.[1]

The most common procedures performed are chorionic villus sampling (CVS), amniocentesis and cordocentesis.[2]

Since 1983, in embryonic period, the most useful diagnostic procedure is CVS performed either transcervically (TC-CVS) or transabdominally (TA-CVS).

All techniques are performed under continuous ultrasound monitoring and following nondirective genetic-obstetric counseling and informed written consent.

More recently, to avoid genetic diseases and voluntary termination of pregnancy (TOP) women can utilize before pregnancy and using in vitro fertilization and intracytoplasmatic injection (IVF-ICSI) the preimplantation genetic diagnosis (PGD).[3,4]

Even if in the past, coelocentesis, early amniocentesis between 12th and 14th week of gestation, vaginal lavage to obtain fetal cells were described as prenatal invasive procedures during the embryonic period, nowadays these techniques are completely abandoned.

In this chapter we would like to give the updated practical recommendations and the most appropriate techniques in invasive prenatal procedures such as CVS and PGD for clinicians and patients when deciding on their reproductive choices available in the embryonic period.

GENETIC-OBSTETRIC COUNSELING

Genetic-obstetric counseling must be performed before any invasive procedure by doctors' who are expert in genetics. Possibly, the counseling must be performed in the preconceptional period or before procedures in order to suggest and offer to the patients the best information about their reproductive choices.[5]

Counseling must always be informative and nondirective[1] and should include:

- The genetic risks of diseases
- The possibility of screening, diagnosis, prognosis and therapy
- Embryo fetal, maternal and neonatal risks following invasive prenatal procedures, diagnostic limits, success and failure rates and time to obtain a diagnosis
- Methods of all invasive procedures
- Other possible techniques and laboratory diagnostic clarifications in case of doubts
- Choice options of fetal-neonatal therapy as well as discussion of the possibility of performing voluntary TOP in pathologic cases.

It is suggested to obtain a written informed consent form signed by the patient at the end of the counseling session.

ULTRASOUND AND PRENATAL INVASIVE TECHNIQUES

All invasive prenatal procedures would not be possible to perform if in the past years there had not been an impressive enhancement of the ultrasonographic equipment.

Each invasive prenatal procedure must be performed under continuous ultrasound monitoring in order to find the best spot for the instrument insertion and the sampling itself.

Ultrasonographic monitoring must be performed before the invasive prenatal procedure in order to define the pregnancy, the viability and the number of fetuses, the gestational age, the placenta location, the amniotic fluid pocket, the umbilical cord insertion and to avoid possible concomitant uterine adnexal pathologies.[6]

EMBRYONIC INVASIVE DIAGNOSTIC PROCEDURES CHORIONIC VILLUS SAMPLING–PREIMPLANTATION GENETIC DIAGNOSIS

The most common invasive technique used in perinatal centers is CVS, either TC-CVS or, mostly utilized, TA-CVS.[7]

The transabdominal route is preferable because it can be performed at any period of pregnancy[8] (from 10th to 40th week of pregnancy), it is generally better accepted by women since it is faster to perform and implies lower fetal loss and infection risks, less risk of vaginal bleeding, better privacy and easier reproducibility.[9]

In order to avoid the voluntary termination of pregnancy, PGD on the embryo or on the blastocyst can be employed.[4]

The techniques used depend on the disease, whether they are performed before or during pregnancy, on the clinician's experience and hands-on skills, on the capacity of the laboratory and on the patient's choice. Women usually prefer the simplest technique which provides a result as early as possible.

Chorionic Villus Sampling

Indications of Chorionic Villus Sampling

Karyotype analysis for chromosomal risks: Even if in several countries the maternal age solely (≥35 years) is still employed as an indication for fetal karyotype study, the most appropriate indication is an abnormal screening test following first trimester combined testing [fetal nuchal translucency ultrasound measurement and dosages of free-β-human chorionic gonadotropin (hCG) and pregnancy-associated plasma protein-A (PAPP-A)] and, more recently, following cell-free DNA [noninvasive prenatal screening (NIPS)] from maternal blood sampling.

Other indications for fetal karyotype study are a previous child with a chromosomal anomaly and ultrasound detection of fetal structural abnormalities in first trimester of pregnancy.[1]

Deoxyribonucleic acid analysis for: Increased risk for single gene diseases with a known DNA mutation, risk for X-chromosomal inheritance and for autosomal recessive diseases such as thalassemia, cystic fibrosis, Duchenne muscular dystrophy, mental retardation, etc.[1]

Errors of Metabolism[1]

Transabdominal chorionic villus sampling technique (TA-CVS): The most commonly employed procedure is TA-CVS by free-hand technique. The free-hand insertion can be done tangentially (Fig. 9.1) or obliquely (Fig. 9.2) to the ultrasound scanner using a 20- or a 18-gauge spinal needle under continuous ultrasound monitoring.[9,10]

Several operators report insertion of the needle into the biopsy rigid adaptor as a guide.[6]

We prefer the free-hand approach using a 20-gauge needle connected to a 2-mL syringe to aspirate chorionic villi by an up-and-down movement because it proves to be less painful for patients and it also allows reaching the shortest route between the maternal abdomen and the chorion site as well as easy correction of the needle trajectory.[11-13]

Neither local anesthesia nor antibiotic treatment is usually required and the sampling is performed in an outpatient facility. In a few cases antispastics can be administered.

Sampling failure is very rare but it can occur in 1–2% cases. The quantity and quality of the chorionic villi

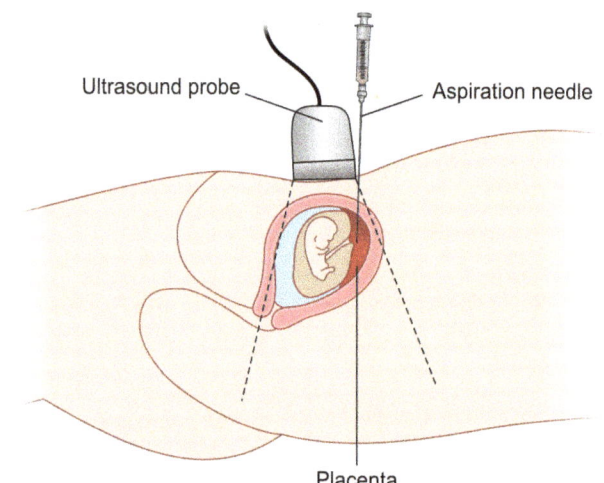

Fig. 9.1: Transabdominal chorionic villus sampling (TA-CVS) and tangentional free-hand insertion of the needle.

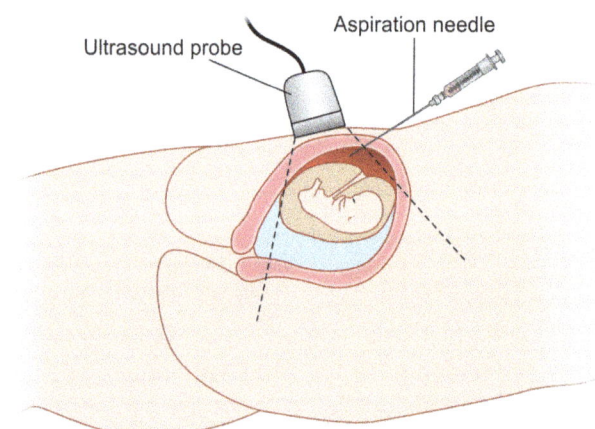

Fig. 9.2: Transabdominal chorionic villus sampling (TA-CVS) and oblique free-hand insertion of the needle.

should be visually controlled by the clinician and usually 10–20 mg of tissue is sufficient for all analysis.

In a few cases maternal intestinal loops can be placed above the uterus so it may be useful to exert mild pressure with the screen probe in order to move the uterus a bit aside and then introduce the needle in the placenta.

In case of retroverted uterus and completely posterior placenta (2–3% of cases) transvaginal manipulation of the uterus by the assistant may be required in order to introduce the needle in the placenta and obtain the sufficient amount of chorionic villi.[14]

All procedures are performed in a sterile area and the needle and syringe must be heparinized to avoid clots, the maternal abdomen must be cleansed with antiseptic solution beforehand. The screen probe must also be in a sterile drape or a glove.

Transcervical chorionic villus sampling technique (TC-CVS): Placenta location by ultrasound and careful disinfection of the vagina must be done before introducing a flexible polyethylene catheter (Fig. 9.3) with an aluminum mandrel connected to a syringe for aspiration[15] or a rigid biopsy forceps[16] in the cervical canal introduced in chorion frondosum (Fig. 9.4) between 10 weeks and 14 weeks of gestation under continuous ultrasound monitoring. In several cases a tenaculum can prove useful for the traction of the cervix and straightening out the uterus to permit a better introduction.

The instruments should not be introduced more than twice and if insufficient chorionic tissue is sampled, it is recommended to use a new sterile device.

Local anesthesia, antibiotics of hospitalization are not necessary and only in a few cases tocolytics can be administered.

Sampling failure is very rare but it is reported to occur in 2–4% of samplings. The sufficient quantity of tissue should be visually controlled by the clinician and may vary from 10 mL to 20 mL for all genetic or chromosomal analyses.

Timing and Risks of Chorionic Villus Sampling

Even if in the past, several procedures were performed in an earlier period of pregnancy before the 9th week of gestation, CVS must be performed following 10 weeks of gestation because several fetal abnormalities such as limb reduction and oromandibular defects were described if performed before the 10th week.[17-19] Therefore, the most appropriate timing is 11–12 weeks.

The additional fetal loss rate following the procedure depends on the clinician's experience and a meta-analysis study reports to be very low, varying between 0,2 and 0,5%, the same as the one reported for the amniocentesis at 16 weeks.[20-22] The fetal risk is higher in early period and in older women.[23]

It is better not to introduce the instruments more than twice. In Rh-negative patients with a negative Coombs test, RH alloimmunization can be caused by CVS. In such cases anti-D immunoglobulins prophylaxis is mandatory. In women already immunized CVS is contraindicated.

It is advisable to perform the procedure after a reasonable period of tutoring under the guiding of a senior

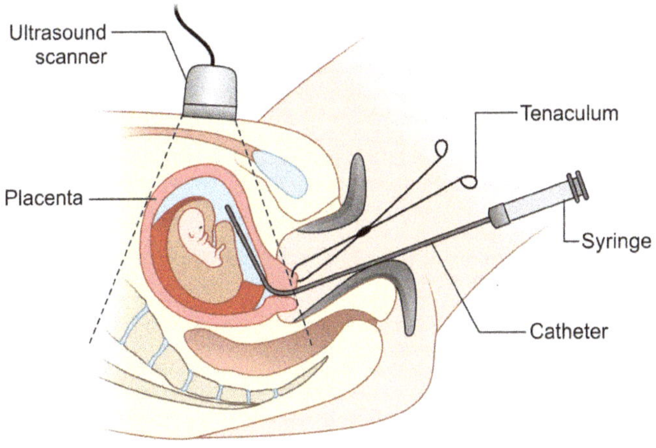

Fig. 9.3: Transcervically chorionic villus sampling (TC-CVS) and catheter introduction.

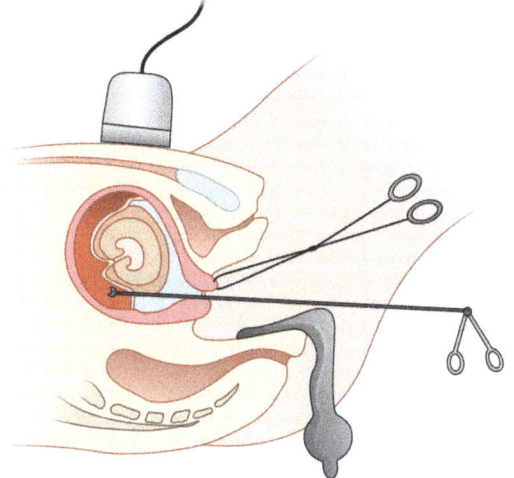

Fig. 9.4: Transcervically chorionic villus sampling (TC-CVS) and rigid biopsy forceps introduction.

clinician.[24] In order to monitor the capacity of sampling success and to have less fetal losses, the clinician must have performed at least 100–200 procedures each year.[25]

Laboratory Analysis of Chorionic Villus Sampling

Prenatal samplings can be analyzed using traditional karyotype, DNA-PCR, quantitative fluorescent PCR or chromosomal molecular analysis, and for single gene diseases.

Traditional karyotype: Metaphase analysis of cultured chorionic tissue and direct analysis of cytotrophoblastic metaphases following CVS is still used in prenatal centers.[26]

In 1–2% several cell lines with different chromosomal kits can be present, this is called mosaicism. Two different types of mosaicism exist: the true chromosomal mosaicism in which case the fetus and the placenta have two chromosomal kits and the so-called "confined placental mosaicism" with two cell lines presents only in the placenta but not in the fetus. In order to distinguish the two cases, further analysis by amniocentesis or fetal blood sampling is required.[27]

Quantitative fluorescent polymerase chain reaction (QF-PCR): Recently quantitative fluorescent-PCR can be used for analysis of the most common trisomies and for X chromosomes and Y chromosomes, but, in few cases this test results in more false positives and false negatives.[28] QF-PCR must be confirmed by metaphase long culture analysis and ultrasound examination.

Chromosomal molecular analysis: Array comparative genetic hybridization (aCGH) or microarray analysis permits to ascertain submicroscopic chromosomal deletions and duplications. Up till now, targeted, mixed arrays and genome-wide can be utilized in prenatal diagnosis for the detection of 6% of aberrations in traditional normal karyotype and also in fetal malformations following ultrasound.[29]

Microarray techniques can also increase the detection rate of aberrations in CVS following abnormal screening combined test or following nuchal translucency thickness more than or equal to 3, 5 mm and congenital cardiac problems.[30,31] Finding a variant of uncertain significance (VOUS) may make genetic counseling difficult.

Sampling for single gene defects: DNA-polymerase chain reaction amplification (DNA-PCR) analysis is the technique of choice for genetic single gene or Mendelian diseases such as thalassemia, cystic fibrosis, Tay-Sachs disease, etc. with very high analysis accuracy and very low misdiagnosis rate is reported.[32-34]

It is preferable to obtain the DNA by CVS rather than by amniocentesis because of lower contamination probability and better analysis results. Variable Number Tandem Repeat (VNTR) analysis can be added to avoid maternal contamination and misdiagnosis.[35]

Training and Audit of Chorionic Villus Sampling

In the era of declining rates of invasive prenatal procedures due to the decrease of natality, screening tests and the onset of NIPS by cell-free DNA the importance of training and tutoring of fellow and maintaining the skill expertise is fundamental.[36-38]

At least 30–100 amniocenteses and 50–200 CVS are recommended yearly in order to maintain the manual skills of clinicians. Prenatal centers must create a database for annual monitoring of the sampling procedures and consider all parameters such as failure, success, repetition of procedure, fetal risks, analysis accuracy as well as number of birth defects.[22]

Tutoring fellows in TA-CVS is simpler if they are already expert in ultrasonography and amniocentesis which is generally easier to acquire as a skill, rather than TC-CVS.[36]

A training period of 2–3 weeks with an adequate number of invasive prenatal procedures and in a center with an expert senior tutor is recommendable, with teaching in vivo instead of using a model, a mannequin or simulators.[24]

Performing procedures must be centralized in centers so that they are of a considerable number in order to maintain the skill and thus reduce the fetal loss risk and complications. The expertise of all operators must also be controlled regularly by an annual audit that should be reported during the counseling of the patients.[14]

Preimplantation Genetic Diagnosis

Preimplantation genetic diagnosis (PGD) is a very early form of prenatal diagnosis prior to the implantation of the embryo in the uterus and involves testing to avoid the transmission of specific genetic or chromosomal birth defects.[39]

It was performed for the first time by Alan H Handyside in 1989 in UK.[40] This technique also aims to bypass the obvious issue of voluntary termination of pregnancy (TOP) because it allows to select and transfer in the maternal uterus only the healthy embryos obtained in vitro by assisted reproductive techniques (IVF-ICSI).[41]

The technique involves the biopsy of a single or more cells from oocytes or from embryos, at the 3rd day cleavage stage (Fig. 9.5) or at the 5th day from trophoblastic cells of blastocysts (Fig. 9.6).[42]

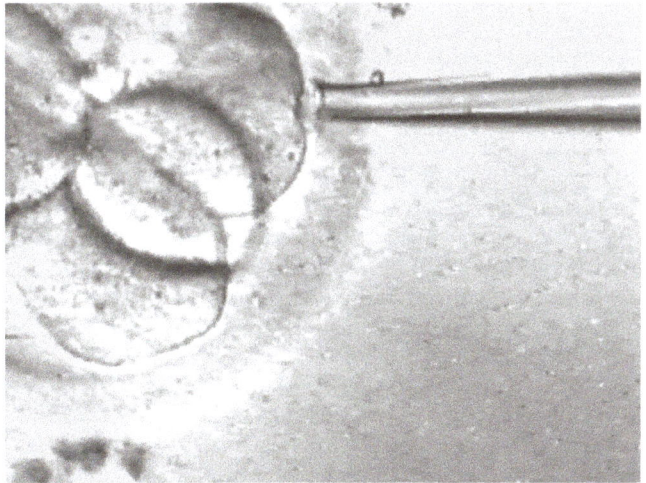

Fig. 9.5: Single cell biopsy from embryo at 3rd day cleavage.

Preimplantation genetic diagnosis is used for genetic diagnosis of autosomic recessive disorders such as thalassemia, cystic fibrosis, Tay-Sachs disease, spinal amiotrophy, etc.[43] and for women at risk for chromosomal disorders, mainly for advanced maternal age, recurrent pregnancy loss and repeated IVF failure, severe sperm factors, carrier of chromosomal rearrangement, and in the last indications it is named "preimplantation genetic screening (PGS)".[44,45]

The biopsied cells are analyzed by DNA-PCR. In the past, the analysis was performed by multiplex polymerase chain reaction for single gene defects and by fluorescent in situ hybridization for chromosomal anomalies.

At present time the most accurate analyses are the whole-genome amplification and genome-wide technologies.[39]

The success rate of analysis is high even if in a few cases a diagnosis may not be available due to DNA amplification problems or contamination. The success of PGD is strongly influenced by maternal age, IVF, quality of embryo culture and biopsy, and also by molecular diagnosis.

The PGD can also be employed for HLA compatibility by human leukocyte antigen matching in case of bone marrow transplantation after birth even if these techniques raise some ethical problems and controversies.[46]

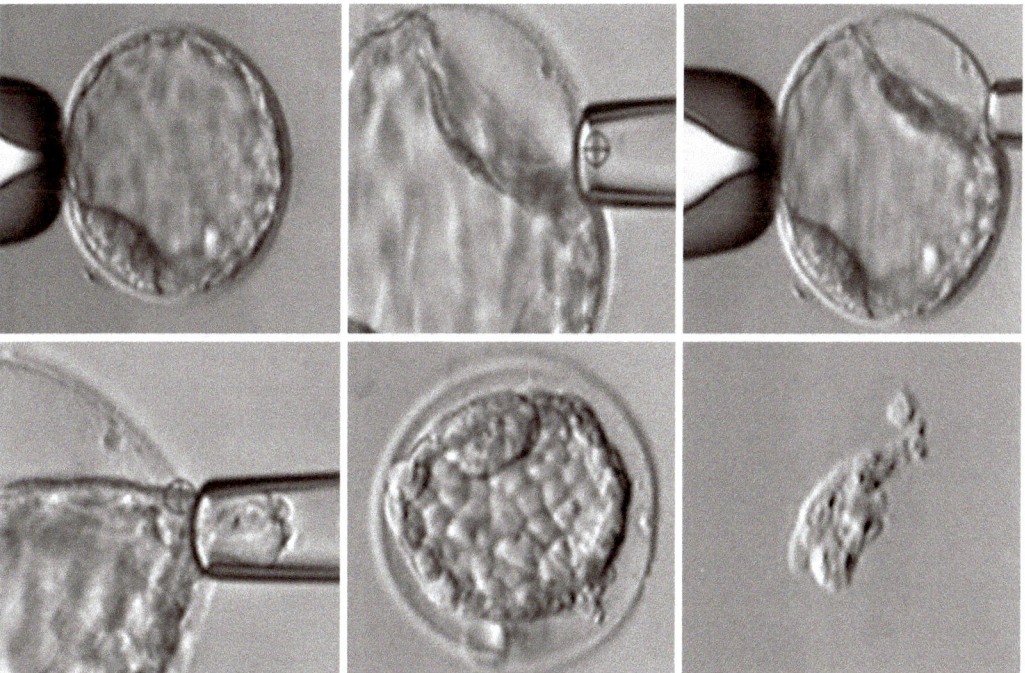

Fig. 9.6: Blastocyst removal at 5th day from trophoblastic cells.

REFERENCES

1. Milunsky A, Milunsky JM (Eds). Genetic Disorders and the Fetus, 6th edition. Chichester: Wiley-Blackwell; 2010.
2. Monni G, Zoppi MA, Axiana C, et al. Changes in the approach for invasive prenatal diagnosis in 35,127 cases at a single center from 1977 to 2004. Fetal Diagn Ther. 2006;21(4):348-54.
3. Kuliev A, Rechitsky S, Verlinsky O, et al. Preimplantation diagnosis of thalassemias. J Assist Reprod Genet. 1998;15(5):219-25.
4. Traeger-Synodinos J. Preimplantation genetic diagnosis. Best Pract Res Clin Obstet Gynecol. 2017;39:74-88.
5. Cao A, Cossu P, Monni G, et al. Chorionic villus sampling and acceptance rate of prenatal diagnosis. Prenat Diagn. 1987;7(7):531-3.
6. Ghi T, Sotiriadis, A, Calda P, et al. ISUOG Practice Guidelines: invasive procedures for prenatal diagnosis in obstetrics. Ultrasound Obstet Gynecol. 2016;48:256-68.
7. Brambati B, Lanzani A, Tului L. Transabdominal and transcervical chorionic villus sampling: efficiency and risk evaluation of 2,411 cases. Am J Med Genet. 1990;35(2):160-4.
8. Monni G, Olla G, Rosatelli C, et al. Second-trimester placental biopsy versus amniocentesis for prenatal diagnosis of beta-thalassemia. N Engl J Med. 1990;322(1):60-1.
9. Monni G, Olla G, Cao A. Patient's choice between transcervical and transabdominal chorionic villus sampling. Lancet. 1988;7(8593):1057.
10. Brambati B, Terzian E, Tognoni G. Randomized clinical trial of transabdominal versus transcervical chorionic villus sampling methods. Prenat Diagn. 1991;11(5):285-93.
11. Monni G, Ibba RM, Lai R, et al. Early transabdominal chorionic villus sampling in couples at high genetic risk. Am J Obstet Gynecol. 1993;168(1 Pt 1):170-3.
12. Monni G, Ibba RM, Zoppi MA. Prenatal Genetic Diagnosis through Chorionic Villus Sampling. In: Milunsky A, Milunsky JM (Eds). Genetic Disorders and the Fetus, 6th edition. Hoboken: Wiley-Blackwell; 2010. pp. 160-93.
13. Monni G, Pagani G, Stagnati V, et al. How to perform transabdominal chorionic villus sampling: a practical guideline. J Matern Fetal Neonatal Med. 2016;29(9):1499-505.
14. Monni G, Iuculano A. Re: ISUOG Practice Guidelines: invasive procedures for prenatal diagnosis. Ultrasound Obstet Gynecol. 2017;49(3):414-5.
15. Ward RH, Modell B, Petrou M, et al. Method of sampling chorionic villi in first trimester of pregnancy under guidance of real time ultrasound. Br Med J (Clin Res Ed). 1983;286(6377):1542-4.
16. Monni G, Ibba RM, Olla G, et al. Chorionic villus sampling by rigid forceps: Experience with 300 cases at risk for thalassemia major. Am J Obstet Gynecol. 1987;156(4):912-4.
17. Firth HV, Boyd PA, Chamberlain P, et al. Severe limb abnormalities after chorion villus sampling at 56-66 days' gestation. Lancet. 1991;337(8744):762-3.
18. Monni G, Ibba RM, Lai R, et al. Limb-reduction defects and chorion villus sampling. Lancet. 1991;337(8749):1091-2.
19. Froster UG, Jackson L. Limb defects and chorionic villus sampling: results from an international registry, 1992-94. Lancet. 1996;347(9000):489-94.
20. Tabor A, Alfirevic Z. Update on procedure-related risks for prenatal diagnosis techniques. Fetal Diagn Ther. 2010;27(1):1-7.
21. Akolekar R, Beta J, Picciarelli G, et al. Procedure-related risk of miscarriage following amniocentesis and chorionic villus sampling: a systematic review and meta-analysis. Ultrasound Obstet Gynecol. 2015;45(1):16-26.
22. Wulff CB, Gerds TA, Rode L, et al. Risk of fetal loss associated with invasive testing following combined first trimester risk screening for Down syndrome: a national cohort of 147,987 singleton pregnancies. Ultrasound Obstet Gynecol. 2016;47(1):38-44.
23. Monni G, Ibba RM, Lai R, et al. Transabdominal chorionic villus sampling: fetal loss rate in relation to maternal and gestational age. Prenat Diagn. 1992;12(10):8150-20.
24. Monni G, Pagani G, Illescas T, et al. Training for transabdominal villous sampling is feasible and safe. Am J Obstet Gynecol. 2015;213(2):248-50.
25. Monni G, Zoppi MA. Improved first-trimester aneuploidy risk assessment: an evolving challenge of training in invasive prenatal diagnosis. Ultrasound Obstet Gynecol. 2013;41(5):486-8.
26. Jackson LG, Zachary JM, Fowler SE, et al. A randomized comparison of transcervical and transabdominal chorionic-villus sampling. The U.S. National Institute of Child Health and Human Development Chorionic-Villus Sampling and Amniocentesis Study Group. N Engl J Med. 1992;327(9):594-8.
27. American College of Obstetricians and Gynecologists. ACOG Practice Bulletin No. 88, December 2007. Invasive prenatal testing for aneuploidy. Obstet Gynecol. 2007;110(6):1459-67.
28. Test and Technology Transfer Committee, American College of Medical Genetics, 9650 Rockville Pike, et al. Technical and clinical assessment of fluorescence in situ hybridization: an ACMG/ASHG position statement.I. Technical considerations. Test and Technology Transfer Committee. Genet Med. 2000;2(6):356-61.
29. Wapner RJ, Martin CL, Levy B, et al. Chromosomal microarray versus karyotyping for prenatal diagnosis. N Engl J Med. 2012;367(23):2175-84.
30. Jansen FA, Blumenfeld YJ, Fisher A, et al. Array comparative genomic hybridization and fetal congenital heart defects: a systematic review and meta-analysis. Ultrasound Obstet Gynecol. 2015;45(1):27-35.
31. Grande M, Jansen FA, Blumenfeld YJ, et al. Genomic microarray in fetuses with increased nuchal translucency and normal karyotype: a systematic review and meta-analysis. Ultrasound Obstet Gynecol. 2015;46(6):650-8.
32. Rosatelli C, Falchi AM, Tuveri T, et al. Prenatal diagnosis of beta-thalassemia with the synthetic-oligomer technique. Lancet. 1985;1(8423):241-3.
33. Rosatelli MC, Tuveri T, Scalas MT, et al. Molecular screening and fetal diagnosis of β-thalassemia in the Italian population. Hum Genet. 1992;88:590-2.

34. Saiki RK, Bugawan TL, Horn GT, et al. Analysis of enzymatically amplified beta-globin and HLA-DQ alpha DNA with allele-specific oligonucleotide probes. Nature. 1986;324(6093):163-6.
35. Batanian JR, Ledbetter DH, Fenwick RG. A simple VNTR-PCR method for detecting maternal cell contamination in prenatal diagnosis. Genet Test. 1998;2(4):347-50.
36. Lo YM, Chan KC, Sun H, et al. Maternal plasma DNA sequencing reveals the genome-wide genetic and mutational profile of the fetus. Sci Transl Med. 2010;2(61):61ra91.
37. Monni G, Zoppi MA, Iuculano A, et al. Invasive or noninvasive prenatal genetic diagnosis? J Perinat Med. 2014;42(5):545-8
38. Odibo AO, Dicke JM, Gray DL, et al. Evaluating the rate and risk factors for fetal loss after chorionic villus sampling. Obstet Gynecol. 2008;112(4):813-9.
39. Palini S, De Stefani S, Primiterra M, et al. Pre-implantation genetic diagnosis and screening: now and the future. Gynecol Endocrinol. 2015;31(10):755-9.
40. Handyside AH, Pattinson JK, Penketh RJ, et al. Biopsy of human preimplantation embryos and sexing by DNA amplification. Lancet. 1989;1(8634):347-9.
41. Monni G, Peddes C, Iuculano A, et al. From Prenatal to Preimplantation Genetic Diagnosis of β-Thalassemia. Prevention Model in 8748 Cases: 40 Years of Single Center Experience. J Clin Med. 2018;7(2).pii:E35.
42. Scott RT Jr, Upham KM, Forman EJ, et al. Cleavage-stage biopsy significantly impairs human embryonic implantation potential while blastocyst biopsy does not: a randomized and paired clinical trial. Fertil Steril. 2013;100(3):624-30.
43. Monni G, Cau G, Usai V, et al. Preimplantation genetic diagnosis for beta-thalassemia: the Sardinian experience. Prenat Diagn. 2004;24(12):949-54.
44. De Wert G, Dondorp W, Shenfield F, et al. ESHRE task force on ethics and Law22: preimplantation genetic diagnosis. Hum Reprod. 2014;29(8):1610-7.
45. Fiorentino F, Kahraman S, Karadayi H, et al. Short tandem repeats haplotyping of the HLA region in preimplantation HLA matching. Eur J Hum Genet. 2005;13(8):953-8.
46. Tur-Kaspa I, Jeelani R. Clinical guidelines for IVF with PGD for HLA matching. Reprod Biomed Online. 2015;30(2):115-9.

CHAPTER 10

The First Four Weeks: Ultrasound and Doppler Assessment of Normal and Abnormal Implantation

Sanja Kupesic Plavsic

INTRODUCTION

Embryo implantation is the attachment of an embryo during the most favorable endometrial receptivity stage, called "window of implantation" (WOI).[1] The endometrium is a dynamic environment, susceptible to many local and systemic changes, requiring well-orchestrated coordination by the sex steroids, estrogen, and progesterone.[2] It is estimated that implantation failure of euploid blastocysts is responsible for about 40% of early pregnancy loss.[3] Poor synchronization between the blastocyst and the endometrium, inflammatory changes [e.g. chronic endometritis (CE)], alteration of the uterine perfusion, and inadequate uterine peristalsis are potential causes of unsuccessful implantation. This chapter focuses on the ultrasound assessment of the mechanical, inflammatory, and functional changes of the uterine environment which may lead to unsuccessful implantation.

ULTRASOUND AND DOPPLER STUDIES OF THE ENDOMETRIUM

The endometrium is best visualized by two-dimensional (2-D) and three-dimensional (3-D) ultrasound in the sagittal plane and multiplanar imaging, respectively. This specialized mucosa, composed of the superficial and basal layers varies in thickness, echogenicity, composition, and vascularity throughout the menstrual cycle.[4-6]

The ultrasound image of the endometrium during the *menstrual phase* depends on the amount of echogenic endometrial fragments and blood clots between the hyperechogenic lines representing the basal layers (Fig. 10.1). By the end of the menstrual bleeding, the endometrium is typically visualized as a thin and hyperechogenic line, measuring between 1 mm and 3 mm. Due to estrogen effect during the *proliferative phase*, the endometrial thickness and echogenicity of the basal layers increase, and the echogenicity of the functional layer decreases, resulting in a *trilaminar* (multilayered,

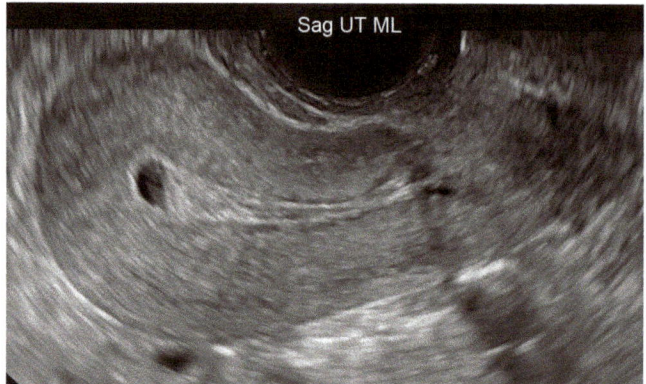

Fig. 10.1: Menstrual phase endometrium; note echogenic endometrial fragments and blood clots between thin basal layers of the endometrium.

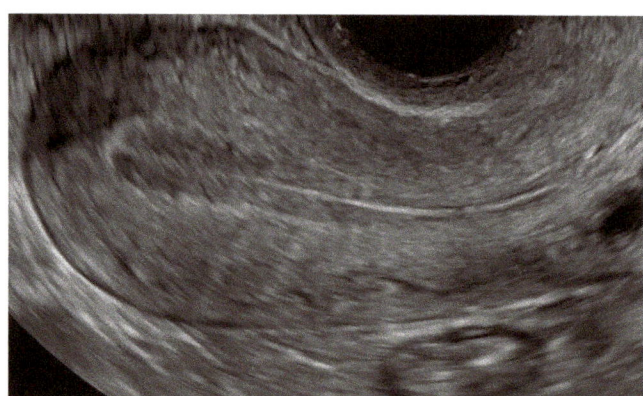

Fig. 10.2: Proliferative, triple-line appearance of the endometrium; note increased echogenicity of the basal layers and decreased echogenicity of the functional layers of the endometrium.

triple-line) appearance (Fig. 10.2).[7] At the end of the proliferative phase, the endometrial thickness ranges between 7 mm and 14 mm.

During the luteal phase, three major types of endometrial pattern are recognized:[8-13]

1. The *early secretory phase* (from postovulatory days 1 to 5), characterized by progressive thickening of the outer hyperechogenic lines caused by progesterone-induced glycoprotein secretion; the endometrium has

a *ring-like* appearance with thick, bright basal layers, and pale, but still recognizable middle line (Fig. 10.3)
2. The *mid-secretory phase* (from postovulatory days 6 to 10), recognized as *homogeneously echogenic* (secretory transformed) endometrium (Fig. 10.4)
3. The *late-luteal* or *pseudodecidualization phase* (from postovulatory days 11 to 14, for nonconception cycles), and *decidualization phase* in pregnant patients, with nidatory human chorionic gonadotropin (hCG) signal from the embryo], with the same appearance as the mid-secretory endometrium.

Interestingly, throughout the luteal phase, the endometrial thickness does not significantly change compared to the periovulatory phase.[6,7]

The endometrium receives blood from the spiral arteries (Fig. 10.5). The endometrial flow is highly dependent upon the uterine, arcuate, and radial artery blood flow.[14] Spiral artery blood flow velocity waveforms are characterized by lower velocity and lower impedance to blood flow than are those observed in the uterine arteries.[14,15] Color Doppler literature hypothesizes that the features of endometrial blood flow may be used to predict the implantation success rate and reveal unexplained infertility problems.[16] Quantification of the endometrial volume by 3-D ultrasound in combination with blood flow studies contributes to the assessment of the endometrial receptivity and may have a potential to predict the pregnancy rates in assisted reproductive techniques (ART).[17] Digital volume storage allows retrospective analysis of the volumes and independent review by a discipline expert in 3-D ultrasound. De-identified datasets may be efficiently used for training purposes.[18]

Future research is focused on identifying endometrial receptivity biomarkers that may reliably predict endometrial receptivity. Simultaneously, the use of 3-D ultrasound technology is directed toward efficient detection of the various causes of implantation failure.[18,19]

Uterine Cavity Defects and Implantation

Intracavitary pathology encompasses both congenital uterine anomalies and acquired intracavitary conditions, such as submucous and intracavitary fibroids, endometrial polyps, and intrauterine adhesions. Visualization of the coronal plane and surface rendering of the uterine cavity by 3-D ultrasound has revolutionized early detection of congenital uterine anomalies by instantaneous visualization of the uterine cavity, myometrium, and fundus (Fig. 10.5).[20,21] By providing multiple tomographic sections of the uterine cavity, the acquired intracavitary lesions have also become visible.[22] Assessment of the uterine

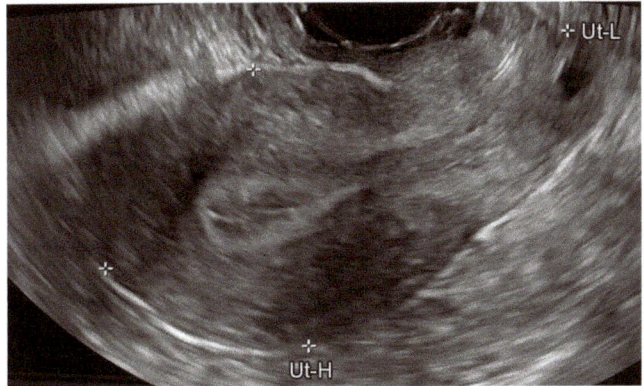

Fig. 10.3: Early secretory ring-like appearance of the endometrium with thick, bright basal layers, and pale, but still recognizable middle line.

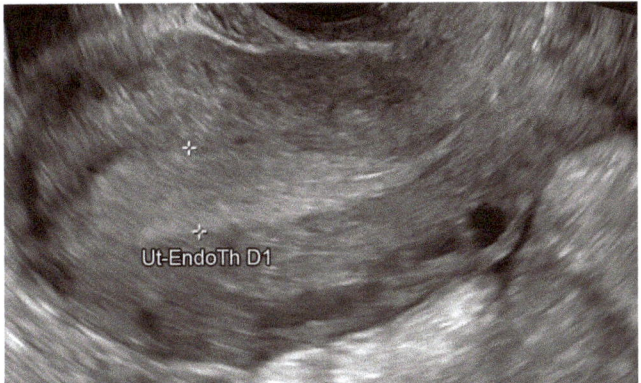

Fig. 10.4: Secretory transformed, uniformly echogenic endometrium.

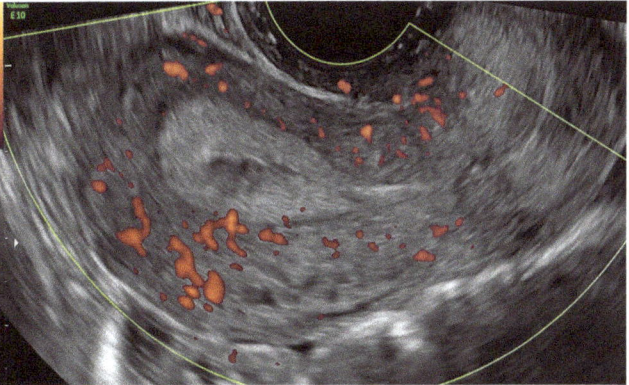

Fig. 10.5: Power Doppler image of the uterine circulation; the endometrial flow is dependent upon the uterine, arcuate, and radial artery blood flow.

cavity can be improved by distension of the uterine cavity with the injection of a small amount of sterile saline [2-D and 3-D saline infusion sonography (SIS) or hysterosonography].[23] 3-D ultrasound and SIS are sensitive diagnostic modalities for the detection of congenital uterine anomalies and intracavitary lesions, highly comparable to MRI and hysteroscopy (Figs. 10.6 to 10.8).

Kupesic et al.[20,21] compared the women with untreated septate uteri versus women who had undergone hysteroscopic metroplasty and found that untreated women had a significantly worse prognosis of pregnancy outcome. Depending on location and size, the acquired intracavitary conditions can also lead to reduced implantation potential

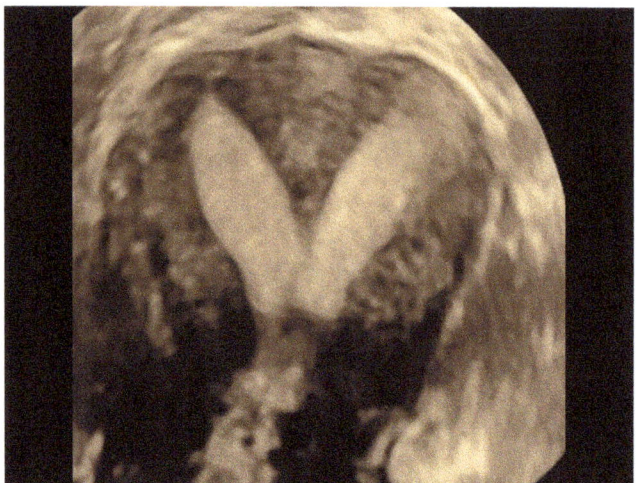

Fig. 10.6: 3-D ultrasound of the septate uterus; coronal plane clearly outlines the convex shape of the uterine fundus and thick septum dividing the upper half of the uterine cavity.

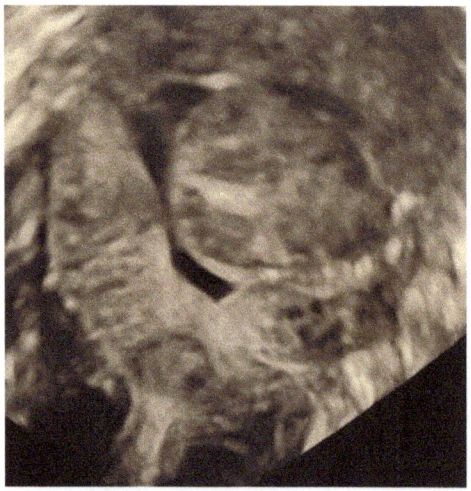

Fig. 10.7: 3-D saline infusion sonography of the intracavitary fibroid.

and recurrent implantation failure.[22] Data from the literature indicate that hysteroscopic metroplasty and hysteroscopic removal of the submucosal or intracavitary fibroids and endometrial polyps have a beneficial effect on implantation and pregnancy rates.[24,25]

Inflammatory Disease and Implantation

Inflammatory factors are commonly associated with implantation failure. Transvaginal B-mode and color or power Doppler ultrasound has a potential to detect chronic inflammatory changes on a routine scan before or during the infertility procedure. Many times patients are unaware of the chronic inflammatory process but can recall one or more episodes of pelvic pain and vaginal discharge.[26] Because of the same echogenicity as surrounding bowel, fallopian tubes could not be visualized by ultrasound unless filled with fluid. Transvaginal sonography is accurate in the identification of the hydrosalpinges by evaluating the structure of the tubal wall and luminal contents. Careful observation may reveal a thin-walled, fluid-filled mass adjacent and medial to the ovary, with incomplete, thin tubal septations, and hyperechogenic "knots" visualized in a transverse section, representing mucosal folds.[27] By conventional 2-D ultrasound, hydrosalpinx can often be mistaken for a multilocular or paraovarian cyst. Color Doppler studies are particularly useful in patients with the complex appearance of the pelvic inflammatory disease (PID) when pseudopapillomatous structures are protruding into the cystic counterpart.[26,27] High vascular resistance and/or absence of blood flow, typical for this PID stage is helpful for differentiating hydrosalpinx from the ovarian neoplasm. 3-D ultrasound features such as multiplanar view and surface rendering contribute to better delineation of the inflammatory conglomerates, providing a unique opportunity to "see through" the slices of the tortuous hydrosalpinx (Fig. 10.9).[28]

Meta-analyses have demonstrated a significant reduction in pregnancy rates and an increase in the probability of spontaneous abortion in in vitro fertilization (IVF) and embryo transfer (ET) patients with hydrosalpinges.[29,30] The mechanism that causes the implantation failure is not fully understood but implies a mechanical leakage of the fluid into the uterine cavity causing a "mechanical washout" of the embryos, embryotoxicity of the hydrosalpingeal fluid and endometrial alterations, including changes of the endometrial environment and increased peristalsis.[31-34] Numerous studies confirmed the benefit of preventative

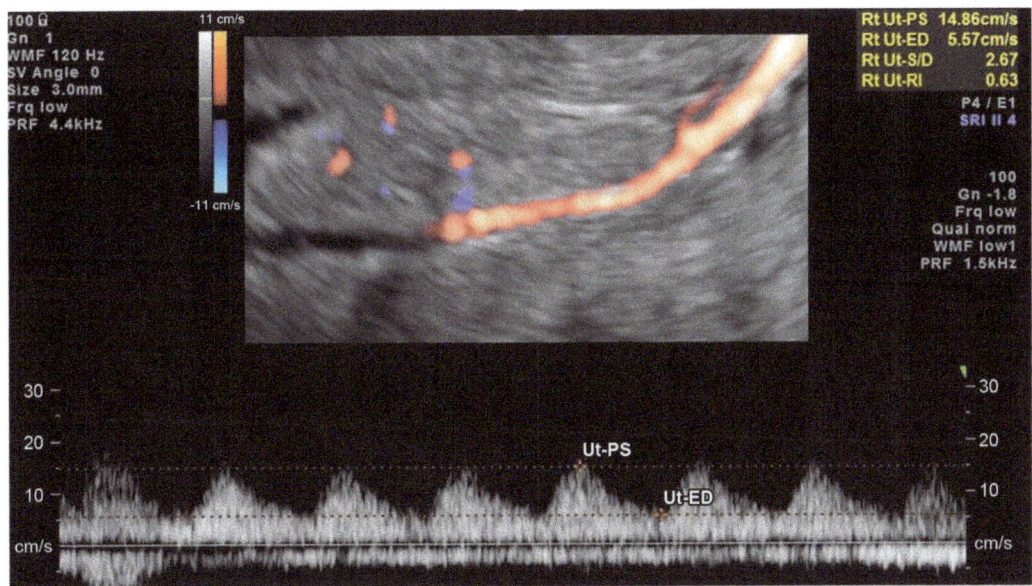

Fig. 10.8: Saline infusion sonography of the endometrial polyp. Color Doppler reveals moderate to high vascular impedance of the feeder vessel (RI 0.63).

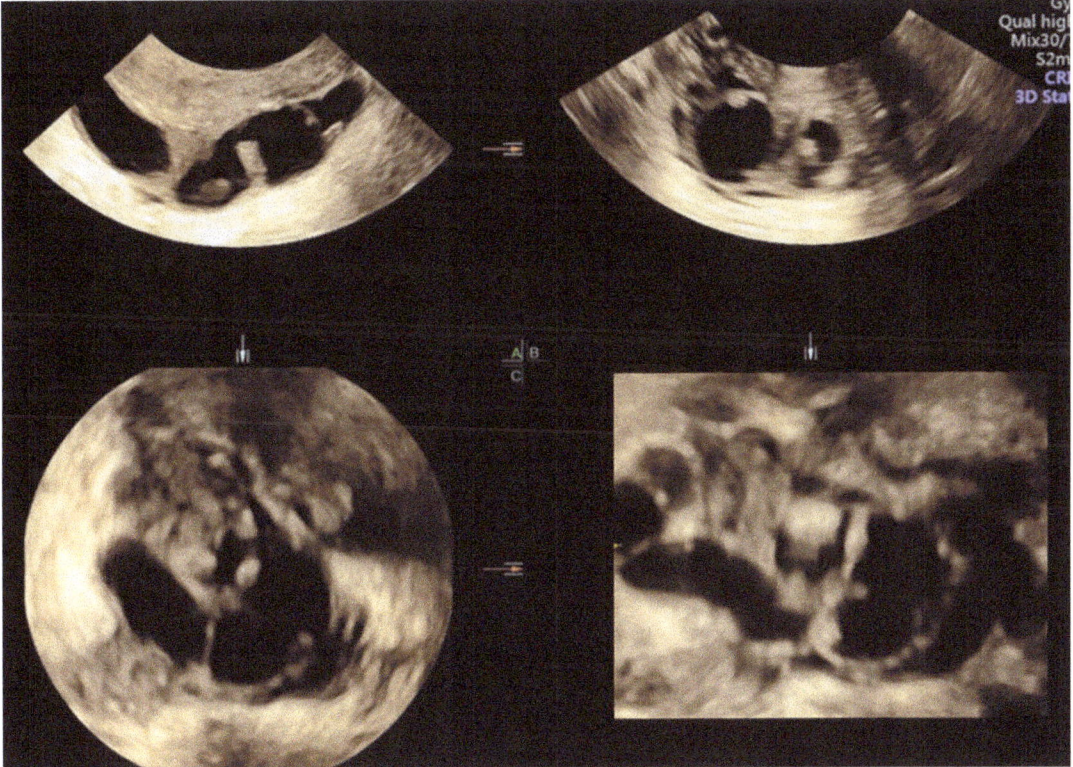

Fig. 10.9: Multiplanar view and surface rendering of hydrosalpinx. Note thick incomplete septations and pseudopapillomatous structures protruding into the fluid-filled fallopian tube.

salpingectomy for patients with hydrosalpinges undergoing IVF or ET.[35,36] These observations emphasize the importance of ultrasound detection of the chronic sequelae of PID in infertile patients undergoing ART.

Chronic inflammation of the endometrium, CE, is usually asymptomatic or has vague symptoms, such as leukorrhea, pelvic pain, and abnormal uterine bleeding.[37] CE is demonstrated in between 10% and 11% of the patients undergoing hysterectomy for benign gynecologic conditions.[38] Romero et al.[39] reported that 15% of infertile women undergoing IVF or ET are diagnosed with CE, with the prevalence rate as high as 42% in patients with recurrent implantation failure. Similar results were reported by Zolghadri et al.[40] who hysteroscopically and histologically confirmed endometritis in 57.8% of women with a history of three or more recurrent pregnancy losses. The exact mechanism through which CE affects embryo implantation is likely to be associated with the dysregulation of cytokines.[41] Most frequent etiological factors of CE are common bacteria seen in bacterial vaginosis,[42] followed by *Mycoplasma and Ureaplasma urealyticum*.[43,44] The conclusion of these studies is that IVF candidates with repeated unexplained implantation failure may benefit from hysteroscopic evaluation and biopsy of the uterine cavity.[45] In this respect, preconceptional antibiotic treatment could produce positive changes in future pregnancy outcomes, even when biopsies are negative for microbiological culture.[46]

Adenomyosis and Implantation

Adenomyosis is a heterogeneous entity, and thus, its appearance on imaging is highly variable. Implantation failure and subfertility associated with adenomyosis is likely to be associated with the structural and functional alterations of the junctional zone (JZ).[47] The JZ is a region of the inner myometrium, where radial arteries divide into two to three spiral arteries from which the basal arterioles divide off to supply the basal layer of the endometrium. Being not only structurally but functionally different from the outer myometrium, the JZ seems to be the origin of the uterine peristaltic activity.

The sonographic findings of adenomyosis involve alterations of the myometrium, JZ, and myometrial vascularity. Recently Arya and Kupesic[48] reported on the following ultrasound features of adenomyosis:

- The heterogeneous appearance of myometrium
- Asymmetrical uterine wall thickening (anteroposterior asymmetry), in particular, when the disease is focal
- Loss of endometrium-myometrium border caused by glands invasion of the myometrium
- Echogenic linear striations fanning out from the endometrial layer represent hyperplastic reaction caused by the invasion of the endometrial glands into the subendometrial tissue
- A random scattering of myometrial vessels demonstrated by color Doppler ultrasonography (Fig. 10.10)[48]

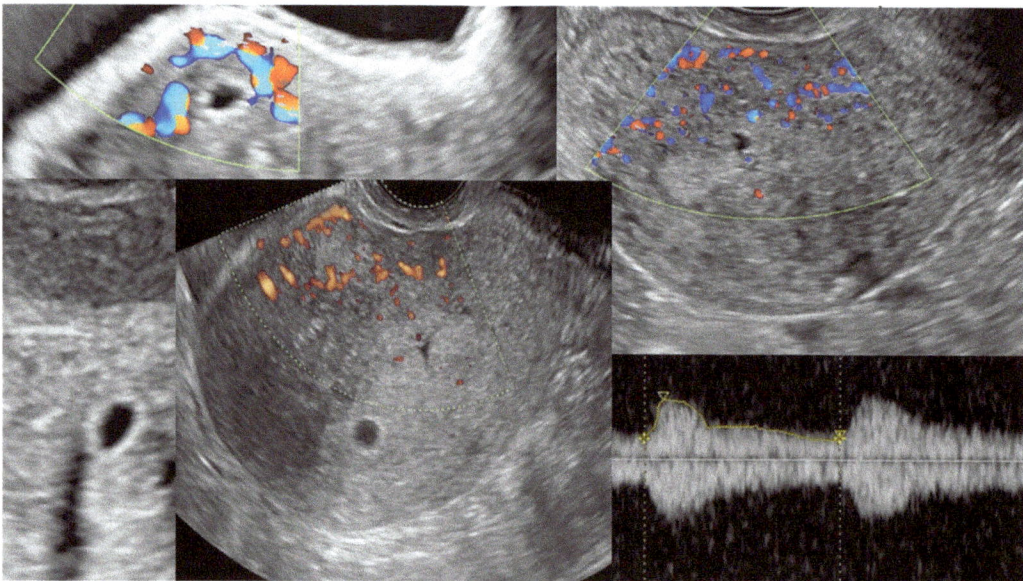

Fig. 10.10: Sonographic and color/power Doppler features of adenomyosis; note anteroposterior asymmetry and heterogeneous appearance of the myometrium, loss of endometrium–myometrium border, presence of myometrial cysts, and random scattering of myometrial vessels.

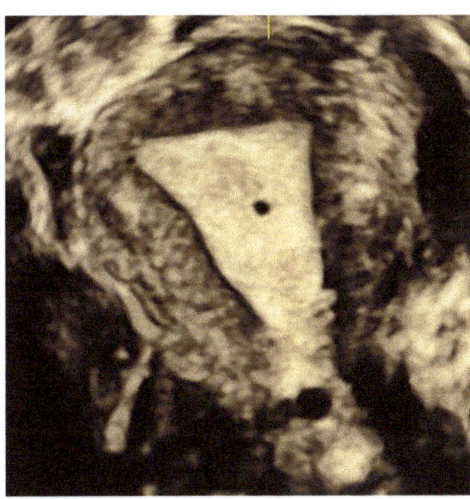

Fig. 10.11: 3-D ultrasound image of a thick JZ and a small cystic lesion within the central portion of the endometrial cavity in a patient with adenomyosis.

- The increased thickness of the JZ (hypoechoic halo surrounding the endometrial layer), best visualized in the coronal plane by 3-D ultrasound. The JZ thickness from 8 mm to 12 mm is reported to be associated with adenomyosis (Fig. 10.11).[49]

Altered uterine peristaltic activity which may affect sperm transport and blastocyst nidation, abnormal decidualization, and increased levels of intrauterine free radicals are the most commonly reported causes of infertility treatment failures in patients with adenomyosis.[47-49] Patients with sonographic findings of adenomyosis show significantly higher miscarriage rate (66.7% vs. 21%, p <0.04), and significantly lower clinical pregnancy rate than controls.[50,51] Maubon et al.[52] found that patients with the average JZ thickness more than or equal to 7 mm on MRI had an implantation failure of 95.8% compared to 37.5 % in those with JZ of less than 7 mm. Further studies are needed to assess the impact of adenomyosis on infertility and association between adenomyosis and pregnancy complications, (e.g. preterm birth).[53]

Hormonal Changes and Implantation

Polycystic ovary syndrome (PCOS) is a common cause of infertility and the most common endocrine disorder affecting approximately 5–18% of reproductive-aged women.[54,55] The diagnosis is established when two or more of the following criteria are met—oligo- and/or amenorrhea, clinical or biochemical androgen excess, and polycystic ovarian appearance on ultrasound. PCOS patients with oligo-amenorrhea have a threefold risk of endometrial cancer.[56]

Impaired follicle maturation and anovulation lead to chronic estrogen exposure and progesterone deficient state of the endometrial lining.[57] Progesterone resistance causes estrogen receptor dominance during the secretory phase, resulting in the creation of an inflammatory milieu which may compromise the implantation.[57-59]

It is well-documented that patients with hyper- and hypothyroidism are at increased risk of infertility and adverse pregnancy outcome, and that untreated hypothyroidism is associated with lower implantation rates in IVF or ET cycles.[60-62] A meta-analysis by Velkeniers et al.[63] demonstrated that women with subclinical hypothyroidism and/or thyroid autoimmunity treated with thyroxine show improved fertilization, implantation and live birth rates, as well as decreased risk of miscarriage.

Despite evidence of prolactin decidual production, its systemic effect on implantation events is not yet determined.[64] Future research is focused on assessing prolactin levels in the endometrial secretome of patients undergoing ovarian stimulation to determine its role as local mediator during the implantation process.[64,65]

The obesity is a well-studied modifiable risk factor for poor pregnancy outcomes in ART. Bellver et al.[66] demonstrated the effect of increasing the recipient body mass index (BMI) on the success of the IVF or ET cycles using oocyte donors with BMI less than 25 kg/m^2; the implantation rate for recipients with BMI more than or equal to 30 kg/m^2 was significantly lower than in recipients with BMI less than 30 kg/m^2 (30.9% vs. 40%, p < 0.001). Further controlled studies are needed to confirm the negative impact of obesity on embryo implantation.

Assessment of Uterine Receptivity

The assessment of endometrial receptivity continues to challenge clinicians from the field of ART who are focused on identifying the most specific markers of successful implantation. Noninvasive studies of endometrial receptivity based on ultrasound and Doppler evaluation of the endometrial pattern, volume and flow indices continue to show inconsistent and controversial findings.[17,67-71] Future efforts are directed toward the creation of an integrated scoring system combining the endometrial thickness, volume, echotexture, subendometrial peristalsis, JZ thickness, and uterine vascularity assessment for determination of endometrial receptivity.[72]

Recent advancement in technology resulted in the development of the microarray technology which allows identification of the "transcriptomic signature of the WOI."[73] Improved understanding of the effect of ovarian induction on the endometrial molecular alterations causing premature secretory changes and altered differentiation of the glandular and stromal cells is crucial for the implementation of the individualized approach to the IVF or ET treatment.[74] Initial studies on the use of the "endometrial receptivity array" (ERA) in patients with recurrent pregnancy failure show improved pregnancy outcomes after personalized ET of the euploid embryos.[75-79] It is hoped that future studies of the luteal phase support, uterine fluid proteomics, induction of decidualization by increasing the secretion of cytokines, growth factors and interleukins, and implementation of the stem cell and gene therapy will contribute to better understanding of the molecular regulation of the endometrial receptivity, leading to a tailor-made infertility treatment.[67,68,80-88]

REFERENCES

1. Ruiz-Alonso M, Galindo N, Pellicer A, Simón C. What a difference two days make: "personalized" embryo transfer (pET) paradigm: A case report and pilot study. Hum Reprod. 2014;29(6):1244-7.
2. Fox C, Morin S, Jeong JW, et al. Local and systemic factors and implantation: what is the evidence? Fertil Steril. 2016;105(4):873-84.
3. Harton GL, Munné S, Surrey M, et al. Diminished effect of maternal age on implantation after preimplantation genetic diagnosis with array comparative genomic hybridization. Fertil Steril. 2013;100(6):1695-703.
4. Kupesic S. The first four weeks assessed by transvaginal color Doppler (Editorial). J Perinat Med. 1996;24:301-17.
5. Janssen H, Kupesic Plavsic S. Ultrasound imaging of the menstrual cycle. Donald School Journal Ultrasound Obstet Gynecol. 2009;3(4):41-7.
6. Kupesic Plavsic S. Pelvic Ultrasound Pearls. In: Kupesic Plavsic S, (Ed). Color Doppler, 3D and 4D ultrasound in Obstetrics, Gynecology and Infertility. New Delhi: Jaypee Brothers Medical Publishers; 2011. pp. 256-348.
7. Kupesic Plavsic S. Normal Anatomy of the Female Pelvis. In: Stephenson S, Dmitrieva J, (Eds). Diagnostic Medical Sonography: Obstetrics and Gynecology, 4th edition. South Holland: Wolters Kluwer; 2018. pp. 75-126.
8. Lessey BA, Castelbaum AJ, Buck CA, et al. Further characterization of endometrial integrins during the menstrual cycle and in pregnancy. Fertil Steril. 1994;62(3):497-506.
9. Genbacev OD, Prakobphol A, Foulk RA, et al. Trophoblast L-selectin-mediated adhesion at the maternal-fetal interface. Science. 2003;299(5605):405-8.
10. Apparao KB, Murray MJ, Fritz MA, et al. Osteopontin and its receptor alphavbeta (3) integrin are coexpressed in the human endometrium during the menstrual cycle but regulated differentially. J Clin Endocrinol Metab. 2001;86(10):4991-5000.
11. Evans J, Salamonsen LA. Inflammation, leukocytes and menstruation. Rev Endocr Metab Disord. 2012;13(4):277-88.
12. Takano M, Lu Z, Goto T, et al. Transcriptional cross talk between the forkhead transcription factor forkhead box O1A and the progesterone receptor coordinates cell cycle regulation and differentiation in human endometrial stromal cells. Mol Endocrinol. 2007;21(10):2334-49.
13. Gellersen B, Brosens IA, Brosens JJ. Decidualization of the human endometrium: mechanisms, functions, and clinical perspectives. Semin Reprod Med. 2007;25(6):445-53.
14. Kurjak A, Kupesic-Urek S, Schulman H, et al. Transvaginal color Doppler in the assessment of ovarian and uterine perfusion in infertile women. Fertil Steril. 1991;56(5):870-3.
15. Kupesic S, Kurjak A. Uterine and ovarian perfusion during the periovulatory period assessed by transvaginal color Doppler. Fertil Steril. 1993;60(3):439-43.
16. Kupesic S, Kurjak A. The assessment of uterine and ovarian perfusion in infertile patients. Eur J Obstet Gynecol. 1997;71(2):151-4.
17. Kupesic S, Bekavac I, Bjelos D, et al. Assessment of endometrial receptivity by transvaginal color Doppler and three-dimensional power Doppler ultrasonography in patients undergoing in vitro fertilization procedures. J Ultrasound Med. 2001;20(2):125-34.
18. Kupesic S. Three-dimensional ultrasound in reproductive medicine. Ultrasound Rev Obstet Gynecol. 2005;5(4):304-15.
19. Kurjak A, Zodan T, Kupesic S. Three-dimensional sonoembryology of the first trimester. In: Kurjak A, Kupesic S (Eds). Clinical Application of 3-D Sonography. New York, London: Parthenon Publishing; 2000. pp. 109-21.
20. Kupesic S, Kurjak A. Diagnosis and treatment outcome of the septate uterus. Croat Med J. 1998;39(2):185-90.
21. Kupesic S, Kurjak A, Skenderovic S, et al. Screening for uterine abnormalities by three-dimensional ultrasound improves perinatal outcome. J Perinat Med. 2002;30(1):9-17.
22. Kupesic S, Kurjak A, Ujevic B. B-mode, color Doppler and three-dimensional ultrasound in the assessment of endometrial lesions. Ultrasound Rev Obstet Gynecol. 2001;1:50-71.
23. Kupesic Plavsic S. New Imaging Diagnostics. In: Simón CL, Giudice LC (Eds). The Endometrial Factor: A Reproductive Precision Medicine Approach. Florida: CRC Press; 2017. pp. 15-36.
24. Coughlan C, Ledger W, Wang Q, et al. Recurrent implantation failure: definition and management. Reprod Biomed Online. 2014;28(1):14-38.
25. Bosteels J, Weyers S, Puttemans P, et al. The effectiveness of hysteroscopy in improving pregnancy rates in subfertile women without other gynaecological symptoms: a systematic review. Hum Reprod Update. 2010;16(1):1-11.

26. Kupesic S, Kurjak A, Pasalic L, et al. The value of transvaginal color Doppler in the assessment of pelvic inflammatory disease. J Ultrasound Med Biol. 1995;21(6):733-8.
27. Bekavac I, Kupesic S, Kurjak A. Color Doppler in the assessment of patients with pelvic inflammatory disease. Gynaecol Perinatol. 2000;9(3):77-82.
28. Kupesic Plavsic S, Kurjak A, Baston K. Pelvic inflammatory disease. In: Kupesic Plavsic (Ed). Color Doppler, 3D and 4D ultrasound in Obstetrics, Gynecology and Infertility. New Delhi: Jaypee Brothers Medical Publishers;2011. pp. 89-95.
29. Zeyneloglu HB, Arici A, Olive DL. Adverse effects of hydrosalpinx on pregnancy rates after in vitro fertilization-embryo transfer. Fertil Steril. 1998;70(3):492-9.
30. Camus E, Poncelet C, Goffinet F, et al. Pregnancy rates after IVF in cases of tubal infertility with and without hydrosalpinx: meta-analysis of published comparative studies. Hum Reprod. 1999;14(5):1243-9.
31. Mukherjee T, Copperman AB, McCaffrey C, et al. Hydrosalpinx fluid has embryotoxic effects on murine embryogenesis: a case for prophylactic salpingectomy. Fertil Steril. 1996;66(5):851-3.
32. Granot I, Dekel N, Segal I, et al. Is hydrosalpinx fluid cytotoxic? Hum Reprod. 1998;13(6):1620-4.
33. Sharara FI. The role of hydrosalpinx in IVF: simply mechanical? Hum Reprod. 1999;14(3):577-8.
34. Aboulghar MA, Mansour RT, Serour GI. Controversies in the modern management of hydrosalpinx. Hum Reprod Update. 1998;4(6):882-90.
35. Strandell A, Lindhard A, Waldenstrom U, et al. Hydrosalpinx and IVF outcome: a prospective, randomized multicenter trial in Scandinavia on salpingectomy prior to IVF. Hum Reprod. 1999;14(11):2762-9.
36. Strandell A. The influence of hydrosalpinx on IVF and embryo transfer: a review. Hum Reprod Update. 2000;6(4):387-95.
37. Polisseni F, Bambirra EA, Camargos AF. Detection of chronic endometritis by diagnostic hysteroscopy in asymptomatic infertile patients. Gynecol Obstet Invest. 2003;55(4):205-10.
38. Kiaya K, Yasuo T. Immunohistochemistrical and clinicopathological characterization of chronic endometritis. Am J Reprod Immunol. 2011;66(5):410-5.
39. Romero R, Espinoza J, Mazor M. Can endometrial infection/inflammation explain implantation failure, spontaneous abortion, and preterm birth after in vitro fertilization? Fertil Steril. 2004;82(4):799-804.
40. Zolghadri J, Momtahan M, Aminian K, et al. The value of hysteroscopy in diagnosis of chronic endometritis in patients with unexplained recurrent spontaneous abortion. Eur J Obstet Gynecol Reprod Biol. 2011;155(2):217-20.
41. Boomsma CM, Kavelaars A, Eijkemans MJ, et al. Endometrial secretion analysis identifies a cytokine profile predictive of pregnancy in IVF. Hum Reprod. 2009;24(6):427-35.
42. Bouet PE, El Hachem H, Monceau E, et al. Chronic endometritis in women with recurrent pregnancy loss and recurrent implantation failure: prevalence and role of office hysteroscopy and immunohistochemistry in diagnosis. Fertil Steril. 2016;105(1):106-10.
43. Fèghali J, Bakar J, Mayenga JM, et al. Systematic hysteroscopy prior to in vitro fertilization. Gynecol Obstet Fertil. 2003;31(2):127-31.
44. Haggerty CL, Totten PA, Astete SG, et al. Mycoplasma Genitalium among women with nongonococcal, nonchlamydial pelvic inflammatory disease. Infect Dis Obstet Gynecol. 2006;2006:30184.
45. Espinoza J, Erez O, Romero R. Preconceptional antibiotic treatment to prevent preterm birth in women with a previous preterm delivery. Am J Obstet Gynecol. 2006;194(3):630-7.
46. Cicinelli E, Matteo M, Tinelli R, et al. Prevalence of chronic endometritis in repeated unexplained implantation failure and the IVF success rate after antibiotic therapy. Hum Reprod. 2015;30(2):323-30.
47. Campo S, Campo V, Benagiano G. Adenomyosis and Infertility. Reprod Biomed Online. 2012;24(1):35-46.
48. Arya, S, Kupesic Plavsic S. Sonographic features of adenomyosis. Donald School J Ultrasound Obstet Gynecol. 2017;11(1):76-81.
49. Exacoustos C, Brienza L, Di Giovanni A, et al. Adenomyosis: three-dimensional sonographic findings of the junctional zone and correlation with histology. Ultrasound Obstet Gynecol. 2011;37(4):471-9.
50. Chiang CH, Chang MY, Shiau CS, et al. Effect of sonographically diffusely enlarged uterus without distinct uterine masses on the outcome of in vitro fertilization—embryo transfer. J Assist Reprod Genet. 1999;16(7):369-72.
51. Thaluri V, Tremellen KP. Ultrasound diagnosed adenomyosis has a negative impact on successful implantation following GnRH antagonist IVF treatment. Hum Reprod. 2012;27(12):3487-92.
52. Maubon A, Faury A, Kapella M, et al. Uterine junctional zone at magnetic resonance imaging: a predictor of in vitro fertilization implantation failure. J Obstet Gynaecol Res. 2010;36(3):611-8.
53. Juang CM, Chou P, Yen MS, et al. Adenomyosis and risk of preterm delivery. Br J Obstet Gynaecol. 2007;114(2):165-9.
54. Dor J, Itzkowic DJ, Mashiach S, et al. Cumulative conception rates following gonadotropin therapy. Am J Obstet Gynecol. 1980;136(1):102-5.
55. Cermik D, Selam B, Taylor HS. Regulation of HOXA-10 expression by testosterone in vitro and in the endometrium of patients with polycystic ovary syndrome. J Clin Endocrinol Metab. 2003;88(1):238-43.
56. Zhang G, Li X, Zhang L, et al. The expression and role of hybrid insulin/insulin-like growth factor receptor type 1 in endometrial carcinoma cells. Cancer Genet Cytogenet. 2010;200(2):140-8.
57. Savaris RF, Groll JM, Young SL, et al. Progesterone resistance in PCOS endometrium: A microarray analysis in clomiphene citrate-treated and artificial menstrual cycles. J Clin Endocrinol Metab. 2011;96(6):1737-46.
58. Burney RO, Talbi S, Hamilton AE, et al. Gene expression analysis of endometrium reveals progesterone resistance and candidate susceptibility genes in women with endometriosis. Endocrinology. 2007;148(8):3814-26.

59. Gregory CW, Wilson EM, Apparao KB, et al. Steroid receptor coactivator expression throughout the menstrual cycle in normal and abnormal endometrium. J Clin Endocrinol Metab. 2002;87(6):2960-6.
60. Negro R, Schwartz A, Gismondi R, et al. Increased pregnancy loss rate in thyroid antibody negative women with TSH levels between 2.5 and 5.0 in the first trimester of pregnancy. J Clin Endocrinol Metab. 2010;95(9):E44-8.
61. Scoccia B, Demir H, Kang Y, et al. In vitro fertilization pregnancy rates in levothyroxine-treated women with hypothyroidism compared to women without thyroid dysfunction disorders. Thyroid. 2012;22(6):631-6.
62. Fumarola A, Grani G, Romanzi D, et al. Thyroid function in infertile patients undergoing assisted reproduction. Am J Reprod Immunol. 2013;70(4):336-41.
63. Velkeniers B, Van Meerhaeghe A, Poppe K, et al. Levothyroxine treatment and pregnancy outcome in women with subclinical hypothyroidism undergoing assisted reproduction technologies: systematic review and meta-analysis of RCTs. Hum Reprod Update. 2013;19(3):251-8.
64. Mendes MC, Ferriani RA, Sala MM, et al. Effect of transitory hyperprolactinemia on in vitro fertilization of human oocytes. J Reprod Med. 2001;46(5):444-50.
65. Gonen Y, Casper RF. Does transient hyperprolactinemia during ovarian hyperstimulation interfere with conception or pregnancy outcome? Fertil Steril. 1989;51(6):1007-10.
66. Bellver J, Pellicer A, Garcia-Velasco JA, et al. Obesity reduces uterine receptivity: clinical experience from 9,587 first cycles of ovum donation with normal weight donors. Fertil Steril. 2013;100(4):1050-8.
67. Kupesic S, Kurjak A, Vujisic S, et al. Luteal phase defect: comparison between Doppler velocimetry, histologic and hormonal markers. J Ultrasound Obstet Gynecol. 1997;9:105-12.
68. Kupesic S, Kurjak A. The assessment of normal and abnormal luteal function by transvaginal color Doppler sonography. Eur J Obstet Gynecol. 1997;72(1):83-7.
69. Ng EH, Chan CC, Tang OS, et al. The role of endometrial and subendometrial blood flows measured by three-dimensional power Doppler ultrasound in the prediction of pregnancy during IVF treatment. Hum Reprod. 2006;21(1): 164-70.
70. Wu HM, Chiang CH, Huang HY, et al. Detection of the subendometrial vascularisation flow index by three-dimensional ultrasound may be useful for predicting the pregnancy rate for patients undergoing in vitro fertilization-embryo transfer. Fertil Steril. 2003;79(3):507-11.
71. Ng EH, Chan CC, Tang OS, et al. Relationship between uterine blood flow and endometrial and subendometrial blood flows during stimulated and natural cycles. Fertil Steril. 2006;85(3):721-7.
72. Arya S, Kupesic Plavsic S. Preimplantation 3D ultrasound: current uses and challenges. J Perinat Med. 2017;45(6):745-58.
73. Mahajan N. Endometrial receptivity array: Clinical Application. J Hum Reprod Sci. 2015;8(3):121-9.
74. Fatemi HM, Popovic-Todorovic B. Implantation in assisted reproduction: a look at endometrial receptivity. Reprod Biomed Online. 2013; 27(5):530-8.
75. Horcajadas JA, Pellicer A, Simón C. Wide genomic analysis of human endometrial receptivity: New times, new opportunities. Hum Reprod Update. 2007;13(1):77-8.
76. Garrido-Gómez T, Ruiz-Alonso M, Blesa D, et al. Profiling the gene signature of endometrial receptivity: Clinical results. Fertil Steril. 2013;99(4):1078-85.
77. Díaz-Gimen P, Ruiz-Alonso M, Sebastian-Leon P, et al. Window of Implantation Transcriptomic Stratification Reveals Different Endometrial Subsignatures Associated With Live Birth and Biochemical Pregnancy. Fertil Steril. 2017;108(4):703-10.
78. Hashimoto T, Koizumi M, Doshida M, et al. Efficacy of the endometrial receptivity array for repeated implantation failure in Japan: A retrospective, two-centers study. Reprod Med Biol. 2017;16(3):290-6.
79. Tan J, Kan A, Hitkari J, et al. The role of the endometrial receptivity array (ERA) in patients who have failed euploid embryo transfers. J Assist Reprod Genet. 2018;35(4):683-92.
80. van der Linden M, Buckingham K, Farquhar C, et al. Luteal phase support for assisted reproduction cycles. Cochrane Database Syst Rev. 2011;5(10):CD009154.
81. Hannan NJ, Nie G, Rainzcuk A, et al. Uterine lavage or aspirate: which view of the intrauterine environment? Reprod Sci. 2012; 19(10):1125-32.
82. Boomsma CM, Kavelaars A, Eijkemans MJ, et al. Cytokine profiling in endometrial secretions: a non-invasive window on endometrial receptivity. Reprod Biomed Online. 2009;18(1):85-94.
83. Hannan NJ, Stoikos CJ, Stephens AN, et al. Depletion of high-abundance serum proteins from human uterine lavages enhances detection of lower-abundance proteins. J Proteome Res. 2009;8(2):1099-103.
84. Casado-Vela J, Rodriguez-Suarez E, Iloro I, et al. Comprehensive proteomic analysis of human endometrial fluid aspirate. J Proteome Res. 2009;8(10):4622-32.
85. Scotchie JG, Fritz MA, Mocanu M, et al. Proteomic analysis of the luteal endometrial secretome. Reprod Sci. 2009;16(9):883-93.
86. Hannan NJ, Stephens AN, Rainczuk A, et al. 2D-DiGE analysis of the human endometrial secretome reveals differences between receptive and nonreceptive states in fertile and infertile women. J Proteome Res. 2010;9(12):6256-64.
87. Cakmak H, Taylor HS. Implantation failure: molecular mechanisms and clinical treatment. Hum Reprod Update. 2011;17(2):242-53.
88. Cheong Y, Boomsma C, Heijnen C, et al. Uterine secretomics: A window on the maternal-embryo interface. Fertil Steril. 2013; 99(4):1093-99.

CHAPTER 11

Ultrasonographic Evaluation of Embryonic Cardiac Development

Gwang Jun Kim

INTRODUCTION

The heart is the first functional organ in human embryo, and starts to beat by 4 weeks of development.[1]

At around 18–19 days after fertilization [4 weeks 4 days to 4 weeks 5 days of gestational age (GA)], the heart begins to form. This process begins with the formation of two cardiac tubes that merge to form the single tubular heart. The single cardiac tube shows five distinctive serial regions: from tail to head, these are the sinus venosus, primitive atrium, primitive ventricle, bulbus cordis and the truncus arteriosus (Fig. 11.1). Simultaneously, the cardiac tube begins looping within pericardial cavity. The sinus venosus is final collecting point of fetal venous circulation and develops into the posterior part of the right atrium, the sinoatrial node and the coronary sinus.[2]

The primitive atrium develops into two separate atria. The primitive ventricle develops primarily into the left ventricle (LV) and the bulbus cordis forms part of the right ventricle. Septa form within the atria and ventricles to separate the left and right sides of the heart.[2]

The embryologic truncus arteriosus develops into the paired arterial trunks; the ascending aorta and pulmonary artery.[3,4]

Over the last decade, good quality of serial histological sections[4] and scaled reproductions of human embryos has been reported.[5]

On imaging, Preeta D et al. showed human cardiac developmental process using high-resolution magnetic resonance imaging (MRI) and episcopic fluorescence imaging.[6]

Recently, progressive advances in medical ultrasonography, especially high frequency transvaginal ultrasonography and the color Doppler equipment allow access to the developing embryonic human heart.

Embryo crown-rump length (CRL) at 2 mm shows a discernible heartbeat. At this time, the embryonic heart is in the cardiac tube stage. Embryo CRL at 5 mm shows distinct differential movements of the ventricles and atria (13th Carnegie stage, 6[4] gestational weeks). At 7th gestational weeks, an interventricular septum can be visualized in the embryonic heart. Although a heartbeat can be detected and gross cardiac structures are visualized early in gestation, visualization of some embryologically important intracardiac structures, such as the endocardial cushion, atrioventricular (AV) foramen, or AV valves are still limited, even with the latest high-end equipment.

Cineloop function and color Doppler provide some valuable information about morphology and function of the developing embryonic heart.

In scanning human embryo, safety issues should be kept in mind. Examination time should be kept as short as possible. Output levels should be kept as low as is reasonably achievable. Thermal and mechanical effects can be produced by diagnostic ultrasound. Mechanical effects have been demonstrated in tissues containing gas. However, the fetus does not produce or retain gas and mechanical effects are not a concern.

For the human embryo, a temperature elevation more than 1.5°C can be hazardous. Under temperature index (TI) less than 1.0, temperature elevation in soft tissue (such as an embryo) caused by ultrasonographic examination with a usual mode (2D, 3D) does not

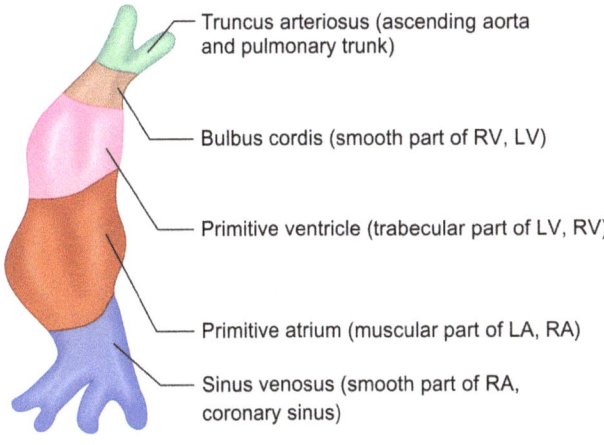

Fig. 11.1: Tubular heart.

increase by more than 1.5°C. However, narrow color box examination and concentrated pulsed-wave Doppler can cause temperature elevation more than 1.5°C during a long examination time. For the evaluation of embryonic heart using ultrasonography, keep the principle of "as low as reasonably achievable (ALARA)" and the least use of color Doppler and pulsed Doppler should be applied in a short period of the examination time.

CARNEGIE STAGE 9 (19–21 DAYS OF CONCEPTION, 5 GESTATIONAL WEEKS), CRL 2 MM

Morphologic Changes

- Paired endocardial tube
- The heart begins to develop near the head of the embryo (cardiogenic region)
- The heart starts to beat and pump blood at around day 21 or 22.

Ultrasonographic Findings

The length of embryo (green) is measured 2.2 mm. The heart is a paired tube form (Fig. 11.2A). Heartbeat can be detected in an embryo measuring more than over 2 mm. At this stage, the yolk sac (yellow ring) is much larger than the tiny embryo (green ring). The red dot is beating cardiac tube (Figs. 11.2B and C).

CARNEGIE STAGE 10 (22–23 DAYS OF CONCEPTION, 5 WEEKS 1–3 DAYS OF GESTATION), CRL 2.5 MM

Morphologic Changes

- Single primitive cardiac tube
- The two endocardial tubes descend into the thoracic cavity, where they begin to fuse into a single primitive cardiac tube. Cardiac tube fusion is complete at about 22 days
- The cardiac tube continues stretching and by day 23, cardiac looping begins.

Ultrasonographic Findings

The heart structure appears as a single beating echogenic dot.

CARNEGIE STAGE 11–12 (23–26 DAYS OF CONCEPTION, 5 WEEKS 2–5 DAYS OF GESTATION), CRL 3–3.5 MM

Morphologic Changes

- Looping cardiac tube
- Cardiac tube looping is occurring inside the pericardial sac
- Neural crest cells migrate from rhombomere 6, 7 to pharyngeal arch 3.

Ultrasonographic Findings

In this ultrasound image, CRL is 3 mm and the heartbeat is more evident. Inside of the beating cardiac tube, more echogenic thick region and a less echogenic thin region can be differentiated (Figs. 11.3A to C). The more echogenic region is presumably a primitive ventricle. At this stage, the heartbeat occurs simultaneously in the entire cardiac tube. Yellow ring is the yolk sac. Pink dot is looping cardiac tube.

CARNEGIE STAGE 13 (28 DAYS OF CONCEPTION, 6 WEEKS OF GESTATION), (9.5 DAYS OF RAT EMBRYO), CRL 4.5 MM

Morphologic Changes

- Primitive ventricles and primitive atria
- Interventricular, interatrial septation budding

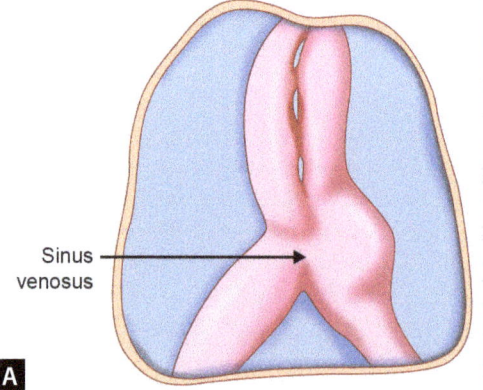
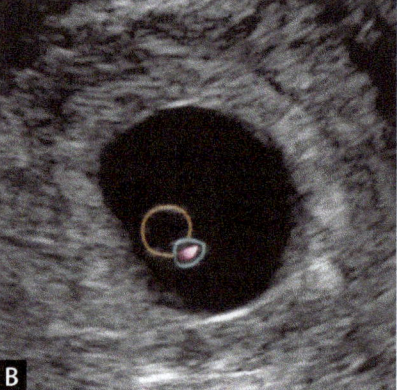
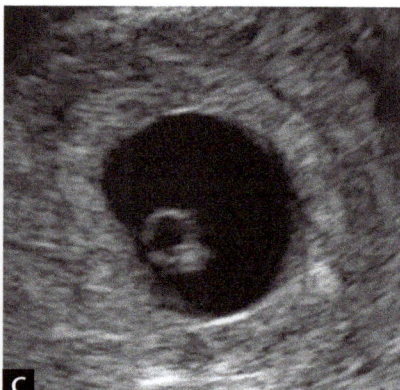

Figs. 11.2A to C: Ultrasonographic findings of Carnegie stage 9.

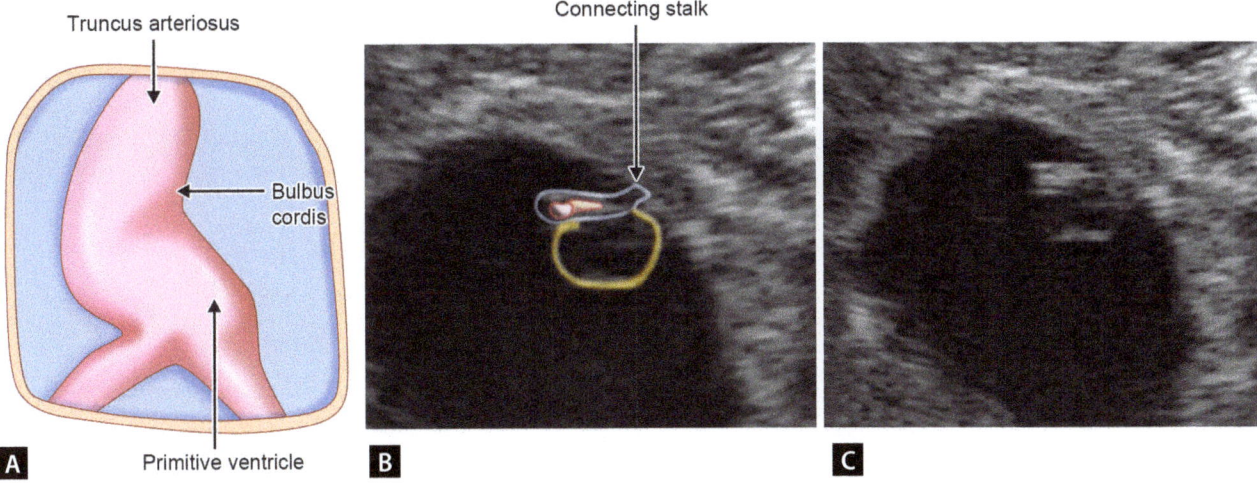

Figs. 11.3A to C: Ultrasonographic findings of Carnegie stage 11-12.

- Interventricular foramen
- Single undivided truncus arteriosus.

Primitive ventricles and primitive atria are discernible. Interventricular, interatrial septation starts. A common AV canal is present. The interventricular foramen is present. Truncus arteriosus is a single undivided state.

Ultrasonographic Findings

In this ultrasound image (Figs. 11.4A to C), CRL is 3 mm. The heart occupies nearly the whole thorax and protrudes ventrally. Primitive ventricles (ventral thick region, pink colored) and primitive atria (dorsal thin region, yellow colored) are now discernible and cardiac contractions are divided into systolic and diastolic. Atrial size is larger than ventricular size. Pericardial effusion can be detected.

Due to trabeculation of the wall, the ventricle appears hyperechogenic and thicker than the atria (Figs. 11.4C and D).

CARNEGIE STAGE 14 (32 DAYS OF CONCEPTION, 6 WEEKS 4 DAYS OF GESTATION), 10 DAYS OF RAT EMBRYO, CRL 6 MM

Morphologic Changes

- Primitive endocardial cushion
- Atrial spine
- Septum primum
- Atrioventricular canal.

At the end of the 6 weeks of gestation, primitive endocardial cushions appear.

Histologically the atrial spine is observed at this stage and fuses with the inferior AV cushion. The septum primum can be observed at the end of 6th weeks of gestation. Later, the septum secundum develops as an infolding of the dorsal wall of the right atrium.[6]

Large endocardial cushions seen prominently at the center of the cardiac loop.

The AV canal is divided by the endocardial cushions.[6]

CARNEGIE STAGE 15 (36 DAYS OF CONCEPTION, 7 WEEKS 1 DAY OF GESTATION), 11.5 DAYS OF RAT EMBRYO, CRL 8 MM

Morphologic Changes

- Large atria compare to ventricles
- Left ventricle is larger and thicker than right ventricle
- Ostium primum
- Apposing AV endocardial cushion
- Truncal cushion.

The atria are relatively large compared to the ventricles. Both right and left atria communicate through the ostium primum. The left ventricle is larger and thicker than the right. The AV endocardial cushions are apposing.[5] The main cardiac walls are formed between day 27 and day 37. Truncal cushions are observed in the form of swellings.[6]

Ultrasonographic Findings

Ventricles and atria are clearly differentiated on ultrasonography (Figs. 11.5A to F). The heart appears as a mass protruding from the embryo. Left and right ventricles can be divided by an incomplete interventricular septum. Left ventricle shows a thicker and brighter echo due to prominent ventricular wall trabeculations (upper chamber

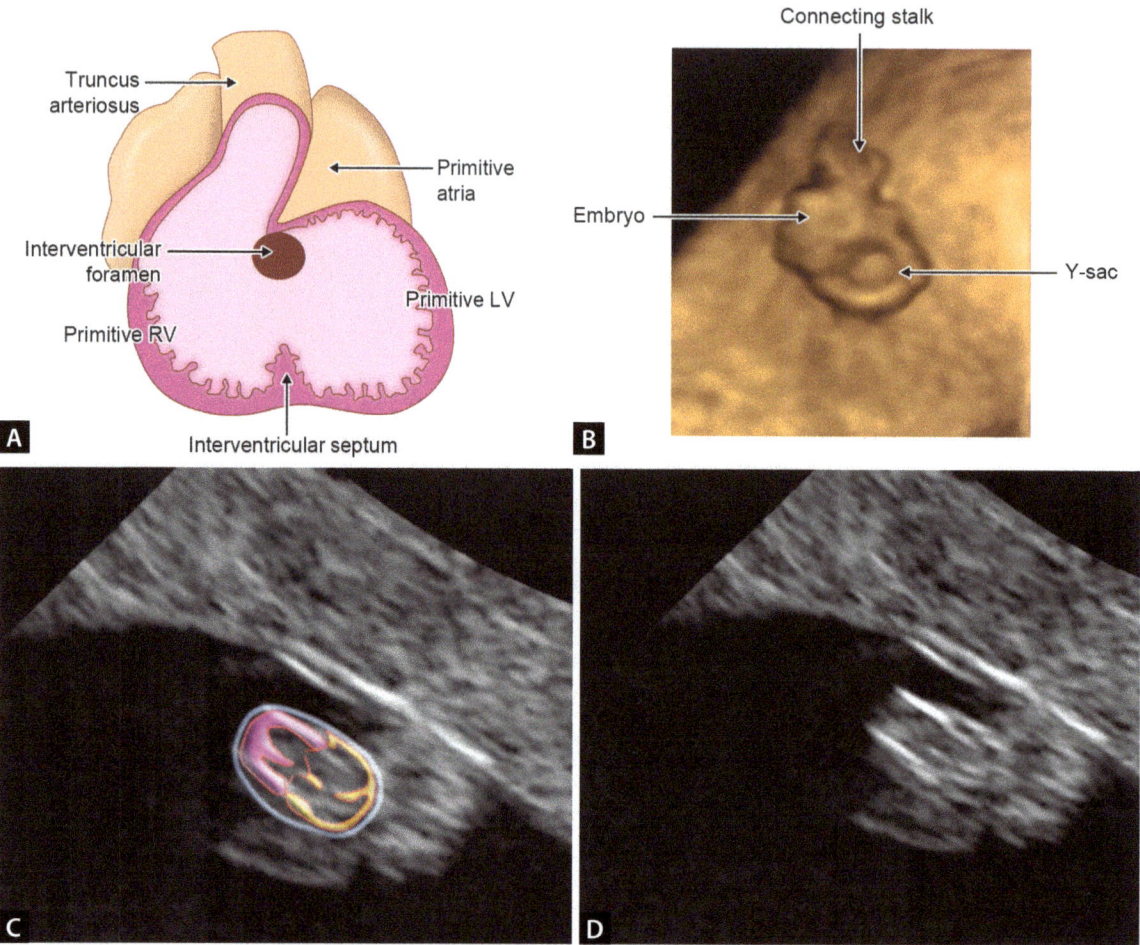

Figs. 11.4A to D: Ultrasonographic findings of Carnegie stage 13.

on Figs. 11.5D and F, long red arrow). Endocardial cushion is located in the center of the heart (short yellow arrow).

CARNEGIE STAGE 16 (40 DAYS OF CONCEPTION, 7 WEEKS 6 DAYS OF GESTATION), CRL 10 MM

Morphologic Changes

- Separate right and left AV canals
- Complete atrial septum primum
- Vena cava valve
- Interventricular foramen
- Three layered cardiac wall.

Atrioventricular endocardial cushions separate the right and left AV canals. Atrial septum primum is complete. The right horn of the venous sinus is incorporated into the right atrial wall and the venous valves are emerging.[5]

The lower part of the ventricular myocardium develops into a trabecular tissue.[5] Interventricular foramen persists. Atrial contraction time is shorter than ventricular contraction time.

The cardiac wall presents three layers: endocardium, myocardium and epicardium.[5] Early outflow septation begins.

Ultrasonographic Findings

Crown-rump length of the embryo is 10 mm. Ventricles and atria are readily differentiated. Ventricles are becoming hyperechoic and thicker as trabeculations of ventricular wall evolve. Interventricular septum is detected, but interventricular foramen is not evident on ultrasonography. Long red arrow indicates umbilical cord and short yellow arrow indicates allantoic cyst (Figs. 11.6A to D).

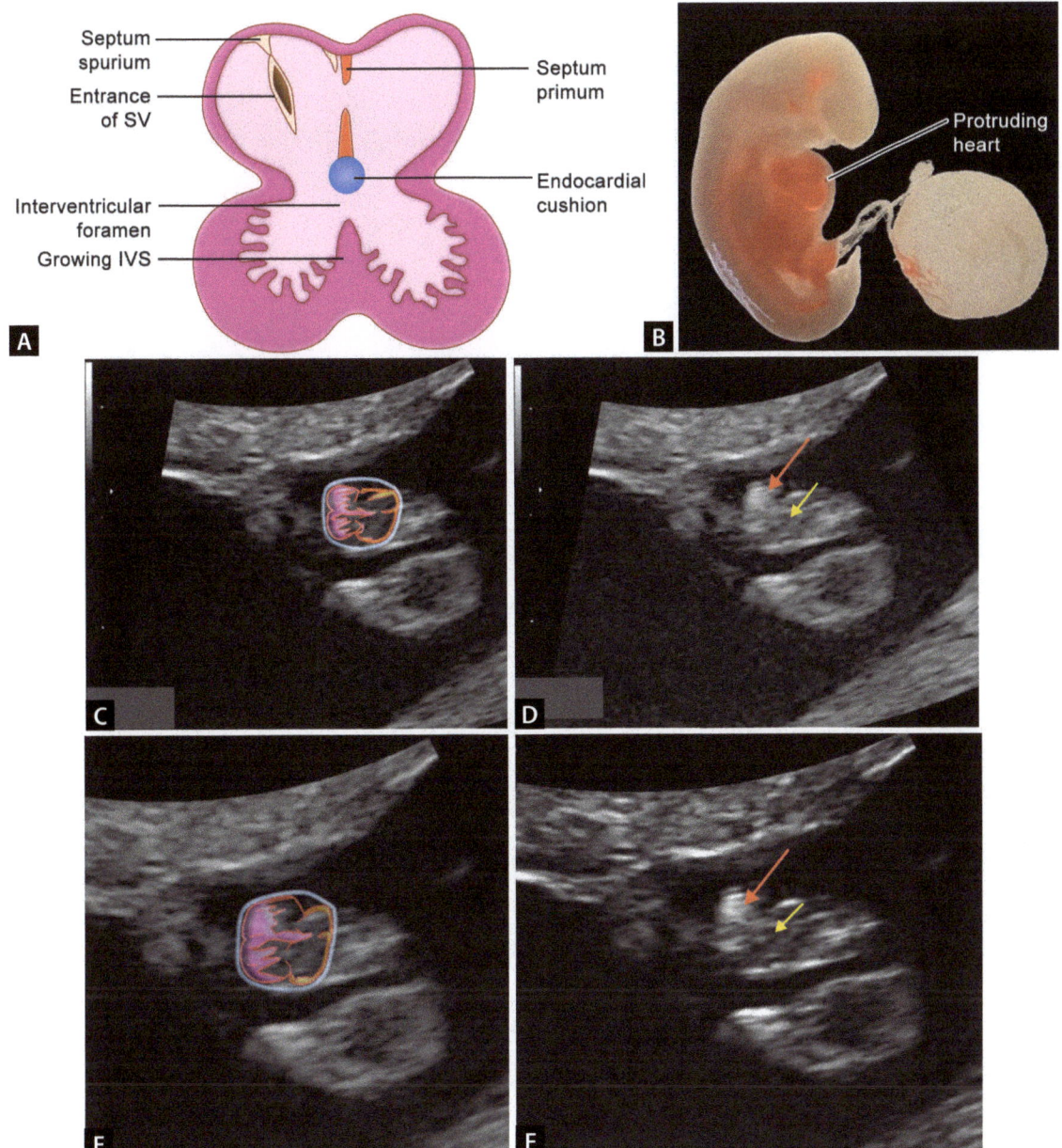

Fig. 11.5A to F: (A) Sinus venosus (SV); (B) Embryo (same developmental stage); (C and D) Systolic phase; (E and F) Diastolic phase.

CARNEGIE STAGE 17 (42 DAYS OF CONCEPTION, 8 WEEKS OF GESTATION) 12.5 DAYS IN THE RAT EMBRYO, CRL 11 MM

Morphologic Changes

- Ostium primum closed
- Separate AV canals
- Interventricular foramen
- Separation of truncus arteriosus.

Ostium primum has been completely closed by the septum primum. The septum secundum starts to appear.[5] The AV canals are completely separated.

Atrioventricular junction is developing, but interventricular foramen exists.

Truncus arteriosus is undergoing septation into aorta and pulmonary artery, starting distally and extends proximally.[2,7]

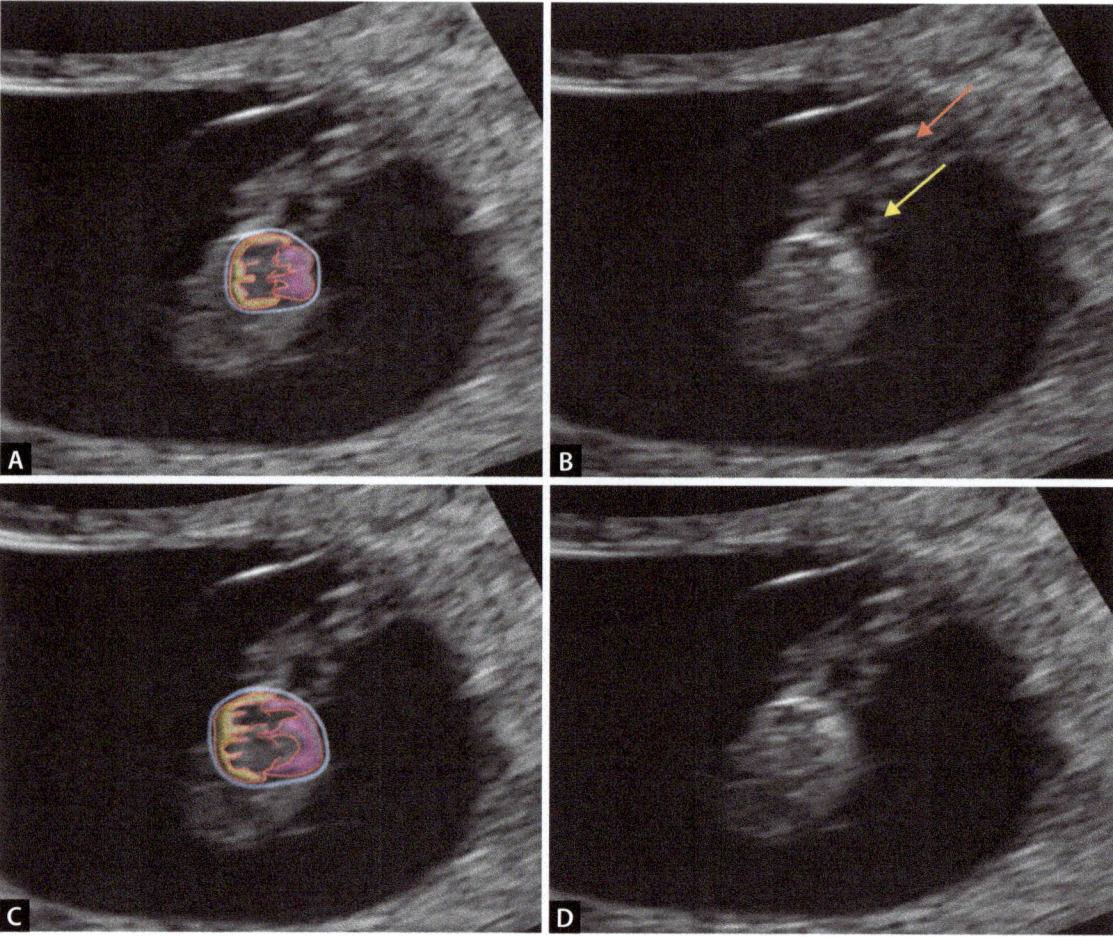

Figs. 11.6A to D: (A and B) Systolic phase; (C and D) Diastolic phase.

CARNEGIE STAGE 18 (44 DAYS OF CONCEPTION, 8 WEEKS 2 DAYS OF GESTATION), 13 DAYS IN THE RAT EMBRYO, CRL 13 MM

Morphologic Changes

- Complete muscular interventricular septum
- Ostium primum closed
- Endocardial cushion fusion
- Developing AV valves, semilunar valves.

The interventricular septum is complete, but the interventricular foramen is still present.[5] Completion of muscular interventricular septum growth, but inlet ventricular septum is incomplete. Ostium primum is closed as septum primum attaches to superior endocardial cushion.[5]

The tricuspid and mitral valves appear as small rounded prominence of reticular gelatinous tissue. The semilunar valves are distinguishable on histologic section.[5]

Now, the heart is four chambered organ.

Ultrasonographic Findings (Figs. 11.7A to E)

Embryo length is 13 mm. Atrial size is larger than that of the ventricle. Small thick echogenic ventricles contracting on Figure 11.6B. Valve movements are not evident on ultrasonography.

CARNEGIE STAGE 19–21 (48–52 DAYS OF CONCEPTION, 8 WEEKS 2–5 DAYS OF GESTATION) 13.5 ED IN THE RAT EMBRYO, CRL 16–23 MM

Morphologic Changes

- Complete interventricular septum
- Interventricular foramen closed
- Separate outflow tract (aorta and pulmonary trunk).

Membranous and inlet portion of interventricular septum are complete and the interventricular foramen is closed.[5]

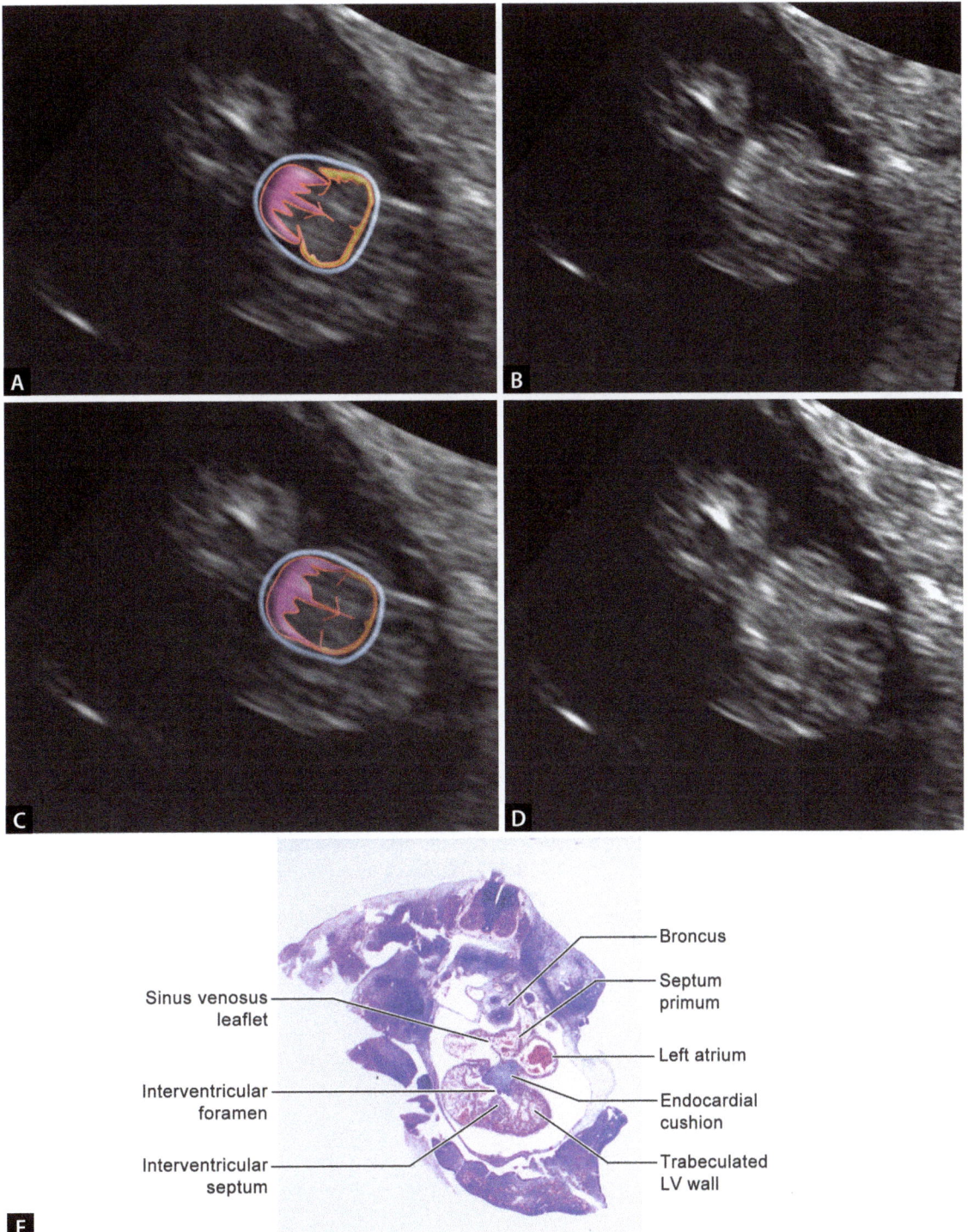

Figs. 11.7A to E: (A and B) Systolic phase; (C and D) Diastolic phase; (E) Histologic section from rat embryo of same developmental stage (13 ED of rat).
(ED: embryonic day means postconception day).

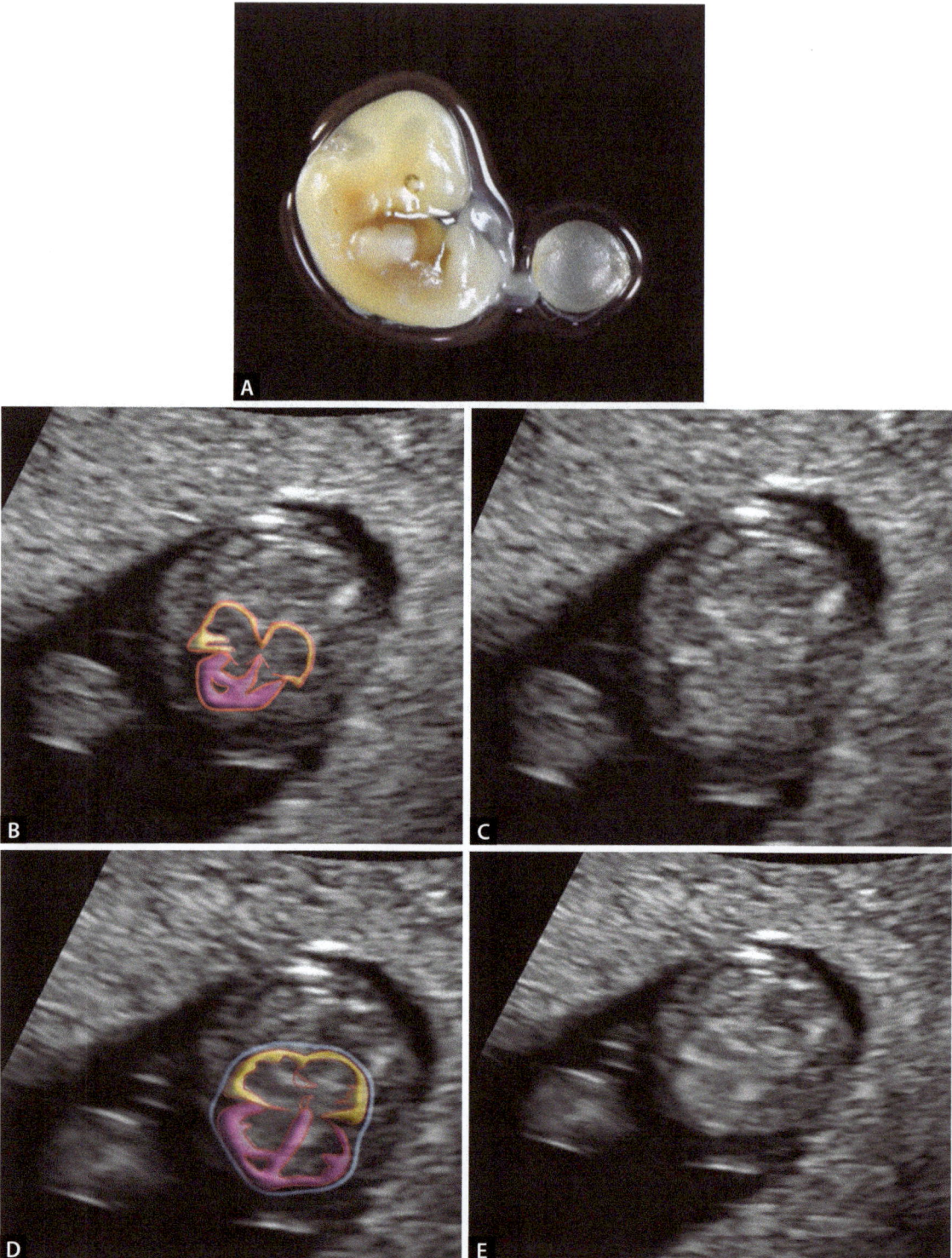

Figs. 11.8A to E: (A) Embryo (CRL 20 mm); (B and C) Systolic phase; (D and E) Diastolic phase.

At the end of 8 weeks of gestation, separate aortic and pulmonary outflows were observed.[8]

Ultrasonographic Findings

Ultrasonographic images of CRL 19 mm embryo are shown in Figures 11.8A to E. Atria and ventricles are more readily discernible and four heart chambers are differentiated.

The CRL of this embryo is 22 mm (Figs. 11.9A and B). Blue flow indicates right ventricular outflow (pulmonary artery flow) (Fig. 11.9C). Diastolic and systolic flows are clearly detected with the color Doppler ultrasound (Fig. 11.9D).

CARNEGIE STAGE 22 (54 DAYS OF CONCEPTION, 9 WEEKS 1 DAY OF GESTATION), 14.5 ED IN THE RAT EMBRYO, CRL 26 MM

Morphologic Changes

- Complete interventricular septum
- Foramen ovale

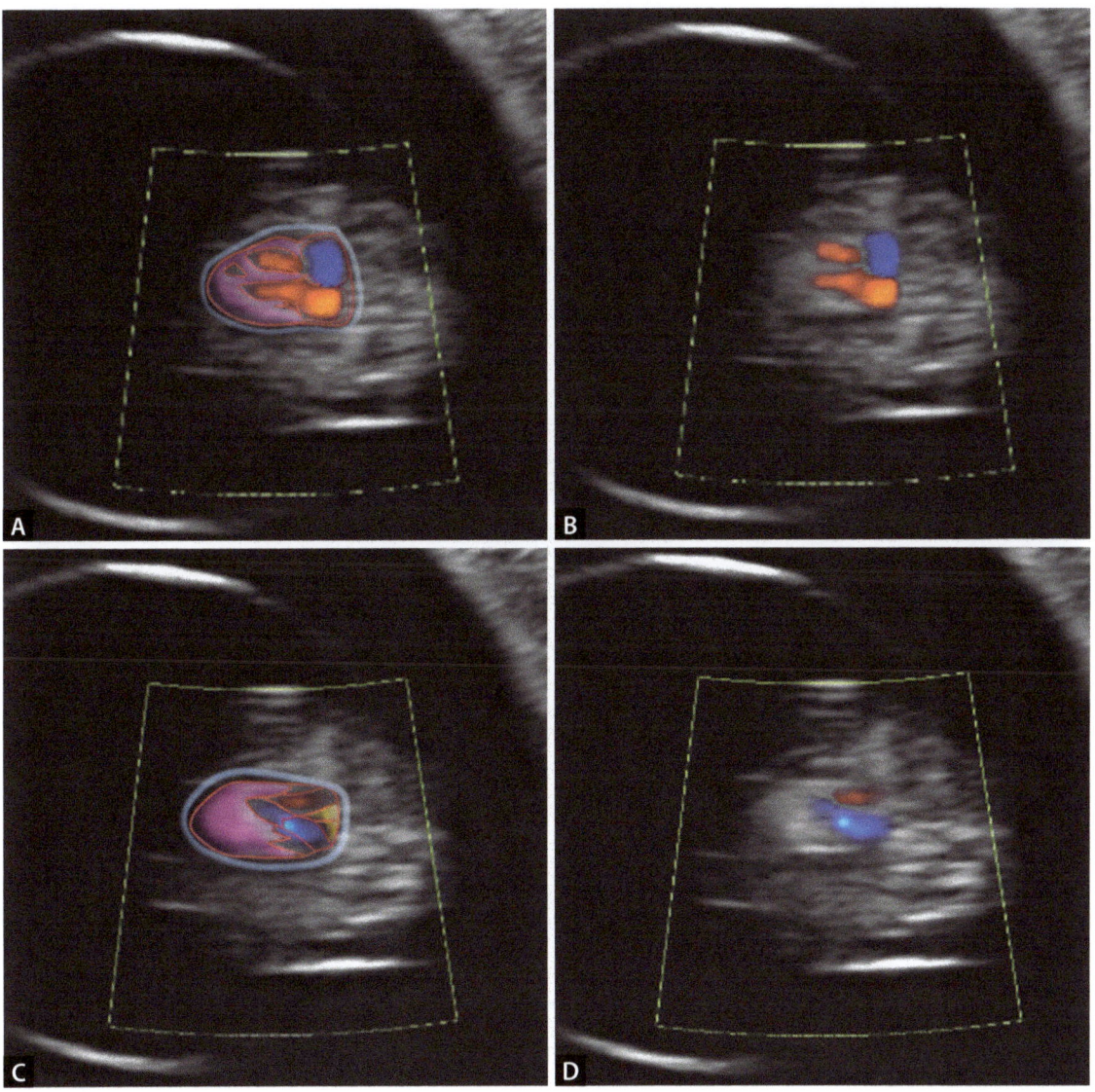

Figs. 11.9A and D: (A and B) Four chamber plane (diastolic phase); (C and D) Four chamber plane (systolic phase).

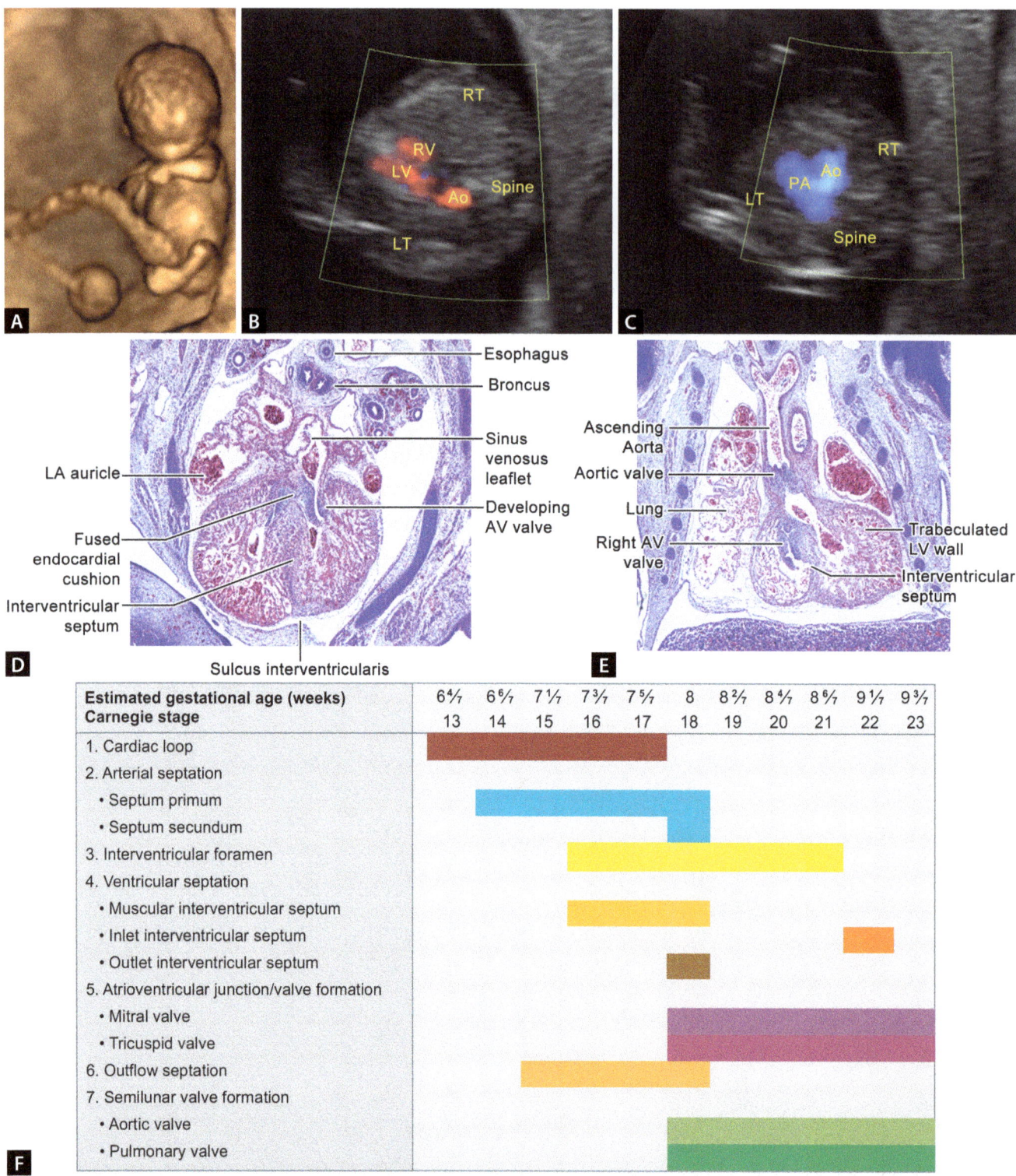

Figs. 11.10A to F: (A) Image of the same embryonic stage; (B) Four chambered heart; (C) Three vessel view (diastolic phase); (D) Histologic section from rat embryo of the same developmental stage (14 ED of rat); (E) Histologic section from rat embryo of same developmental stage (14 ED of rat); (F) Development time course of human cardiac morphogenesis.
Source: Redrawn from the Preeta D, Elaine L, Anita K, et al. A high-resolution magnetic resonance imaging and episcopic fluorescence image capture atlas. Circulation. 2009;120:343-51.

- Coronary circulation
- All definite major cardiac structure identified
- The inlet and membranous portions of the ventricular septum fully closed[6]
- Foramen ovale communicates the two atrial cavities[5]
- Coronary arteries with their main branches can be identified on histologic slides.[5]

Ultrasonographic Findings

The ultrasonographic findings of Carnegie stage 22 are shown in Figures 11.10A to F.

REFERENCES

1. Moorman A, Webb S, Brown NA, et al. Development of the heart: (1) formation of the cardiac chambers and arterial trunks. Heart. 2003;89(7):806-14.
2. Anderson RH, Webb S, Brown NA, et al. Development of the heart: formation of the ventricular outflow tracts, arterial valves, and intrapericardial arterial trunks. Heart. 2003;89(9):1110-8.
3. Orts-Llorca F, Puerta Fonolla J, Sobrdo J. The formation, septation and fate of the truncus arteriosus in man. J Anat. 1982;134(Pt 1):41-56.
4. Krishnan A, Samtani R, Dhanantwari P, et al. A detailed comparison of mouse and human cardiac development. Pediatr Res. 2014;76(6):500-7.
5. Arraez-Aybar LA, Turrero-Nogues A, Marantos-Gamarra DG. Embryonic cardiac morphometry in Carnegie stages 15-23, from the Complutense university of Madrid Institute of Embryology Human Embryo Collection. Cells Tissues Organs. 2008;187(3):211-20.
6. Preeta D, Elaine L, Anita K, et al. A high-resolution magnetic resonance imaging and episcopic fluorescence image capture atlas. Circulation. 2009;120:343-51.
7. Streeter GL. Developmental horizons in human embryos: description of age group XV, XVI, XVII, and XVIII, being the third issue of a survey of the Carnegie collection. Contrib Embryol. 1948;32:133-203.
8. Grant RP. The embryology of ventricular flow pathways in man. Circulation. 1962;25:756-79.

CHAPTER 12

Preimplantation Genetic Diagnosis

Elitza Markova-Car, Krešimir Pavelić

INTRODUCTION

Preimplantation genetic diagnosis (PGD) or preimplantation genetic screening (PGS) is a very early form of prenatal diagnosis that allows embryos to be tested for genetic disorders before pregnancy has begun.[1] The rationale behind the method lies in the removal of cells from early embryos and a genetic analysis of these cells before being transferred to the uterus. The procedure offers an advantage for couples with genetic disorders whose offspring has an increased risk of a specific genetic condition by helping in the delivery of a healthy baby or the prevention of repeated spontaneous abortions.[2] As a result, PGS has developed as a valuable tool for enhancing pregnancy success with assisted reproductive technologies.[3] In fact, PGD may possibly be offered for any disorder for which the molecular testing can be performed.

BIOPSY TECHNIQUES

The diagnostic material for PGD is generally collected at three different stages of embryo development. These include first and second polar body biopsy, blastomere biopsy at cleavage stage, and trophectoderm (TE) tissue biopsy at blastocyst stage.[2] Each of these approaches has some advantages and limitations.[1] For example, biopsies of the first and second polar bodies nowadays are not common practice as only a maternally-inherited disease can be analyzed, and the obtained genetic material is small, which increase possibilities of amplification errors in polymerase chain reaction (PCR) experiments, contaminations, and allele dropout (ADO) during the PCR. However, polar body biopsy has no or minimum risk effect on embryo development and the lack of mosaicism.[2,4] Cleavage stage embryo biopsy, whereby 1 or 2 blastomeres are removed from a 6- to 8-cell embryo, retains some advantages over polar body biopsy as maternally- and paternally-inherited disorders can be diagnosed. Nevertheless, disadvantages, such as a small amount of the genetic material, remain and the high risk of mosaicism exists, which appears to be a possible cause of misdiagnoses.[2,4] In the blastocyst stage, multiple cells can be biopsied, which leads to decreased amplification errors and an improvement of the result accuracy. Development of sequential culture medium facilitated application of TE biopsy in clinical practice by enabling successful culture of embryos to the blastocyst stage and improving pregnancy outcome after blastocyst transfer.[4] However, mosaicism also occurs in blastocysts but to a lesser extent than in cleavage stage embryos, and the aneuploidy rate is significantly lower in this stage in comparison with early stage embryos.[2] Despite its significance and contribution to routine clinical procedures, PGD requires testing in an aggressive manner, which may disturb the embryo and compromise the clinical outcome. Therefore, the development of potential noninvasive approaches that might play an important role in the future are of interest and require further investigation.[2]

Molecular genetics and chromosomal analysis methods have also developed and currently include the PCR, fluorescence in situ hybridization (FISH), and comprehensive chromosome screening platforms such as the array comparative genomic hybridization (aCGH), single nucleotide polymorphism (SNP) microarray as well as next-generation sequencing (NGS)[4] (Table 12.1).

USE OF POLYMERASE CHAIN REACTION

The PCR protocol was used for the first clinical application of PGD in 1990 for gender determination of embryos for X-linked diseases.[5] Accordingly, the PCR method has become one of the most important molecular diagnostic techniques especially useful for monogenic diseases. The first reports of PCR use for single gene defects were for well-known monogenic diseases such as cystic fibrosis and thalassemia.[6] In general, PCR is a very powerful tool for the exponential amplification of short DNA fragments starting with a very small quantity, which opens up the possibilities for analyzing single-cell genetic content.

However, dealing with a limited DNA amount in a PCR reaction is challenging and leads to a number of hitches, including contaminations, amplification failure, and ADO (extreme preferential amplification of one allele or complete absence of one allele) in heterozygous samples.[1] Sources of contamination are numerous, and commonly used precautions can be undertaken to overcome this problem. On the other hand, ADO can lead to misdiagnoses especially for compound heterozygous or autosomal dominant conditions, while ADO should not lead to the transfer of an affected embryo in autosomal recessive disorder if both partners carry the same mutation. Therefore, for monogenic diseases, ADO appeared to be a complication for accurate PGD.[1] Accordingly, several variants and improvements of PCR have developed in an attempt to overcome these problems. For instance, to improve sensitivity and specificity, nested PCR was introduced where two consecutive rounds of PCR are applied. A more sensitive detection method, fluorescent PCR, was also developed and has helped in ADO detection because of its higher resolution and higher accuracy. In particular, fluorescent PCR is very precise in fragment sizing because it uses a laser system for automated fragment analysis with different fluorescent molecules.[1,6]

Another PCR strategy, multiplex PCR, has been adopted for simultaneous amplification of two or more DNA templates by using combinations of unrelated primer sets in a single PCR assay in the attempt to overcome the limitations of single-cell PCR. In addition, linked markers can be used for ADO detection as there is low possibility of ADO occurring at a series of different adjacent loci.[1] Microsatellite markers or SNP markers may well be used for linked markers. In multiplex PCR, both the mutation and the polymorphic markers are amplified together to increase the diagnostic accuracy.[7] Moreover, a substantial benefit of multiplex PCR is the possibility of using linked markers for diagnosis, and this strategy was applied for cystic fibrosis, fragile X syndrome, and Duchenne muscular dystrophy deletion carriers. Besides, in some of these cases, ADO might be detected as well.[6] Consequently, multiplex PCR with linked markers in combination with fluorescent PCR has become a method of choice in the diagnosis of different ailments.[6] For instance, a fluorescent one-step multiplex PCR technique based on the co-amplification of CAG repeats and three different polymorphic microsatellites was developed at the single-cell level for PGD of Huntington disease.[8] Moreover, the authors have used the same approach for PGD for other genetic disorders, such

Table 12.1: Comparison of preimplantation genetic diagnosis (PGD) methods.

Method	Diagnostic capabilities and strengths	Limitations
PCR	• Single gene defects	• Contaminations • Amplification failure • ADO
FISH	• Initially, used for sex determination • Identification of aneuploidy • Translocations	• Limited number of chromosomes can be evaluated
qPCR	• Whole chromosome aneuploidy • Allows carrying out of genotyping • Very sensitive and diagnostically accurate	• Unable to detect segmental aneuploidy • Cannot detect mosaicism or translocations
aCGH	• Whole chromosome aneuploidy • Translocations	• Cannot detect mosaicism • Might lead to false positives
SNP microarray	• Whole chromosome aneuploidy • Uniparental disomy • Translocations • More complex and with higher resolution than aCGH	• Unable to detect balanced chromosomal rearrangements • Unable to detect mosaicism
NGS	• Whole chromosome aneuploidy • Translocations • Mosaicism • Mitochondrial copy number • Single gene disorders • High resolution and complexity	• Limited in detection of balanced chromosome translocations

(aCGH: array comparative genomic hybridization; ADO: allele dropout; FISH: fluorescence in situ hybridization; NGS: next generation sequencing; PCR: polymerase chain reaction; SNP: single nucleotide polymorphism; qPCR: quantitative polymerase chain reaction) as cystic fibrosis, spinal muscular atrophy, and Duchenne muscular dystrophy. Interestingly, this methodology can be considered for PGD cycles in which the use of numerous markers are required.[8] For a comprehensive overview of PCR-based strategies used in PGD and summary of the methods used for the reduction and detection of ADO, please refer to related literature.[1,6]

Quantitative or real-time PCR (qPCR or RT-PCR) is a highly sensitive technique in which the fluorescent reporter molecules are used for the quantification and monitoring amplicon accumulation during each cycle of the PCR reaction. Moreover, the technique permits carrying out of genotyping and even single nucleotide can be detected, because fluorescent probes can be directed to either a wild-type or mutant sequence showing the potential of the implementation of this method in PGD.[1] Furthermore, qPCR assay was established for identification of whole chromosome aneuploidy through detection of the copy number of each examined chromosome. The method relies on the comparison of several locus-specific amplified sequences of each chromosome to a reference gene from the same chromosome.[3,4] The technique is highly diagnostically accurate and completed in approximately 4 hours; however, it is unable to detect segmental aneuploidy as well as mosaicism or translocations.[4]

MICROARRAY PLATFORMS

Initially, the FISH was used for sex determination, soon after that for aneuploidy identification through visualization of chromosomal regions, and later in PGD for translocations.[6] However, the FISH allows for a limited number of chromosomes to be evaluated,[3,9,10] therefore, more comprehensive chromosomal screening techniques have been recently developed. For example, aCGH microarray technology is able to test whole chromosome aneuploidy as well as translocations, but its limitation is its inability of mosaicism detection.[4] The method utilizes a PCR library-based whole genome amplification followed by fluorescent DNA labeling, hybridization, and array screening. The amplified DNA from blastomere biopsy is compared to karyotypically normal reference DNA, and both are then hybridized to a microarray with around 3,000–4,000 human DNA fragments probes. The experimental procedure is complete for about 12 hours.[4,7] The method might lead to false positives; nevertheless, TE biopsy with aCGH appeared to be highly sensitive and specific for aneuploidy screening.

Single nucleotide polymorphism microarrays appeared to be more complex and time-consuming than aCGH, even though they have a higher resolution. The SNP array offers genotype information for each sample analyzed in comparison to the human reference genome in the assessment of roughly 300,000 SNPs spaced throughout the genome. The array allows the identification of whole chromosome aneuploidy, uniparental disomy plus approximately 250 common structural chromosome aberrations. Large deletions or duplications, bigger than 50 Mb, can be detected as well.[3,4] However, the technique is limited in the detection of balanced chromosomal rearrangements and is unable to detect mosaicism. In addition, in the case of consanguineous couple, genetic anomalies might not be detected due to the possibility of SNPs being homozygous at every locus.[4]

Interestingly, karyomapping was also developed to screen and compare the genotype of embryos with a reference genome; naturally, that of an affected family member. Therefore, karyomapping is typically used to assess embryos for single conditions that affect essentially their family. The technique utilizes genome-wide linkage analysis for the comparison of mother and father SNPs with those of the family members of a known genetic status in order to identify the SNPs alleles' combination linked to a chromosome which carries a gene mutation.[4] In addition, the method appears to be very accurate with no need of design patient/disease specific tests.[4] Furthermore, the karyomap gene chip has been used in PGD to avoid monogenic disease as well as chromosomal anomalies, simultaneously.[11,12] Recently, the karyomap gene chip was used for monogenic disease PGD and PGS for exploring aneuploidy incidence in embryos from couples carrying monogenic diseases and the effect of embryo aneuploidy screening in monogenic disease PGD.[11] In particular, blastocysts were analyzed using the karyomap gene chip technique and, among embryos diagnosed as normal for monogenic diseases, 26.5% (approximately 1/4) were found to be aneuploidy and could not be transferred, demonstrating the requirement and importance of embryo aneuploidy screening in PGD for monogenic diseases. Therefore, the advantage of the karyomapping technology-based monogenic PGD is the ability to simultaneously implement embryo aneuploidy screening.[11]

NEXT GENERATION SEQUENCING

Next generation sequencing is generally a massive parallel sequencing that has significantly reduced the cost of human genome sequencing. Accordingly, in the field of PGD and PGS, this method might have certain contributions to the improvement of the genetic assessment of embryos before their transfer to the uterus.[13] NGS assay for PGS utilizes whole genome DNA amplification followed by DNA fragmentation and library preparation, where DNA fragments are fused to designated adapters.[3,4] Library preparation is followed by emulsion PCR or bridge PCR steps, depending on the NGS platform that has been used.[3] Two main NGS platforms are currently in use for PGS, Thermo Fisher Ion PGM from Thermo Fisher Scientific and Illumina MiSeq, both offering targeted clinical applications but employing different sequencing techniques.[3,4,14] In general, NGS is highly complex, possesses high resolution, and testing takes less than 24 hours to perform. MiSeq can detect whole chromosome aneuploidy, mosaicism, mitochondrial copy number, as well as single gene disorders and translocations.[3,4] However, the MiSeq platform is not designed to detect large deletions or duplications (>50 Mb)[3] but rather segmental imbalances of around 14 Mb and more.[4] PGM also allows the identification of whole chromosome aneuploidy, mosaicism, mitochondrial copy number, and single gene mutations. PGM, in contrast to MiSeq, is able to identify large deletions or duplications, and clinically significant deletions or duplications to a resolution of approximately 800 kb to 1 Mb.[3,4] NGS is a powerful technique for comprehensive chromosome screening, though the platform has limited ability to detect balanced chromosome translocations. Nevertheless, NGS-based platforms are becoming the standard of care because of their high accuracy and high throughput.[4]

For example, recent applicability of a commercial NGS-based workflow (MiSeq System from illumina) was evaluated for preimplantation genetic testing for chromosomal structural rearrangement.[15] Indeed, the study demonstrated that NGS was able to diagnose unbalanced reciprocal translocation/inversion products with the same efficiency as aCGH. In addition, using the karyotype of reciprocal translocation/inversion carriers, the size of predicted segmental aneuploidies could be calculated and used for the prediction of NGS implementation before treatment proceeding, which is important in counseling couples before beginning the treatment.[15] The potential of NGS was also shown in analyzing couples with an increased risk of autosomal recessive disorders.[16] Targeted NGS was undertaken for carriers screening of autosomal recessive lethal disorders in consanguineous and nonconsanguineous couples with one or more affected children. The study has shown that NGS-based gene panel sequencing of selected genes involved in lethal autosomal recessive disorders appeared to be a valuable tool for the detection of carrier status in families that have experienced early child death and/or multiple abortions. Therefore, these might now be used for prenatal and preimplantation genetic diagnosis for families in whom causative variants could be identified.[16]

CONCLUSION

The PGD methods will surely continue to develop in favor of an improved diagnostic precision and affordable cost for patients. However, before proceeding with PGD, patients need proper genetic counseling on the possible risks and clinical outcomes. Namely, each diagnostic platform might have some error rate and not all available technologies offer equal diagnostic capabilities. The choice of a diagnostic platform needs to be personalized to fit the patients' as well as clinical needs.

ACKNOWLEDGMENTS

We acknowledge the Croatian Science Foundation project "5709–Perspectives of maintaining the social state: toward the transformation of social security systems for individuals in personalized medicine", University of Rijeka research grant 13.11.1.1.11, and the project "Research Infrastructure for Campus-based Laboratories at University of Rijeka", co-financed by European Regional Development Fund (ERDF).

REFERENCES

1. Thornhill AR, Snow K. Molecular diagnostics in preimplantation genetic diagnosis. J Mol Diagn. 2002;4:11-29.
2. Milachich T. New advances of preimplantation and prenatal genetic screening and noninvasive testing as a potential predictor of health status of babies. Biomed Res Int. 2014;2014:306505.
3. Brezina PR, Anchan R, Kearns WG. Preimplantation genetic testing for aneuploidy: what technology should you use and what are the differences? J Assist Reprod Genet. 2016;33:823-32.
4. Sullivan-Pyke C, Dokras A. Preimplantation Genetic Screening and Preimplantation Genetic Diagnosis. Obstet Gynecol Clin North Am. 2018;45:113-25.
5. Handyside AH, Kontogianni EH, Hardy K, et al. Pregnancies from biopsied human preimplantation embryos sexed by Y-specific DNA amplification. Nature. 1990;344:768-70.
6. Sermon K. Current concepts in preimplantation genetic diagnosis (PGD): a molecular biologist's view. Hum Reprod Update. 2002;8:11-20.
7. Lee VCY, Chow JFC, Yeung WSB, et al. Preimplantation genetic diagnosis for monogenic diseases. Best Pract Res Clin Obstet Gynaecol. 2017;44:68-75.
8. Peciña A, Lozano Arana MD, García-Lozano JC, et al. One-step multiplex polymerase chain reaction for

preimplantation genetic diagnosis of Huntington disease. Fertil Steril. 2010;93:2411-2.
9. Jobanputra V, Sobrino A, Kinney A, et al. Multiplex interphase FISH as a screen for common aneuploidies in spontaneous abortions. Hum Reprod. 2002;17:1166-70.
10. Northrop LE, Treff NR, Levy B, et al. SNP microarray-based 24 chromosome aneuploidy screening demonstrates that cleavage-stage FISH poorly predicts aneuploidy in embryos that develop to morphologically normal blastocysts. Mol Hum Reprod. 2010;16:590-600.
11. Li G, Niu W, Jin H, et al. Importance of embryo aneuploidy screening in preimplantation genetic diagnosis for monogenic diseases using the karyomap gene chip. Sci Rep. 2018;8:3139.
12. Handyside AH, Harton GL, Mariani B, et al. Karyomapping: a universal method for genome wide analysis of genetic disease based on mapping crossovers between parental haplotypes. J Med Genet. 2010;47:651-8.
13. Martín J, Cervero A, Mir P, et al. The impact of next-generation sequencing technology on preimplantation genetic diagnosis and screening. Fertil Steril. 2013;99:1054-61.e3.
14. Liu L, Li Y, Li S, et al. Comparison of next-generation sequencing systems. J Biomed Biotechnol. 2012;2012:251364.
15. Chow JFC, Yeung WSB, Lee VCY, et al. Evaluation of preimplantation genetic testing for chromosomal structural rearrangement by a commonly used next generation sequencing workflow. Eur J Obstet Gynecol Reprod Biol. 2018;224:66-73.
16. Komlosi K, Diederich S, Fend-Guella DL, et al. Targeted next-generation sequencing analysis in couples at increased risk for autosomal recessive disorders. Orphanet J Rare Dis. 2018;13:23.

CHAPTER 13

Vanishing Twin Syndrome

Maria Carla Monni, Ambra Iuculano, Cristina Peddes, Valentina Corda, Giovanni Monni

INTRODUCTION

The vanishing twin syndrome (VTS) was first described by Levi et al.[1] and it is defined as a spontaneous demise of one twin or one gestational twin sac in a multiple pregnancy in the 1st trimester (Figs. 13.1A and B).[2]

The main causes would seem to be chromosomal aberrations of the demised twin (known as a risk of premature abortion) and placental pathologies, probably due to early changes in implantation that would result in an unfit uteroplacental exchange.[3-5]

Other possible mechanisms involved are intrauterine hemorrhages, placental crowding, and chronic maternal diseases such as diabetes during pregnancy and hypertension, which can cause disorders of placenta and uterine environment by themselves.[6-12]

Most cases of VTS are asymptomatic, although some patients report mild vaginal bleeding.[13,14]

The incidence of VTS is estimated to be in about 50% of pregnancies that start with three or more gestational sacs, and about 36% in twin pregnancies,[15] but the exact prevalence in spontaneously conceived pregnancies remains uncertain.[4,16,17] The incidence of VTS in in vitro fertilization (IVF) pregnancies with or without intracytoplasmic sperm injection (ICSI) is 12–30%.[3,18,19]

VANISHING TWIN SYNDROME IN ART PREGNANCIES

Regarding pregnancies following assisted reproductive techniques (ART), the higher the number of embryos transferred at IVF cycles, the higher rate of multiple pregnancies, which is currently estimated at 19.2% in Europe and 43.6% in the USA.[20,21]

The great advances in laboratory protocols, culture media, and incubation techniques have allowed to extend cell culture duration from cleavage-stage to blastocyst-stage and to improve embryo selection in order to reduce the number of transferred embryos into uterine cavity. In fact, until not long ago, cleavage stage was considered to be the standard stage for embryo transfer (ET) because of the still limited knowledge about the stage-specific culture media and the low embryo survival after this stage.[22,23] Despite this, the number of single ET is still relatively low (e.g., 21.4% in 2013 in the United States, 30% in 2010 globally).[21,24] A number of studies have reported that about

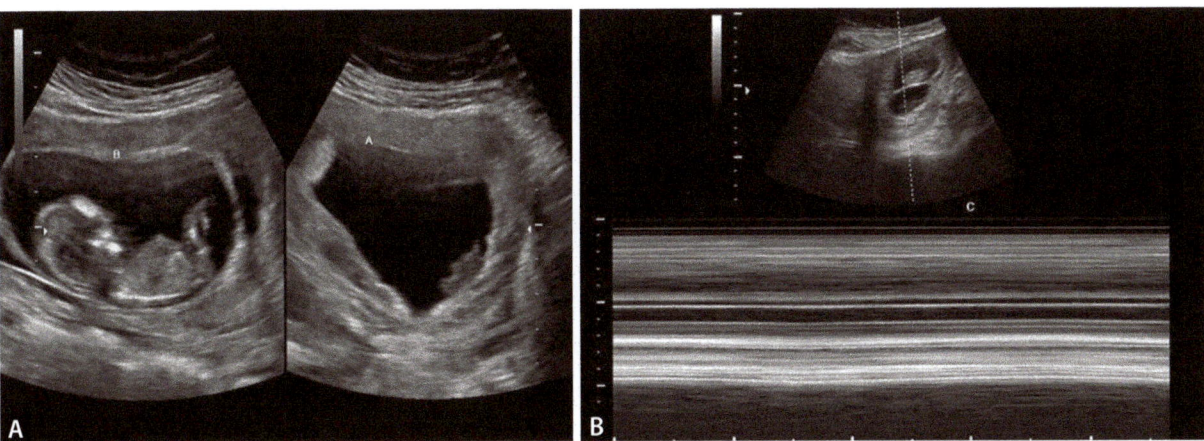

Figs. 13.1A and B: Twin pregnancy of 12 weeks with early spontaneous loss of heartbeat of one twin.
Courtesy: Reprinted with permission of KV Sridevi, Pinnacle Hospital.

one in ten singleton pregnancies after IVF treatment starts as a twin pregnancy.[25] However, it is important to note that most of these studies involve cases of cleavage-stage ET and it would seem that this estimate is significantly lower in case of blastocyst-stage ET.[26,27]

Despite evidence of lower incidence of early VTS in blastocyst-stage ET compared to cleavage-stage ET, it appears that the possible adverse effects on the surviving twins are almost the same in both cases.[27] It is essential to underline the need for single ET in IVF/ICSI cycles in order to reduce risks associated with twin pregnancies, both in case of survival of all fetuses and in case of VTS.

It should also be pointed out that the increased rate of VTS in ART pregnancies is fundamentally due to the increased twin pregnancy rate rather than ART per se. Indeed, according to Marton et al., fetal loss within 14 weeks is statistically greater in spontaneously conceived twin pregnancies than in IVF/ICSI twin pregnancies.[28] Given the close correlation between VTS and chromosomal abnormalities,[29,30] it is likely that the lower incidence of VTS in pregnancies from IVF/ICSI is due to the morphological selection of embryos chosen for transfer to the uterine cavity.

The percentage of VTS in IVF/ICSI pregnancies can also be related to the transfer of intermediate quality embryos,[30] to laboratory techniques,[31] and to artificial modifications of the endometrium.[32] Even though a mildly thick endometrium with a triple-line pattern is correlated with a good implant outcome, the decidualized endometrium has an important role as a biosensor of embryo quality, and its interaction with an inadequate quality embryo can influence the appearance of a VTS.[33]

Furthermore, as already known, adverse obstetric outcomes in ART pregnancies, such as abortion in singletons and twin pregnancies, have been found to be more related to the status of infertility/subfertility per se, to advanced maternal age, and to chronic pathologies linked to advanced maternal age, rather than to ART. In fact, these can determine low oocyte quality and, consequently, low embryonic quality too.[31,34]

The high frequency of VTS in IVF/ICSI pregnancies and its possible effects on embryos[3] have become the subject of numerous debates among ART experts in recent years. Despite conducting numerous studies, results are contradictory.

Some studies conclude that VTS is associated with adverse obstetric outcomes for the remaining survivor,[19,34-39] while other show that similar obstetric events are also present in IVF/ICSI singletons.[2]

So far, the fundamental differences among existing studies must be considered, such as maternal lifestyle characteristics; the type of study performed (e.g., case-control, cohort study); chorionicity which often is not evaluated; and gestational age at fetal death that is not always limited to the 1st trimester.

Vanishing twin syndrome seems to be associated with adverse outcomes affecting the remaining survivor both in spontaneously conceived pregnancies and ART pregnancies,[34,40] including increased risk of low birth weight, preterm birth, small for gestational age, and congenital malformations. However, several studies in this regard cannot exclude the possibility of confounding factors linked to maternal characteristics. A sibling comparison approach (which confronts brothers from the same mother) is useful to assess the importance of maternal factors not yet evaluated that remain stable among deliveries (Fig. 13.2).[41]

In 2017, a study by Magnus et al. evaluated the association between VTS and adverse events at birth in singleton ART pregnancies. More than 20,000 singleton ART pregnancies were included in this survey based on the Medical Birth Registry of Norway, containing information about all births after 16 weeks of gestation since 1984. This study concluded that pregnancies with VTS had higher incidence of low birth weight and small for gestational age compared to other singleton pregnancies following ART. This data was also evaluated among siblings, thus limiting maternal confounding factors.[15]

Multiple pregnancies involve an increased risk of adverse outcomes at birth due in part to placentation[42]

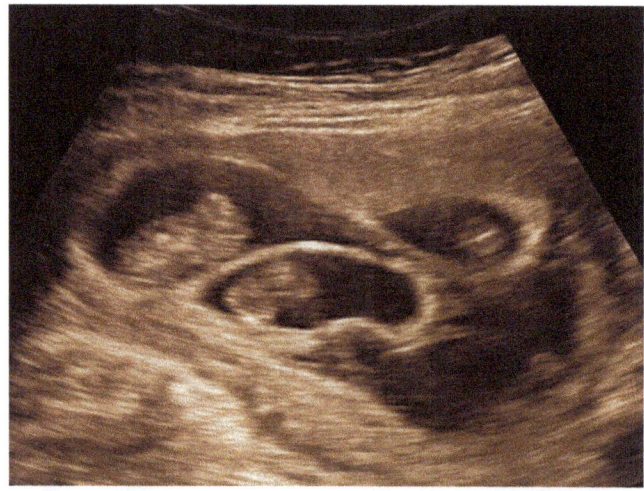

Fig. 13.2: Trichorionic triamniotic triplets with a partially demise of one twin at 9 weeks.
Courtesy: Reprinted with permission of KV Sridevi, Pinnacle Hospital.

and it is possible that related consequences explain this data in singleton ART pregnancies with VTS. It appears that complications in pregnancies with VTS can be attributed to the absorption of necrotic fetoplacental tissues which can lead to an increased release of cytokines and prostaglandins with consequent determination of an inflammatory process.[37] The cytokines released by the missing twin can affect the placental function and influence the growth of the surviving fetus.[40]

A recent review carried out on behalf of the Embryology Special Interest Group for Early Pregnancy[43] suggested that the increase in adverse obstetric outcomes can be attributed to the placental crowding, that is an early alteration of the implant that would result in a uterus-placental insufficiency.

Chasen et al. observed that this altered placental growth would also be at the base of the increased rate of pre-eclampsia during pregnancies with VTS.[44]

The characteristics of the adverse events detected in the study conducted by Magnus et al. were similar to those of reduced growth in case of maternal smoking during pregnancy. They can be indicators of a uterine environment which can determinate long-term health effects. In fact, children with low birth weight or small for gestational age are at higher risk of chronic diseases such as asthma and allergies, neuronal disorders, and metabolic dysfunctions related to cardiovascular disease.[45]

In a meta-analysis published by Sun et al. in 2017 on ART pregnancies, more than 400 cases of VTS were compared with nearly 3,000 singleton control pregnancies: no difference was found between the two groups regarding duration of pregnancy, rate of preterm birth, low birth weight, and rate of small for gestational age.[3]

EFFECTS OF VANISHING TWIN SYNDROME ON SURVIVING TWIN

Considering the numerous studies reporting the presence of adverse pregnancy outcomes in case of VTS, it is important to clarify some aspects.

First of all, the stage of pregnancy when fetal death occurred is not defined in some of these studies although it is closely related to the prognosis of VTS.[19]

The loss of a twin in the 2nd trimester is associated with an increased risk for the surviving twin in terms of growth restriction, premature delivery, and perinatal mortality compared to the 1st trimester VTS. This is most likely linked to the fact that an inflammatory response occurs after one twin demise because cytokines and prostaglandins released from fetoplacental necrotic tissues increase with pregnancy advancing and fetus growing.[46]

The meta-analysis by Sun et al. included studies which defined VTS as the disappearance of one empty gestational twin sac. In these cases, the gestational sac is smaller when compared to a gestational sac containing an embryo with cardiac activity. Hence, fetoplacental necrotic tissues are of less quantity and therefore the absorption of inflammatory substances is lower. If this hypothesis is correct, obstetric implications in case of VTS with confirmed embryonic cardiac activity could be worse as compared to VTS with an empty gestational sac (Fig. 13.3).

In addition, Sun's meta-analysis does not take into account some maternal characteristics that are known to influence studied outcomes, such as body mass index, weight gain during pregnancy, and presence of maternal diseases during pregnancies affecting placental function.

A number of studies[19,46,47] suggest that, in case of late VTS, the greater amount of fetoplacental tissues requires longer elimination time and this can result in unfavorable obstetric outcomes. After VTS is manifested, we can observe placental remodeling which can result in greater blood supply to the demised twin decomposition products and thereafter in temporary reduction of blood toward the surviving twin, with induction of a relative placental insufficiency at the base of a possible intrauterine growth restriction.[28]

There are other meta-analyses of adverse obstetric outcomes in case of VTS, but they also take into account

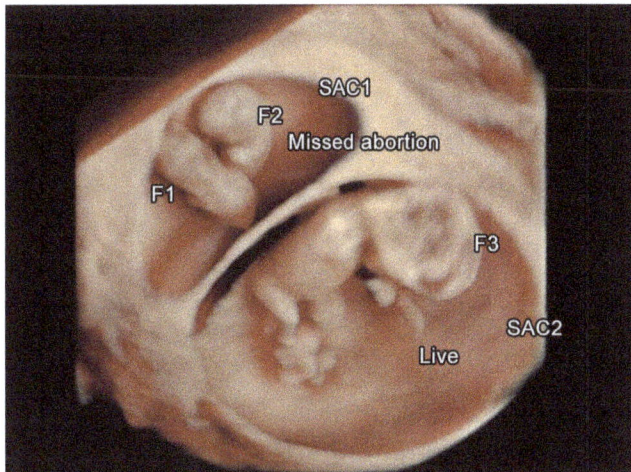

Fig. 13.3: HDlive imaging of bichorionic biamniotic triplets at 13 weeks with spontaneous heartbeat interruption of the two fetuses in the monochorionic sac at 9 weeks.
Courtesy: Reprinted with permission of KV Sridevi, Pinnacle Hospital.

spontaneously conceived monochorionic twin pregnancies (excluded by Sun's study) which notoriously involve a greater incidence of adverse obstetric outcomes.[48-50]

In conclusion, we notice an association between VTS and obstetric outcomes of the surviving twin but it is currently not well-defined.

As regarding other possible VTS complications, it is necessary to mention the case report by Dällenbach et al. describing a rare case of repeated and potentially fatal hemorrhages during pregnancy caused by fetoplacental tissues believed to originate from a VTS diagnosed early in the first trimester.[51]

Early ultrasound scan showed a dichorionic twin pregnancy with both fetal heart pulses. An early embryonic loss of one of the twins occurred in the 1st trimester (Fig. 13.4).

Ultrasound scan was performed at 25 and 27 weeks of gestation when a mild vaginal bleeding occurred. An intense arteriovenous flow of low impedance was detected with Doppler sonography distant from the apparently normal placenta of the surviving fetus. An urgent cesarean section was performed after a severe 27-week hemorrhage with hypovolemic shock. Heavily bleeding fragments were found in the correspondence of the intense flow area seen on ultrasound. The removal of these tissues was sufficient to stop the profuse bleeding and to prevent hysterectomy. They clinically corresponded to necrotic placental retained products with dilated vessels, later confirmed histologically.

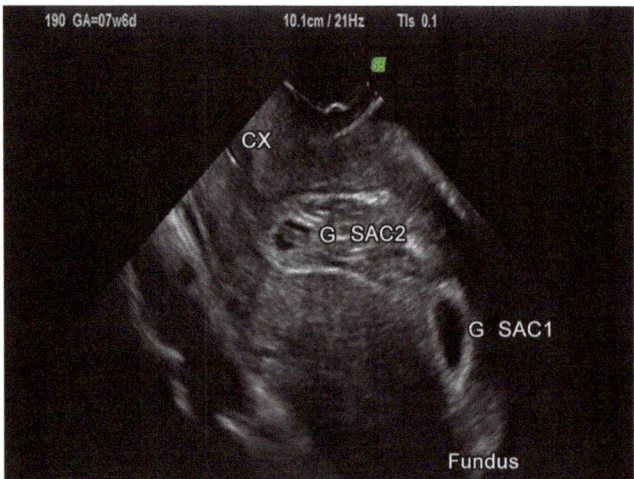

Fig. 13.4: Early ultrasound scans at 6 weeks with one sac low implantation and less chorionic fluid. Absent cardiac activity was found in a repeated scan after one week.
Courtesy: Reprinted with permission of KV Sridevi, Pinnacle Hospital.

Probably the subinvolution of the disappeared twin tissues led to the development of an arteriovenous fistula that determined the ultrasound evidence during pregnancy. Although rare, this complication must be considered in case of bleeding in pregnancies with VTS.

INFLUENCE OF VANISHING TWIN SYNDROME ON MATERNAL SERUM MARKERS

Vanishing twin syndrome can influence the measurement of maternal serum markers used in association with fetal nuchal translucency (NT) and maternal age for 1st trimester prenatal screening of aneuploidies in singleton pregnancies.[52]

Controversial results were reported in previous studies; some authors found differences in measurements of serum markers between pregnancies started as singleton and those of singleton pregnancies following VTS. This is probably related to the well-known differences of the serum marker levels between singleton and twin pregnancies, and the 1st trimester screening must be adjusted for twin pregnancy and chorionicity in order to not reduce its reliability.[52]

First trimester screening is one of the most effective methods for screening of Down syndrome (trisomy 21), with a detection rate of 90% and a false-positive rate less than 5%. It also allows the identification of a large portion of the other major aneuploidies such as trisomies 13 and 18, triploidies, and different aneuploidies of sex chromosomes.[53] The dosed markers for this screening are pregnancy associated plasma protein (PAPP-A) and free beta-human chorionic gonadotropin (β-hCG).

Second trimester screening has that same purpose and uses additional maternal serum markers—alpha-fetoprotein (AFP), dimeric inhibin A (DIA), and unconjugated estriol (uE3).

Chasen et al. reported in their study of 41 cases of VTS that no changes in PAPP-A and free β-hCG if VTS occurs more than 4 weeks before the 1st trimester screening; however, if VTS occurs less than 4 weeks before both markers are altered.[54]

Gjerris et al. evaluated the same parameters in IVF pregnancies and found no differences as compared to pregnancies started as singleton.[55]

Spencer et al. found an increase in PAPP-A of about 30% and levels of free β-hCG almost unchanged on a large sample of pregnancies with VTS of a measurable crown-rump length (CRL) embryo in the 1st trimester;

while there was difference in case of VTS of an empty gestational sac as compared to singleton pregnancies.[53]

In 2015, Huang et al. published a study about the impact of VTS on screening both in 1st and 2nd trimester in spontaneously conceived twin pregnancies. PAPP-A, AFP, and DIA in 2nd trimester were increased, while free β-hCG in 1st trimester, uE3 in 2nd trimester, and total hCG remained unchanged.[52]

The low impact of the demise of a twin on free β-hCG levels is not surprising given its very rapid clearance (< 24 hours).[53] On the other hand, high PAPP-A values similar to those seen in twin pregnancies were observed up to 8 weeks after the disappearance of one twin.[56]

Previous studies of the increase of PAPP-A were contradictory. This is probably due to the differences in studied populations, like gestational age at blood sampling for the 1st trimester screening, period between the disappearance of one embryo and the blood sampling, lack of discernment between VTS of an embryo with measurable CRL and an empty twin sac. The study of Chasen's group was criticized about the failure to correct the results for IVF (64% of pregnancies in VTS group were obtained with IVF).[53]

Several studies' results support the recommendation to exclude PAPP-A from the screening algorithm and employ NT measurement only or associated with free β-hCG for pregnancies with VTS.[57]

Second trimester screening of pregnancies with VTS may be inaccurate, therefore, it is currently not recommended.[52]

INFLUENCE OF VANISHING TWIN SYNDROME ON NIPS

Noninvasive prenatal screening (NIPS) also appears to be influenced by VTS, particularly those using methods that can evaluate total DNA but cannot determine the presence of additional haplotypes.

These last methods allow the determination of the number of copies of fetal chromosomes by comparing the absolute number of the sequences read in chromosomes in question (e.g. chromosome 21) and a reference number, deducing a fetal trisomy when this number is greater than a certain threshold value.[58] Therefore, by counting the high frequency of chromosomal abnormalities in VTS, Down syndrome can lead to false positive results when non-determination of additional haplotypes method is used.

Furthermore, in case of VTS with gender discrepancy, an incorrect sex identification can be observed (e.g., when a male fetus VTS occurs, a female fetus can be identified as a male fetus in case of NIPS). This is particularly important for diseases such as X-linked monogenic disorders.[59]

The use of a new analysis approach based on single nucleotide polymorphisms (SNP) seems to reduce this potential source of false positives. Indeed, this method allows detecting the presence of any twins not previously found thanks to the identification of additional fetal haplotypes.

The presence of additional fetal haplotypes in case of singleton pregnancy may therefore suggest a VTS. In these cases there are several diagnostic options: NIPS repetition, wait-and-see approach, follow-up diagnostic tests to exclude trisomies and, finally, the use of invasive tests (chorionic villus sampling and amniocentesis) that have to be evaluated regarding other indications and risks for the mother and the fetus.[60] Once the possibility of trisomy is discarded, the possibility of a VTS with an early disappeared embryo cannot be ruled out.

Most VTS occur in the 1st trimester, so the clinical diagnosis largely depends on the age of the first obstetric ultrasound and the time of fetal disappearance.[61] For this reason, in case of NIPS it is advisable to perform an early ultrasound scan to determine the fetus number and to identify the presence of VTS (Figs. 13.5 and 13.6).

In fact, the high incidence of VTS means that this possibility must not be neglected in case of positive NIPS result. This is particularly important seeing the increased incidence of twin pregnancies in developed countries, which in turn is fundamentally linked to the increased maternal age and the consequent use of ART techniques.[62] As already mentioned, twin pregnancy rate is higher in ART pregnancies and consequently the VTS rate increased too. This seems indirectly confirmed also by the significantly higher maternal age in case of NIPS with demonstrated VTS.

The weight of VTS on false positives at NIPS is still controversial.

The cumulative risk of false positives at NIPS is 1%.[63] The risk of aneuploidy in VTS is about 60%,[64,65] and about 0.11% of NIPS are calculated to be cases of VTS with chromosomal abnormalities. According to other authors, this estimate is 0.42–0.6%.[58] However, VTS would appear to be in 42.1% of confirmed false positive NIPS results.[58,66]

Furthermore, it is still unclear for how long fetal DNA remains in maternal blood after twin disappearance in case of VTS. This time interval is probably related to the quantity of placental tissues from the demised twin and to the gestational age at the time of disappearance. Some studies about singleton pregnancies have shown

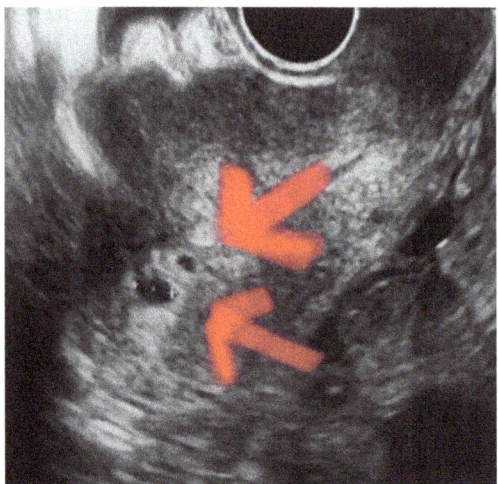

Fig. 13.5: Early ultrasound scans at 6 gestational weeks with one vanishing gestational twin sac.

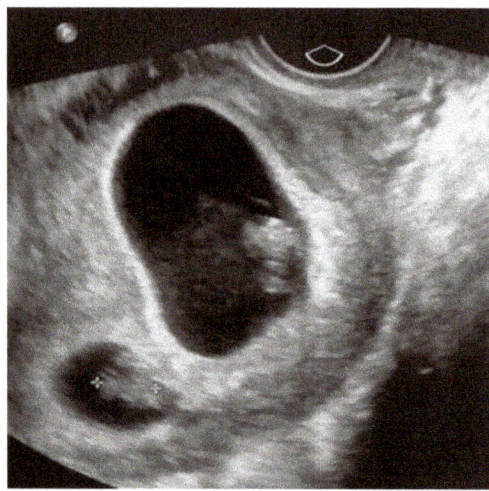

Fig. 13.6: Twin pregnancy of 8 weeks with early spontaneous loss of cardiac activity of one of the two twins.

that levels of circulating fetal DNA are five times greater at the time of spontaneous abortion as compared to evolutionary pregnancies at the same gestational age.[67] These values remain increased up to 7 days after diagnosis of abortion. Furthermore, this effect is more pronounced in spontaneous abortions with chromosomal abnormalities than in those with normal karyotype.[68] Because of this, it is likely that, in multiple pregnancies with VTS, NIPS results for the surviving twin are strongly compromised immediately after the disappearance of the vanishing twin. In several studies concerning the impact of VTS on NIPS,[58,59] fetal DNA circulating from the demised twin was detected up to 8 weeks after disappearance, suggesting that the reliability of NIPS in these cases is long-term compromised as well as maternal serum markers of 1st and 2nd trimester screening.

The early detection of VTS is undoubtedly important and positive results obtained by non-SNP-based NIPS should be carefully evaluated in order to avoid anxiety in parents and unnecessary and potentially dangerous invasive diagnostic procedures.

INFLUENCE OF VANISHING TWIN SYNDROME ON INVASIVE PRENATAL DIAGNOSIS

Vanishing twin syndrome can be a cause of misdiagnosis in chorionic villus sampling (CVS). Incidence of CVS "false negative" results is very low, approximately less than 1%.

Very few studies are reported in literature[36,69-71] about the association between VTS and misdiagnosis at CVS. They are essentially case reports in which a non-diagnosis of VTS has been ascertained. In these cases, the villus sampling was carried out by residual chorion frondosum coming from a twin or from fetal tissues previously disappeared.

Nowadays, in most cases the first obstetric ultrasound scan is performed between 6 weeks and 8 weeks so that most twin pregnancies with VTS are identified even when they affect only the gestational sac.

Vanishing twin syndrome tissues may no longer be visible when CVS is usually performed, between 11 weeks and 13 weeks. However, as previously mentioned, these tissues may persist for several weeks after the other twin has vanished and they can be inadvertently acquired during the CVS procedure and result in a misdiagnosis (Figs. 13.7A and B).

In case of a dubious result, it is possible to discern VTS from other diagnostic hypotheses by using specific chromosomal markers. In case of VTS, the possibility that these markers are identical is below 25% meanwhile they will be identical if the discrepancy found between karyotypes is due to a poor chromosomal disruption.[69]

Considering that about 70% of twin pregnancies is dizygotic and because of the increase in the incidence of twin pregnancies mentioned above, the possibility of CVS misdiagnosis by VTS is not negligible. Nonetheless, the low series of VTS-related CVS misdiagnosis reported in literature makes this risk reasonably unimportant, but it must be taken into account when a contrasting CVS result occurs.

In 2001, Lloveras et al. published a case report of an amniocentesis performed because of maternal age which

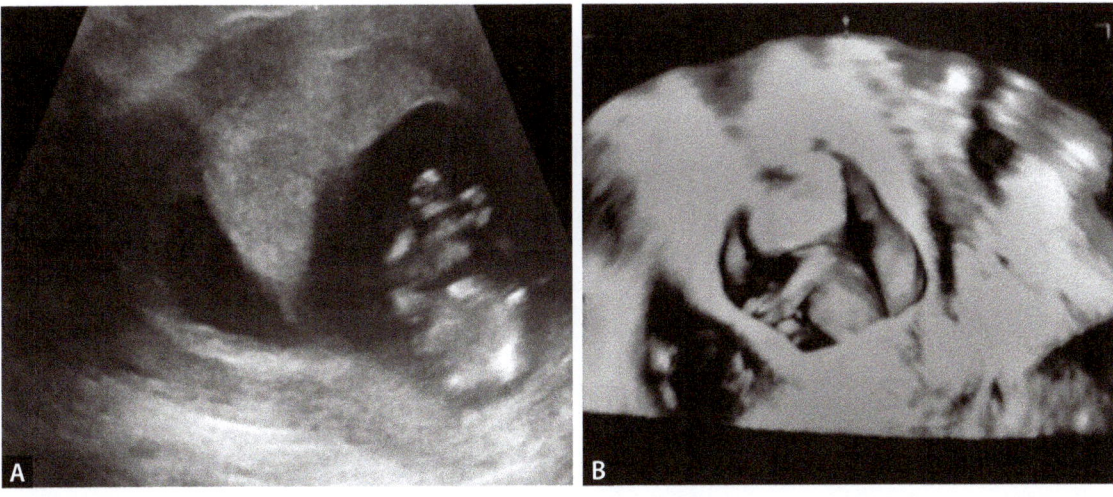

Figs. 13.7A and B: Two-dimensional (2D) and three-dimensional (3D) ultrasound images of 13-week twin pregnancy with one empty gestational twin sac undergoing VTS for maternal age.

showed a karyotype 46,XX in 35 cells and a karyotype 48,XY+8+10 in 3 cells. Subsequent ultrasound scan check throughout all pregnancy resulted in a normal and phenotypically female fetus, which was then confirmed after birth. The small percentage of Y chromosome found at amniocentesis, once excluded technical errors such as maternal contamination and exchange of samples, suggested an early VTS, indirectly supported also by the fact that double trisomies are often aborted in very early age of pregnancy.[72] It is therefore necessary to take VTS into account as a possible cause of mosaicism detected in cells sampled in amniotic fluid.

HOW EARLY CAN THE SUSPICION OF VANISHING TWIN SYNDROME BE POSED?

To find an answer to this question some authors evaluate the growth trend of β-hCG, which is classically used to monitor the progression of an early pregnancy, in order to identify as early as possible couples to be directed toward counseling and appropriate clinical options. A 53% increase of β-hCG in 48 hours was accepted as the minimum increase to identify a physiological intrauterine pregnancy, while lower values are indicated as suspected of an ectopic or non-evolutionary pregnancy. More recent studies suggest that a more stringent cut-off (35%) could minimize errors in the identification of developmental pregnancies.[73,74]

The study of Kelly et al. found an increase of β-hCG in 40 twin pregnancies dosed at 12 and 52 days after induced ovulation and 1 and 3 days after these two samples. The β-hCG increase was significantly higher in evolutionary twin pregnancies than in those with VTS.[75] Brady et al. evaluated the increase in β-hCG dosed at 7 and 22 days after ET and 1 and 7 days after these two samples in all pregnancies obtained from IVF/ICSI in Brigham and Women's Hospital from 1998 to 2010. They found that this increase was significantly lower in pregnancies with VTS when compared to singleton and twin evolutionary pregnancies, and the earlier one of the pregnancies was interrupted, the lower the increase.[76]

Considering that the majority of pregnancies with abnormal growth of β-hCG result in non-evolutionary pregnancy, the possibility of VTS should not be omitted in the evolutionary ones in order to carry out a possible early diagnosis (Figs. 13.8A to D).

CONCLUSION

To date, the evidence of the short- and long-term effects of VTS on the surviving fetus is discordant. The incidence of this event can be reduced by correcting maternal predisposing factors and reducing the risk of twin pregnancies obtained from ART techniques by the improvement of embryo selection techniques which are able to allow single ET. Early detection of VTS and monitoring of fetal and placental residues disappearance are crucial for the prognosticating of VTS possible effects on the surviving twin. The use of noninvasive screening techniques such as maternal serum markers and NIPS remains controversial.

Meticulous ultrasound monitoring of the alive twin for the entire pregnancy is mandatory to identify possible adverse obstetric outcomes.

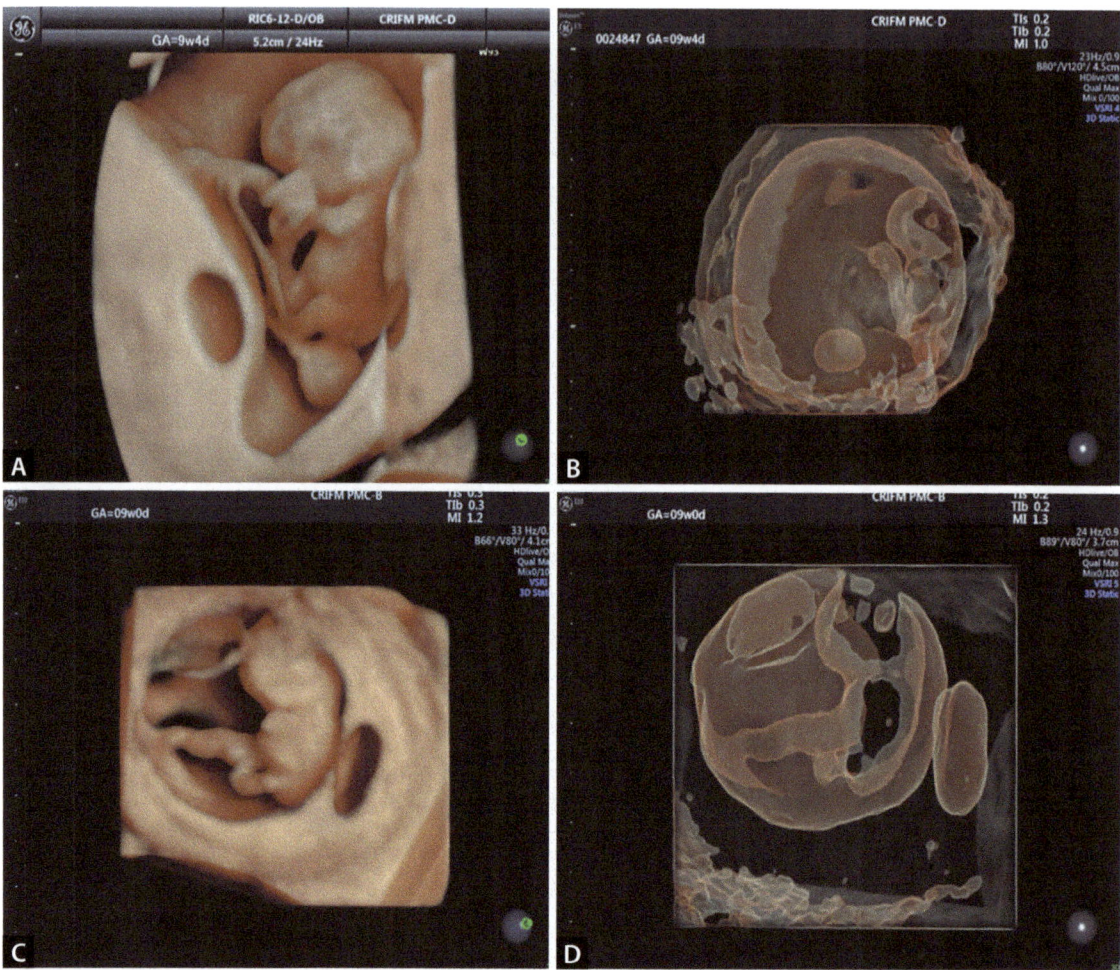

Figs. 13.8A to D: HDlive and three-dimensional (3D) HD silhouette images of two 10-weeks twin pregnancy with one partially demised empty gestational twin sac.
Courtesy: Reprinted with permission of RK Pooh, Clinical Research Institute of Fetal Medicine PMC.

REFERENCES

1. Levi S. Ultrasonic assessment of the high rate of human multiple pregnancy in the first trimester. J Clin Ultrasound. 1976;4:3-5.
2. La Sala GB, Villani MT, Nicoli A, et al. Effect of the mode of assisted reproductive technology conception on obstetric outcomes for survivors of the vanishing twin syndrome. Fertil Steril. 2006;86:247-9.
3. Sun L, Jiang LX, Chen HZ. Obstetric outcome of vanishing twins syndrome: a systematic review and meta-analysis. Arch Gynecol Obstet. 2017;295:559-67.
4. Landy HJ, Keith L. The vanishing twin: a review. Hum Reprod Update. 1998;4:177-83.
5. Patrizio P, Bianchi V, Lalioti MD, et al. High rate of biological loss in assisted reproduction: it is in the seed, not in the soil. Reprod Biomed Online. 2007;14:92-5.
6. Barton SE, Missmer SA, Hornstein MD. Twin pregnancies with a 'vanished' embryo: a higher risk multiple gestation group? Hum Reprod. 2011;26:2750-3.
7. Greenwold N, Jauniaux E. Collection of villous tissue under ultrasound guidance to improve the cytogenetic study of early pregnancy failure. Hum Reprod. 2002;17:452-6.
8. Jauniaux E, Van Oppenraaij RH, Burton GJ. Obstetric outcome after early placental complications. Curr Opin Obstet Gynecol. 2010;22:452-7.
9. Oloyede OA, Iketubosin F, Bamgbopa K. Spontaneous foetal reduction and early pregnancy complications in multiple pregnancies following in vitro fertilisation. Int J Gynaecol Obstet. 2012;119:57-60.
10. Pinborg A, Wennerholm UB, Romundstad LB, et al. Why do singletons conceived after assisted reproduction technology have adverse perinatal outcome? Systematic review and meta-analysis. Hum Reprod Update. 2013;19:87-104.
11. Rizzo G, Capponi A, Pietrolucci ME, et al. First trimester placental volume and three dimensional power Doppler ultrasonography in type I diabetic pregnancies. Prenat Diagn. 2012;32:480-4.
12. Loeken MR. Advances in understanding the molecular causes of diabetes induced birth defects. J Soc Gynecol Investig. 2006;13:2-10.

13. De Sutter O, Bontinck J, Schutysers V, et al. First trimester bleeding and pregnancy outcome in singletons after assisted reproduction. Hum Reprod. 2006;21:1907-11.
14. Jauniaux E, Elkazen N, Leroy F, et al. Clinical and morphological aspects of the vanishing twin phenomenon. Obstet Gynecol. 1988;72:577-81.
15. Magnus MC, Ghaderi S, Morken NH, et al. Vanishing twin syndrome among ART singletons and pregnancy outcomes. Hum Reprod. 2017;32(11):2298-304.
16. Depp R, Macones GA, Rosenn MF, et al. Multifoetal pregnancy reduction: evaluation of foetal growth in the remaining twins. Am J Obstet Gynecol. 1996;174:1233-8.
17. Sampson A, de Crespigny LC. Vanishing twins: the frequency of spontaneous foetal reduction of a twin pregnancy. Ultrasound Obstet Gynecol. 1992;2:107-9.
18. Gjerris AC, Tabor A, Loft A, et al. First trimester prenatal screening among women pregnant after IVF/ICSI. Hum Reprod Update. 2012;18:350-9.
19. Pinborg A, Lidegaard O, la Cour Freiesleben N, et al. Consequences of vanishing twins in IVF/ICSI pregnancies. Hum Reprod. 2005;20:2821-9.
20. Kupka MS, D'Hooghe T, Ferraretti AP, et al. European IVF-Monitoring Consortium (EIM) European Society of Human Reproduction and Embryology (ESHRE). Hum Reprod. 2016;31:233-48.
21. Sunderam S, Kissin DM, Crawford SB, Centers for Disease Control and Prevention (CDC). Assisted reproductive technology surveillance, United States, 2012. MMWR Surveill Summ. 2015;64:1-29.
22. Glujovsky D, Blake D, Farquhar C, et al. Cleavage stage versus blastocyst stage embryo transfer in assisted reproductive technology. Cochrane Database Syst Rev. 2012;7:CD002118.
23. Glujovsky D, Farquhar C. Cleavage-stage or blastocyst transfer: what are the benefits and harms? Fertil Steril. 2016;106(2):244-50.
24. Dyer S, Chambers GM, de Mouzon J, et al. International Committee for Monitoring Assisted Reproductive Technologies world report: assisted reproductive technology 2008, 2009 and 2010. Hum Reprod. 2016;31(7):1588-609.
25. Rudnicki M, Vejerslev LO, Junge J. The vanishing twin: morphologic and cytogenetic evaluation of an ultrasonographic phenomenon. Gynecol Obstet Invest. 1991;31:141-5.
26. Fernando D, Halliday JL, Breheny S, et al. Outcomes of singleton births after blastocyst versus nonblastocyst transfer in assisted reproductive technology. Fertil Steril. 2012;97(3):579-84.
27. Pereira N, Pryor KP, Petrini AC, et al. Perinatal risks associated with early vanishing twin syndrome following transfer of cleavage- or blastocyst-stage embryos. J Pregnancy. 2016;2016:1245210.
28. Márton V, Zádori J, Kozinszky Z, et al. Prevalences and pregnancy outcome of vanishing twin pregnancies achieved by in vitro fertilization versus natural conception. Fertil Steril. 2016;106(6):1399-406.
29. Jauniaux E, Ben-Ami I, Maymon R. Do assisted-reproduction twin pregnancies require additional antenatal care? Reprod Biomed Online. 2013;26:107-19.
30. La Sala GB, Nicoli A, Villani MT, et al. Spontaneous embryonic loss rates in twin and singleton pregnancies after transfer of top- versus intermediate-quality embryos. Fertil Steril. 2005;84:1602-5.
31. Schieve LA, Meikle SF, Ferre C, et al. Low and very low birth weight in infants conceived with use of assisted reproductive technology. N Engl J Med. 2002;346:731-7.
32. Jauniaux E, Farquharson RG, Christiansen OB, et al. Evidence-based guidelines for the investigation and medical treatment of recurrent miscarriage. Hum Reprod. 2006; 21:2216-22.
33. Zhao J, Zhang Q, Li Y. The effect of endometrial thickness and pattern measured by ultrasonography on pregnancy outcomes during IVF-ET cycles. Reprod Biol Endocrinol. 2012;10:100.
34. Evron E, Sheiner E, Friger M, et al. Vanishing twin syndrome: is it associated with adverse perinatal outcome? Fertil Steril. 2015;103:1209-14.
35. Almog B, Levin I, Wagman I, et al. Adverse obstetric outcome for the vanishing twin syndrome. Reprod Biomed Online. 2010;20:256-60.
36. Shebl O, Ebner T, Sommergruber M, et al. Birth weight is lower for survivors of the vanishing twin syndrome: a case-control study. Fertil Steril. 2008;90:310-4.
37. Mansour R, Serour G, Aboulghar M, et al. The impact of vanishing fetuses on the outcome of ICSI pregnancies. Fertil Steril. 2010;94:2430-2.
38. Sun L, Chen Z, Liu J, et al. Obstetric and neonatal outcomes of vanishing twin syndrome. Nan Fang Yi Ke Da Xue Xue Bao. 2014;34:1537-40.
39. Tabanelli C, Ferraretti AP, Feliciani E, et al. Vanishing twins in IVF/ICSI pregnancies: a case-control study. Mol Hum Reprod. 2009;24:i130-i131.
40. Zhou L, Gao X, Wu Y, et al. Analysis of pregnancy outcomes for survivors of the vanishing twin syndrome after in vitro fertilization and embryo transfer. Eur J Obstet Gynecol Reprod Biol. 2016;203:35-9.
41. Frisell T, Oberg S, Kuja-Halkola R, et al. Sibling comparison designs: bias from non-shared confounders and measurement error. Epidemiology. 2012;23:713-20.
42. Oepkes D, Sueters M. Antenatal fetal surveillance in multiple pregnancies. Best Pract Res Clin Obstet Gynaecol. 2017;38:59-70.
43. Van Oppenraaij RH, Jauniaux E, Christiansen OB, et al. Predicting adverse obstetric outcome after early pregnancy events and complications: a review. Hum Reprod Update. 2009;15,409-21.
44. Chasen ST, Luo G, Perni SC, et al. Are in vitro fertilization pregnancies with early spontaneous reduction high risk? Am J Obstet Gynecol. 2006;195,814-7.
45. Murray E, Fernandes M, Fazel M, et al. Differential effect of intrauterine growth restriction on childhood neurodevelopment: a systematic review. BJOG. 2015; 122:1062-72.
46. Bass NH, Oliver JB, Srinivasan M. Persistently elevated AFP and ACHE in amniotic fluid from a normal fetus following the demise of its twin. Prenat Diagn. 1986;6:33-5.

47. Pinborg A, Lidegaard O, Freisleben N, et al. Vanishing twins: a predictor of small-for-gestational age in IVF singletons. Hum Reprod. 2007;22:2707-14.
48. Shek NW, Hillman SC, Kilby MD. Single-twin demise: pregnancy outcome. Best Pract Res Clin Obstet Gynaecol. 2014;28:249-63.
49. Hillman SC, Morris RK, Kilby MD. Co-twin prognosis after single fetal death: a systematic review and meta-analysis. Obstet Gynecol. 2011;118:928-40.
50. Ong SS, Zamora J, Khan KS, et al. Prognosis for the co-twin following single-twin death: a systematic review. BJOG. 2006;113:992-8.
51. Dällenbach P, Pelte MF, Irion O. Life-threatening third-trimester hemorrhage following a vanishing twin phenomenon in early pregnancy. Ultrasound Obstet Gynecol. 2005;26(2):196-7.
52. Huang T, Boucher K, Aul R, et al. First and second trimester maternal serum markers in pregnancies with a vanishing twin. Prenat Diagn. 2015;35(1):90-6.
53. Spencer K, Staboulidou I, Nicolaides KH. First trimester aneuploidy screening in the presence of a vanishing twin: implications for maternal serum markers. Prenat Diagn. 2010;30:235-40.
54. Chasen ST, Perni SC, Predanic M, et al. Does a "vanishing twin" affect first-trimester biochemistry in Down syndrome risk assessment? Am J Obstet Gynecol. 2006;195:236-9.
55. Gjerris AC, Loft A, Pinborg A, et al. The effect of a 'vanishing twin' on biochemical and ultrasound first trimester screening markers for Down's syndrome in pregnancies conceived by assisted reproductive technology. Hum Reprod. 2009;24:55-62.
56. Abbas A, Sebire NJ, Johnson M, et al. Maternal serum concentrations of pregnancy associated placental protein A and pregnancy specific B1 glycoprotein in multifetal pregnancies before and after fetal reduction. Hum Reprod. 1996;11:900-2.
57. Sankaran S, Rozette C, Dean J, et al. Screening in the presence of a vanished twin: nuchal translucency or combined screening test? Prenat Diagn. 2011;31:600-1.
58. Curnow KJ, Wilkins-Haug L, Ryan A, et al. Detection of triploid, molar, and vanishing twin pregnancies by a single-nucleotide polymorphism-based noninvasive prenatal test. Am J Obstet Gynecol. 2015;212(1):79.e1-9.
59. Masala M, Saba L, Zoppi MA, et al. Pitfalls in noninvasive fetal RhD and sex determination due to a vanishing twin. Prenat Diagn. 2015;35(5):506-8.
60. American College of Obstetricians and Gynecologists. Invasive prenatal testing for aneuploidy. ACOG Practice bulletin no. 88. Obstet Gynecol. 2007;110:1459-67.
61. Manzur A, Goldsman MP, Stone SC, et al. Outcome of triplet pregnancies after assisted reproductive techniques: how frequent are the vanishing embryos? Fertil Steril. 1995;63:252-7.
62. Centers for Disease Control and Prevention ASfRM, Technology SfAR. 2010 Assisted reproductive technology national summary report. Atlanta, GA: US Department of Health and Human Services, Centers for Disease Control and Prevention; 2012.
63. Niles KM, Murji A, Chitayat D. Prolonged duration of persistent cell free fetal DNA from a vanishing twin. Ultrasound Obstet Gynecol; 2018.
64. Lathi RB, Gustin SL, Keller J, et al. Reliability of 46, XX results on miscarriage specimens: a review of 1,222 first-trimester miscarriage specimens. Fertil Steril. 2013;101:178-82.
65. Levy B, Sigurjonsson S, Pettersen B, et al. Genomic imbalance in products of conception: single nucleotide polymorphism chromosomal microarray analysis. Obstet Gynecol. 2014;124:202-9.
66. Hartwig TS, Ambye L, Sorensen S, et al. Discordant noninvasive prenatal testing (NIPT) - a systematic review. Prenat Diagn. 2017;37(6):527-39.
67. Yin A, Ng EH, Zhang X, et al. Correlation of maternal plasma total cell-free DNA and fetal DNA levels with short term outcome of first-trimester vaginal bleeding. Hum Reprod. 2007;22:1736-43.
68. Lim JH, Kim MH, Han YJ, et al. Cell-free fetal DNA and cell-free total DNA levels in spontaneous abortion with fetal chromosomal aneuploidy. PLoS One. 2013;8:e56787.
69. Reddy KS, Petersen MB, Antonarakis SE, et al. The vanishing twin: an explanation for discordance between chorionic villus karyotype and fetal phenotype. Pren Diagn. 1991;1:679-84.
70. Tharapel AT, Elias S, Shulamm LP, et al. Resorbed co-twin as an explanation for discrepant chorionic villus results: non-mosaic 47,XX, + 16 in villi (direct and culture) with normal (46,XX) amniotic fluid and neonatal blood. Prenat Diagn. 1989;9:467-72.
71. Ledbetter DH, Martin AO, Verlinsky Y, et al. Cytogenetic results of chorionic villus sampling: high success rate and diagnostic accuracy in the United States collaborative study. Am J Obstet Gynecol. 1990;146:495-501.
72. Lloveras E, Lecumberri JM, Pérez C, et al. A female infant with a 46,XX/48,XY+8+10 karyotype in prenatal diagnosis: a 'vanishing twin' phenomenon? Prenat Diagn. 2001;21(10):896-7.
73. Barnhart KT, Sammel MD, Rinaudo PF, et al. Symptomatic patients with an early viable intrauterine pregnancy: HCG curves redefined. Obstet Gynecol. 2004;104:50-5.
74. Morse CB, Sammel MD, Shaunik A, et al. Performance of human chorionic gonadotropin curves in women at risk for ectopic pregnancy: exceptions to the rules. Fertil Steril. 2012;97:101-6.
75. Kelly MP, Molo MW, Maclin VM, et al. Human chorionic gonadotropin rise in normal and vanishing twin pregnancies. Fertil Steril. 1991;56:221-4.
76. Brady PC, Correia KF, Missmer SA, et al. Early beta-human chorionic gonadotropin trends in vanishing twin pregnancies. Fertil Steril. 2013;100(1):116-21.

CHAPTER 14

Genomic Editing, Human Enhancement and Transhumanism: A Brief Overview

Kresimir Pavelic, Sandra Kraljevic Pavelic

INTRODUCTION

Recent discussions on preimplantation or intrauterine interventions and prenatal diagnosis on fetuses and babies have opened up serious questions about the purpose and consequences of genetic editing, human enhancement, and designing of babies by means of gene editing. All these questions, especially from the methodological and socio-humanistic point of view, are reflected under the common topic known as transhumanism. In this chapter, we therefore present and discuss the fundamentals of genomic editing (GE) and human enhancement–within the topic of transhumanism.

GENOMIC EDITING

Science is nowadays facing an essential issue how to manage the unprecedented scientific and technological achievements and progress within sociocultural evolution. It can indeed be foreseen that, soon, our survival and well-being are going to depend on the new wisdom that may be attained only through interdisciplinary thinking and interdisciplinary approaches in science, comprising natural, social, and humanistic fields. The so-called "bio-optimists" predict a bright future for humanity if we become able to use our technology to enhance our sense of morality and our capacity for social responsibility. Still, we cannot evaluate the consequences of future major scientific or technological advancements. Instead, the current focus remains limited mainly to research and technologies that are meant to enhance human health or substantially prolong the human lifespan. These are GE and human enhancement approaches that encompass current biomedical technologies and their possible development into enhancement technologies in general.[1]

Genomic editing is a genetic engineering procedure whereby the genetic material, the DNA, is intentionally inserted, cut, modified, or replaced in the genome of any living organism. The purpose of GE is to modify the DNA sequence or genotype of a cell or organism for the purpose of modification. The method is mostly based on the use of "molecular scissors" or enzymes known as nucleases, which create specific double-stranded DNA breaks at certain sites in the genome. The created breaks are repaired with nonhomologous end-joining (NHEJ) or homologous recombination (HR) mechanisms, which result in editing or target mutations.[2] GE also appears in natural processes, without artificial genetic engineering. For example, viruses or subvirus RNA agents[3] are capable of editing the genetic code. Genetic engineering methods used thus far include different approaches; for example, forward genetics methods include different approaches to the study of the genetic basis of phenotype, including mutation induction or insertional mutagenesis methods, where a new phenotype is first observed and then the underlying genetic base is explored.[4] Also, the study of the gene function through analyses of phenotypic effects can be done through modifications of the DNA in the reverse genetics process in a target organism by means of site-directed mutagenesis, i.e. using a phage or polymerase chain reaction (PCR)-mediated method and short DNA-oligonucleotide sequences containing desired mutations.[2] Another way of studying genes is through recombination-based methods, which use the natural ability of cells to alternate their own and exogenous DNA. Still, these approaches are not completely adequate with regard to efficiency. The engineered nucleases used in GE seem to be a promising approach that enhance the efficiency and increase the accuracy of the reverse genetic procedures.

Genomic editing is possible due to accumulated knowledge on DNA repair mechanisms. The main mechanisms on which GE is based are the NHEJ, which is based on multiple enzymes that directly affect double strand breaks (DSB) in the DNA, and HR, whereby the homology-directed homologous sequence repair in DSB is performed by using a template for repair at the break site. The problem of creating specific DSB-restriction enzymes is that certain restriction endonucleases recognize several pairs of DNA bases as their targets, so it is certain that such base pairs will be present in many locations along the genome and not only at the wanted site of intervention during the eventual GE. This problem was solved with the development of a site-specific DSB procedure through distinct classes of nucleases. Indeed, this method of GE was proclaimed the method of the year in 2011 by the journal *Nature*,[5] and, since then, the following types of nucleases have been continuously developed: meganucleases (MAGE), zinc-finger nucleases (ZFN), transcription activator-like effector-based nucleases (TALEN), and the clustered regularly interspaced short palindromic repeats (CRISPR/Cas) nuclease system.

Meganucleases are a family of endonuclease enzymes that can induce a homologous recombination and are characterized by the ability to recognize and cut off large DNA sequences (12 to 40 pairs of bases).[4,6] MAGE-based GE methods are considerably less toxic to cells in comparison to ZFN-based GE methods, probably due to a stricter recognition of DNA sequences. The MAGE can be engineered to replace or modify almost any wanted DNA sequences in a highly targeted way. MAGE applications are in multiple target sites, individual genetic mutations or one-target site, and multiple genetic mutations or multiple-target sites.[7,8]

Zinc-finger nuclease engineering involves unspecific cuttings of DNA where ZFN contain a zinc finger DNA-binding domain and a DNA-cleavage domain. The zinc ion found in 8% of all human proteins, plays an important role in organizing the ZFN three-dimensional structure. In transcription factors, they are usually located on the protein-DNA interaction side where stabilizing the motif. The C-terminal part of each "finger" is responsible for the specific recognition of the DNA sequence. ZFN are used for genetic engineering of stem cells and for the modification of immune cells for therapeutic purposes.[9,10] For example, ZFN-modified T lymphocytes have been tested within clinical studies for the treatment of glioblastoma and the treatment of AIDS patients.[11]

Transcription activator-like effector nucleases or TALEN are artificially created restriction enzymes obtained through fusion of specific TAL effector DNA-binding domains with a DNA-cleavage domain. DNA-binding domains can be designed to bind almost any desired DNA sequence.[10,12] A study in vitro, for example,[13] successfully studied TALEN-induced mutations of 15 genes in cultured somatic cells and human pluripotent stem cells. The authors were able to demonstrate cell-autonomous phenotypes that point to a number of diseases including insulin resistance, lipodystrophy, or motor-neuron death. Moreover, the first clinical use of TALEN genetically engineered cells was based on the treatment of CD19 + lymphoblastic leukemia cells in an 11-year-old child. TALEN-modified T-cell carriers were designed to "attack" leukemia cells to be resistant to alemtuzumab and to avoid the host immune system after application. The patient's condition improved several weeks after receiving therapy. One year after the treatment, the patient is still in remission.[14] The same approach was further developed[15] and several more similar examples of HIV and hematological malignancies therapy through T-cell GE have been documented so far.[16] Therapeutic examples of ZFN or TALEN GE-based approaches also include GE of X-linked severe combined immunodeficiency (X-SCID) through ex vivo correction of the DNA gene, interleukin 2 receptor subunit gamma (IL2RG) in SCID-X1 patient, hematopoietic stem cells (HSCs), and progenitor cells using ZFNs or a correction of mature lymphoid cells in vitro in induced pluripotent stem cells (iPSCs) derived from SCID-X1.[17] Similarly, a correction of *Xeroderma pigmentosum* cells in vitro with TALEN has been successfully performed.[18]

Further on, CRISPRs are genetic elements, specifically the viral genome DNA sequences, which have been incorporated into the bacterial genome upon bacteria viral infections. Therefore, this system is an important adaptive immunity system of bacteria toward bacteriophage infections. CRISPR-associated proteins, Cas, are involved in the processing of these sequences and they ultimately cut the corresponding homologous viral DNA sequences. CRISPR/Cas (herein after CRISPR) system used for GE is based on the use of a piece of RNA called guide RNA (gRNA), which guides the Cas9 nuclease to a specific position on the DNA sequence.[19] Induced cleavage is subject to the cell's DNA repair mechanisms when wanted corrections of the DNA sequences can be induced in the targeted DNA position.[20] Such CRISPR system has been widely used in diverse genetic studies and is being rapidly developed toward in vivo therapeutic models. Recently, it has also been tested in clinical trials, i.e., therapeutic GE of malignancies[21] or HIV,[22] which has opened up a number of regulatory questions, especially those related to the safety of such a GE approach. Some issues for CRISPR technology at the moment include the delivery and precision of the CRISPR system. Particularly, researchers have been intensively evaluating the "off-target" toxicity, i.e. the alternation of the genome or off-target mutations at the non-target loci. Solutions including an augmentation of the CRIPSR system specificity or a limitation of the Cas nuclease action have been tested so far to circumvent the "off-target" issue.[23]

An extremely wide range of genome-engineered applications documented in the scientific literature so far by means of using engineered nucleases include the research of gene function in plants, animals, and humans as well therapeutic application in vivo with promising results. In particular, a major GE outcome of relevance to human health and longevity is gene therapy. Its main purpose is to replace defective genes with normal alleles at their natural site or to control the symptoms of disease by modifying genes involved in pathological processes. The delivery of genes within gene therapy does not usually require the delivery of the entire gene sequence given that only a small sequence of the gene has to be altered in order to cure or control the disease. The first GE clinical trial for Europe was announced in 2018 for the biotech company CRISPR Therapeutics, which aims to treat patients with sickle cell disease and β thalassemia;[24] however, this has been challenged in a recent paper that proved that CRISPR/Cas technology may induce dangerous and unwanted DNA changes that may initiate malignant processes in cells.[25] There is still much to learn before coming to a conclusive approach for safe GE in humans.

Another application of GE methods may be also envisaged in the field of synthetic biology, which aims to build artificial biological systems either for the purpose of research, medical purposes, or even biosensors and medical devices. The ability of the engineered nuclease to add or remove genomic elements and thus create complex systems is central to this field.[26] Within this field, GE methods can be used, e.g. for the creation of artificial cells and organs with new functions. This may be envisaged in current research of the human microbiome, which is increasingly correlated with systemic human disorders, including bone disease, cancer, or neurodegenerative pathologies. GE in synthetic biology approaches might foster the development of effective microbiota-based therapeutics.[27] However, risks that synthetically engineered DNA from microbes may compromise the wider microbiota environment.

Perspectives and Concerns

What are the perspectives and implications of GE for the future of our civilization? Despite some tangible successes of genetic engineering technologies and GE, specificity and certainty of nuclease procedures are still not adequate for major genome interventions. Detection and understanding of the unwanted, "off-target" events are essential elements for further GE applications in humans. Besides the accuracy of GE processes, a better understanding of the basic recombination and DNA damage-repair mechanisms is also required. The CRISPR and TALEN methods are precise and efficient, cheap, and will probably remain the methods of choice for large-scale GE procedures in the future. In particular, the CRISPR method can help to bridge the current gap between GE studies in animals and humans. This is especially important as mice or other animal models studies failed to be translated into humans[28] and genotype-phenotype relationships have been found not to be reliably inferred by studying a single genetic background of the inbred model animals.[29] The use of CRISPR opens up new opportunities as it is used to produce a mutant in nearly any genetic background.[30] Indeed, CRISPR has been extensively used in animal model, mainly mouse models, including the modification of the fertilized zygote using CRISPR to achieve the desired modifications.[31] It is also possible to apply the CRISPR in xenotransplantation. In a recent study, for example, it was shown that the replacement of pig genes with human genes with CRISPR precision may be seriously evaluated in the production of donor pigs for xenotransplantation.[32] In addition, CRISPR was used to target and eliminate endogenous retroviruses from the pig genome, which reduces the risk of disease transmission and reduces immune barriers.[33] Eliminating these problems may improve the possibility to use pigs as organ donor animals for humans, and the application of this method brings the idea of pig xenotransplantation closer to reality. Still, one might speculate on the real risk of pig retrovirus infection and the necessity to heavily edit the pig genome for the purpose of xenotransplantation as the GE might add to the complexity of a xenotransplant in a still undefined dimension.

Genome editing techniques are so appealing and work very well in the experimental set-up that many socio-humanist scientists believe that GE will potentially contribute to improving the human race or human enhancement (a term which is explained in greater detail in the continuation of the text). In this connection, the problem of designing a baby has also been elaborated by a number of ethical commissions or research institutions.[34,35] It seems that the majority of participants involved in this debate agree that a moratorium on GE research is counterproductive and that other solutions found within a wide social dialogue might generate appropriate guidelines. One suggested approach was a clear distinction between somatic cells and germ cells GE research. Still, research was already conducted on human embryos, providing relevant information on the CRISPR method efficiency at this developmental stage. For example, it was shown that gene targeting and editing has to be done in a certain cell cycle phase as it is associated with DNA synthesis.[36] In its 2017 report, the American National Academy of Sciences and the National Academy of Medicine published a comprehensive GE report recommending clinical testing as GE was identified as a procedure that might one day solve serious health problems assuming that it is undertaken in strict and controlled conditions and under assumptions that issues on efficiency and safety have been adequately resolved.[37] This was an important release as any new, thus potentially dangerous, technology raises abuse concerns, such as for the first serious critics toward research results on infected mice with a modified pox virus that caused their infertility.[38] A potential mass bioterrorist usage of this publicly available research has been subject of debates as the results may be used to create a vaccine resistant to other pox viruses, such as small pox, that can infect people.[39] There is also the ecological fear of the release of an artificially engineered gene into the environment and "wild" populations. This danger is very difficult to evaluate appropriately as it cannot be readily transferred to a laboratory environment. Concerns are present due to the simplicity and low cost of CRISPR technology that can be used for the production of massive weapons of mass destruction, which is especially applicable to nations without strict regulation and ethical standards in the genetic manipulation area. For example, CRISPR and similar GE technologies might be used for mass production of killer mosquitoes.[40] The fears are also related to the risks but also the potential benefits of modification of the human genome and the transfer of these modifications to future generations. This requires some urgent ethical scrutiny. Such modifications could have unwanted and unexpected consequences that could damage not only children but their future offspring, as an alteration of their genes will be contained in their germ cells permanently.[41,42]

HUMAN ENHANCEMENT

Human enhancement (HE) is generally understood as a term describing any attempt to temporarily or permanently alter the existing limitations or disadvantages of the human body, either by natural or artificial means. This also implies technological means of selection or change of human traits and capacities regardless of whether this change results in characteristics that represent the existing human limits.[43]

Human enhancement technologies are not just those intended to treat patients with certain diseases or injuries but also those designed to improve human traits and capacities.[44] Often, HE is used as a synonym for human genetic engineering using nanotechnology, biotechnology, information technology, and cognitive science with the aim of improving human characteristics (memory enhancement, communication skills, senses, multidimensional thinking, psychical, and physical improvement, acceleration of mental and general thinking abilities solving problems).[45] The innovativeness in such an interdisciplinary area is envisaged to be self-catalyzing toward an improvement of human performance. Numerous socio-humanistic issues arise in connection with the application of HE. Particularly, HE has been increasingly identified with the term transhumanism as a controversial ideology and movement that has developed to support the recognition and protection of the rights of citizens to maintain or modify their own intellect and body and to allow them freedom of choice and informed consent to use HE technology for themselves and their children freely. Transhumanism, as defined by More, pursues on the acceleration of the evolution of intelligent life beyond its currently "human form" and "human limitations" by means of science and technology, guided by life-promoting principles and values.[46] The most frequent criticism is that these technologies will be usually practiced with uncontrolled and short-term selfish perspectives ignoring long-lasting consequences on individuals and the rest of society. For example, it may be envisaged that some so-called enhancements, which will create unequal physical and mental benefits, are given to those who can afford this technology or that an unequal approach to such enhancement will arise, which will deepen the difference between those who may or may not have it.[47,48] Unfair competition of those who can apply such technology for the purpose of trading has also been mentioned. It is possible that this technology will disrupt the dynamics of relationships within families and close relationships. Socio-humanist thinkers also often point to the problem of inequality and social disruption. Enhancement of the human body can cause significant changes in everyday situations. For example, sport will change dramatically if enhanced people are allowed to take part in competitions, whereby they will have a tremendous advantage over people who will not have access to such enhancement.[49] Also, no one can exactly know at this point whether enhancements will really be satisfactory for individuals and the society in the long-term. Still, it should be noted that biological or pharmacological enhancements, such as those potentially envisaged by GE and aimed to promote human health, capacities or dramatically extend the life-span, are different from technological enhancements, i.e. development of nanotechnology or further advancements in artificial intelligence. While nanotechnology potentially poses serious and immediate risks to the humanity itself, artificial intelligence may accelerate creation of superintelligence that, on one hand, holds great promises to solving many humanity issues including implementation of nanotechnology but, on the other, may lead human evolution into another direction. Philosopher Nick Bostrom, for example, emphasizes that artificial intellects need not have human-like motives or psyches, which makes their goals potentially radically different or opposite to those of humans. In Bostrom's opinion, the risks of developing superintelligence include the risk of failure to give it a philanthropic goal.[50] Such debates will require a deeper discussion and re-evaluation of the humanity goals and understanding of humans in general.

When evaluating the potential HE impact on economy, it should be mentioned that HE might significantly extend the life span, and adaptive measures for the legal and economic implications of retirement will be necessary in order to compensate for longer retirement or to postpone retirement for several years. If these adaptations are not made and if the longevity is not taken into account, this could negatively affect resources such as energy or available food. Resources are inevitably something that will have to be re-evaluated as well. In addition, if artificial intelligence leaves enough room for human jobs, then candidates with neural enhancements, i.e., those in the form of transplants aimed to increase their abilities, will easily surpass other candidates. Such social injustice is already exaggerated in our society and may be, therefore, a real scenario in the future that is further exacerbated with enhancement opportunities.[51] Accordingly, it is clear that the availability of these methods may be achievable only for certain groups of individuals depending on the socioeconomic situation[52] even in a very optimistic scenario. Also, HE will heavily influence the human identity by acting on self-conception. Taking into account the fact that at this point many do not seriously evaluate these questions, often focusing instead on every-day problems and existence, an enormous area of discussion may be opened up before fostering and implementing HE. Extreme personality changes can affect relationships between individuals, and people will probably have problems with relying or interacting with newly formed individuals who have been subjected to enhancement. Ultimately, a risk is inherently present in these enhancement technologies as well as a certain level of robustness should be achieved to prevent theft and influence (interfere with) human augmentation.[53]

While we have to acknowledge that new and radical technologies are already here and more are to come, it is difficult to envisage that these will necessarily provide all solutions to our problems and morality. It is more likely that they will reflect the state of their creators, 'us-humans', and with this knowledge further developments should be carefully guided.

DESIGNING A BABY WITH GE

The concept of a designed baby (DB) implies a human embryo that is genetically modified, usually following the instructions of a parent or a scientist to obtain the desired properties. This can be achieved with various methods, such as embryonic cells engineering or preimplantation genetic diagnosis. These technologies are the subject of ethical debate, as they imply a concept of genetically modified "superhumans" who will eventually replace the present population.

Modifications of germ cells have been carried out since the 1980s, mainly on animals.[54] A successful embryonic modification requires the knowledge of the exact gene insertion procedure so that the new property can be successfully transmitted to the next generation and maintained in the offspring.[55] GE of the germline DNA will be passed onto further generations if the changes are present through the development of germ cells. Manipulation of the germline genome for the purpose of achieving the desired properties is technically already possible and depends on the medical procedure. For example, the cloning process can be used to create genetically identical organisms. In addition, scientists may use gene therapy vectors to modify target DNA, including the DNA of DBs. This can be easily envisaged in an in vitro fertilization (IVF) environment where the creation of a genetically engineered baby may occur.

Even though these effects can be positive, i.e. the correction of inherited disorders, an inherent risk of possible amplification of negative properties is still a plausible risk at this stage of scientific knowledge. Since the results of such germline genetic manipulations are a complex matter and long-term effects are difficultly observable, it is not easy to evaluate the eventual benefits or enhanced negative effects. It is thus rather questionable whether to allow parents to design their children and to select desired qualities given that the means for human germline GE would be soon available.

Ethical implications and the risks associated with baby designing are already a matter of debates. It is emphasized that DB may be generated through genetic engineering without the exact knowledge on the far-reaching effects on the overall human genes.[56] On the other hand, it is argued that DB can play an important role in counteracting the dysgenic trend. The main ethical issue on DB is that these types of treatment will create changes that can be passed onto future generations so that any mistakes, known and unknown, will be transmitted to their descendants.[55] Therefore, theoretically, a sudden emergence of new diseases and their transfer onto offspring could appear.[57,58] It is therefore not surprising that GE and the transmission of donor mitochondria are the subject of intense controversy and concerns. If a patient is subjected to germline modification, the offspring will be monitored for a long period of time for any adverse consequence. This period may induce very harmful psychological consequences for these persons and the problems can occur at a significantly later moment in life.[59] On a larger scale, genetic modification can strongly impact the gene pool of the entire human race, both in a positive and negative way.[54] GE modifications are, however, ethically and morally more easily acceptable when the patient or a future baby are seriously ill and the treatment may improve the genotype but also the safety of future generations. Used for these purposes, such treatments can fill the gaps that other technologies are unable to solve.[54]

Of course, experimentations with embryonic cells or embryos are ethically overwhelmingly questionable. Some countries allow these experimentations with fertilized egg cells available in excess after IVF.[59] It should be remembered, of course, that the embryo cannot give consent and that these procedures give way to long-lasting and potentially harmful implications. Human embryo editing is currently illegal in many countries. The American National Academy for Science, Engineering and Medicine recently supported the research and interventions into human embryos but only in cases of the prevention of serious illness and conditions as a "last option" when others had failed. Embryonal editing can prevent large numbers of medical problems in the future and it is worth noting that about 10,000 medical conditions are associated with specific mutations, including Huntington's disease, cancer caused by *BRCA* gene mutations, Tay-Sachs disease, cystic fibrosis, sickle cell anemia, and some cases of early Alzheimer's disease. Replacing a mutation on responsible genes could theoretically eradicate these inherited diseases and prevent the transmission onto next generations, so that future family members would not have similar problems.

Some of the dilemmas and fears about human embryo GE can be compared with similar fears and dilemmas present at the very beginning of the application of IVF. These dilemmas are present even today after more than 5 million IVF babies have been born using this wide human reproduction experiment. Some researchers warn about IVF consequences and call for a serious follow-up of IVF conceived babies as longer-term health outcomes for these children may include cardiometabolic problems[60] or even a shorter life-span as suggested by the evolutionist Pascal Gagneux from University of California.[61] Gagneux emphasized that assisted reproduction might lead to biological and social consequences that have not been evaluated enough. Therefore, the embryo GE dilemma on creating a world where children would be considered superior to the other, unedited ones, may be observed from a different angle—is it possible that designed babies may have poorer chances for long-term survival? Both the scientists and ethics share concerns about the accessibility of this procedure. A premise is that any clinical intervention should be available to everyone and society should not create inequality, but should firstly solve issues of safety and long-term outcomes. We must reconcile the fact that new fears arise with each new technology and that these fears may be justifiable or not. Often, these are replaced by some other objective problems during the implementation process that turn the societal outcomes into new, previously unknown directions.

While human embryo GE is prohibited by law in most countries, there are recommendations or guidelines in China for the ban or restrictions in clinical use, but not a statutory prohibition. Indeed, in a very recent paper, by Chinese scientists on a multiple CRISPR, GE of human embryos showed an efficient correction of the Marfan syndrome pathogenic mutation in the *FBN1* gene, which provides instructions for making a large protein called fibrillin-1, with efficacy up to 89% and without detected "off-target" mutations. This research opens the door for

GE in genetic correction at the embryonal stage.[62] This procedure was conducted as a proof of the concept on 18 embryos, but in two embryos unintentional editing occurred as well. It is still unclear whether such procedure might be considered as safe for further IVF procedures and human reproduction.

TRANSHUMANISM AND "THE CULTURE OF LIFE"

Major cultural changes have been elaborated in the socio-humanistic literature; for example, the culture of perfection of society has been viewed as dominant. It implies human ideals of rationality, freedom, equality, and justice. It also includes belief in science. On the other hand, "the culture of life," which is, according to Knorr Cetina,[63] a radically distinct mentality based on the promises of an individual enhancement and life extension. The humanity and humanism are accordingly replaced by, what Knorr Cetina denotes, the "notion of individual life" where individuals feel a need for enhancement of life in general, often fed by biological sciences and promises of life extension and anti-aging approaches, which has major social and economic implications as well.[63] Biological sciences may be identified as the major driving force that inspires ideas on human individual enhancements based on GE, biotechnology, and biology. These ideas are then dependent on knowledge and technologies available for their implementation, such as, e.g. preimplantation genetic diagnosis, screening, germline engineering, GE, pharmacological interventions, and human cloning. Furthermore, bioengineering ought to combine nanotechnology, information science, and cognitive research (NBIC) with the aim of developing devices that enhance and augment biological human nature, often in the direction of prolongation of life span. When assessing NBIC goals, a major question may arise on how to define a sharp distinction between humans and machines/technology and whether this approach will bring true "enhancement" to a human or just partial enhancements with unknown consequences to other human structures. One can speculate that NBIC may lead to performance enhancements, especially in elderly population, such as expanded memory capacity, faster thinking speed, or even enable novel sensor capabilities, i.e., infrared and ultraviolet wavelengths "sight".[64] It may also repair the genetic damage and prevent illnesses. Knorr Cetina thinks that moving to a "culture of life" implies deep societal changes beyond ethical questions of certain scientific disciplines.

The main purpose of transhumanism is a substantial improvement of human intellectual and physiological abilities (Tables 14.1 and 14.2), and the so called "transhumanist parties" have been established in several countries so far. For example, the US transhumanist party supports activities or means to improve the human condition for "as many people as possible, with as much beneficial impact as possible—and without regard for scoring political points or defeating the other side".[65] Even the European Union has acknowledged transhumanism as a new exponential future thinking that has a political aim.[66] It is, therefore, obvious that tremendous changes are going to happen in the next era of our civilization, which will require new, constructive solutions to the challenges of societal transformation. Scientists and thinkers, therefore, increasingly consider the benefits and dangers of newly created technologies and knowledge that can overcome human limitations but also current ethical barriers to their use.[67] Amongst transhumanists, e.g. the fundamental and most common position is finding avenues to transform

Table 14.1: Questions about the rights of transhumans and the ethics expected from them.

Questions	Possible implications of human enhancement
Will those with a higher percentage of prosthetic/techno body parts have fewer rights than biological persons?	Increased capabilities, on one hand, along with decreased human characteristics, on the other, may lead to unknown social relations
Why should a biological cell structure be an adequate criterion for establishing a distinction between human and techno-human alike beings?	Erasing a clear line between human and techno-human beings alike may lead to unknown or unpredictable ethical or moral consequences
What will it mean if life-extending technologies together with reduction of birth rates increase the population of the elderly?	Unknown consequences on the human reproduction and population status, especially health status and evolutionary important premises may arise
How will the political area and social institutions have to change under HE-induced circumstances?	Current systems fail to follow novel societal challenges and novel solutions may fail to protect civilization achievements or philanthropic values
What are the implications for families when relatives—such as siblings, aunts, and uncles are replaced by the simultaneous existence of four or five generations of parents and children?	Unknown implications for development of the human being in early developmental stages (childhood and adolescence) may be due to the loss of current biologically rooted development

Table 14.2: Term explanation.		
Term	**Explanation**	**Literature**
Democratic transhumanism	A political ideology synthesizing liberal democracy, social democracy, radical democracy, and transhumanism	73,76
Extropianism	An early school of transhumanism that promotes critical and creative thinking on emerging technologies as well as management and risks to maximize the benefits and opportunities arising from emerging technologies	77,78
Immortalism	A moral ideology based on radical life extension and technological immortality goals, advocating research and development to ensure such a scenario	79,80,81
Libertarian transhumanism	A political ideology synthesizing libertarianism and transhumanism	82,83
Postgenderism	A social philosophy which seeks for a society without genders through the use of advanced biotechnology and assisted reproductive technologies	84,85
Singularitarianism	A philosophy based on the acknowledgement of an approaching moment in human evolution beyond which technological progress will become incomprehensively rapid and complicated	85,86
Technogaianism	An ecological ideology that aims to use technology to counteract ecocrisis	73,87

humans into beings with abilities that visibly outgrow the original state (posthuman beings).[68] Still, the similarity of the transhumanist vision of changing the future seems influenced by science fiction and is encouraged by numerous supporters or opposed by a wide range of professions, including philosophers and theologians.[69]

One of the aspects of transhumanism, but also scientific advancements in general, is the development of artificial intelligence (AI) tools or AI per se. In its infancy, AI is understood as a prerequisite for the creation of superintelligent devices that can significantly outperform all human intellectual activities. The assumption is that such devices will design novel AI more intelligently. Some argue that the invention of the first superintelligent device will possibly be the last human invention and that development of this field should, therefore, be carefully evaluated.[70] Even though transhumanism shares many elements of humanism, including the respect for science, the commitment to progress, and the appreciation of transhuman existence, it differs from humanism in its commitment to improve attributes that humanists often consider unique to humanity (i.e., intelligence and autonomy) but through technology.[71] Currently, the main purpose of transhumanism is to eliminate aging as well as to "repair" and "improve" intellectual, physiological, and psychological capacities. From a philosophical point, transhumanism is concerned with human race development or even evolution by new and innovative pharmacological and/or technological means into a new, enhanced species. This includes ideas on creating highly intelligent animals or humans with cognitive enhancement.[69,72]

Many transhumanist theorists advocate immediate and often radical implementation of scientific and technological achievements to reduce the severity of an illness, physical inability, and malnutrition throughout the world.[71] The urge for an immediate implementation of scientific and technological achievements is often driven by the fear of not living long enough to benefit from improvements. Since transhumanism deals with the enhancement of the human body on an individual level, many transhumanists actively assess the potential of future technologies and innovative social systems to improve the quality of life in general. Interestingly, transhumanist philosophers claim that no obligatory ethical basis can be found to prevent humans to choose and use a human condition improvement programs. In their view, it is possible and desirable for people to engage in the transhuman phase of existence where individual decisions will drive their own personal enhancements. Transhumanists also strongly support the development of methods of "improvement" of the human nervous system, including the peripheral nervous system or brain as a primary target of transhumanist ambition.[73] In particular, the idea is to "merge" or "connect" the human mind and the computer, going into the direction of "mind uploading" human consciousness to an alternative medium.[74] Transhumanists advocate technologies such as sex-cell screening, nanotechnology, information technology, and cognitive science as well as hypothetical future technologies, such as simulated reality, artificial intelligence, superintelligence, 3D bioprinting, mind up-loading, and cryonic. They believe that people need and must apply these technologies if they are to have better properties than existing human characteristics.[74] Therefore, they encourage the recognition and/or protection of cognitive freedom, morphological freedom, and deceitful liberty as civil liberties in order to allow for a free application of human enhancement technology to themselves and their children.[75] Some distinctive currents of transhumanism are listed in Table 14.2.

Many of these transhumanist ideas have been critically evaluated by a number of philosophers and sociologists[88,89] whereby serious questions beyond the scope of this overview have been raised, including those on ethical issues, societal changes, political context, and future perspectives of our civilization. Indeed, the concept and likelihood of human enhancement and similar issues provoke public controversy, even suggesting that transhumanism is the "latest site for the struggle" of the progressive ideologies of liberalism and socialism.[89] Critics and opponents often see transhumanist goals as a threat to humanistic values. Some authors believe that humanity is already becoming transhuman as a consequence of continuous advances in the medical sector that has changed our species significantly. Some prominent transhumanists also remain sceptical on the technical feasibility in the near future. They speculate that even if it were possible to predict a deep integration of individuals into the machine system, people would remain "biologized" and essential changes to their own form and character would not arise as a consequence of information technology but rather from direct manipulation of their genetics, metabolism or biochemistry.[90]

A current hot topic in the area of HE is the intervention on the embryo development, especially in the phase of early embryogenesis. This means correction of diseases or unwanted traits that interfere with the normal development and life, including corrections of basic properties of the embryo to enhance the human being in the later developmental and life phases. Most common unexpected risks of these processes that can disrupt embryonic development are a subject of debate. Experiments directed toward permanent biological consequences on a person have been acknowledged as a violation of the accepted principles of the Helsinki Declaration, i.e., that biomedical research involving human subjects cannot legitimately be carried out unless the importance of the objective is in proportion to the inherent risk to the subject or concern for the interests of the subject must always prevail over the interests of science and society.[91]

In addition, experimental "enhancement" or GE outputs in a specific species, i.e., rats or mice do not mean automatic transmission of results to a new species, i.e., humans, without further experimentation. It is thus considered that at this point, when the knowledge on "enhancement" procedures, including GE, is still vague, genetic manipulation of people at an early stage of development is not justified.[92] Moreover, some scientists and thinkers believe that advances in science and technology can lead to greater catastrophe than progress. At the same time, they are techno-progressive with caution, and demand for greater security and new ways on traditional availability approach and distribution of scientific data and knowledge.[93] Some emphasize the importance of careful, slow progress and discontinuation of research in potentially dangerous areas, such as HE and GE. Some cautious scientists and thinkers find that the articulate intelligence and robotics represent the possibility of alternative forms of knowledge that can endanger human life.[94] Contrary to that, GE perceived as anything more than a "natural" progression is viewed by some scholars as an expression of our humanity, rather than a "dehumanizing" concept.[1] Ultimately, enhancement may be good for us as current physiological limitations, which we consider to be normal, are only "natural" or "normal" in the context of one human generation and its culture. Many scientists believe that this topic should be, therefore, discussed within a specific socio-historical context of our current civilization. In particular, they think that biological limitations will soon be replaced with new biological, artificial, and mixed carbon/silicon-based technologies. Also, biology is not the only field where perceptive beings with the ability to react and adapt can evolve; computer-based entities and their software may even become sentient in the future and new forms of life may emerge.[1]

LIVING INDEFINITELY LONG

Since its dawn, human civilization has been fascinated by overcoming death. Therefore, it is not surprising that immortality, eternal youth, or at least the perspectives of biblical life have always been a powerful topic of religion and art. Life and death or eternal life are central elements of all religions. Only recently, intensive efforts have been made in modern science to understand and prevent aging and prolong life. An effective anti-aging therapy might, indeed, dramatically change the modern society and a number of debates are ongoing in this field. Although this problem has not been solved today, scientific discoveries provide some intriguing promises for substantial prolongation of the lifespan. Some promises include pharmacotherapy, actions directed toward senescent cells or use of stem cells. An extension of the average lifespan and maximum age has an immense social and political impact and, as expected, opinions on this subject vary. Some models suggest the possibility of extending life to 120 years;[95] others think that such a prolongation of human life is impossible since human lifetime has already reached the biological limit.[96] Westendorp argues that medical advances during the past century and reduced childhood mortality, which remove the pressure of having to produce progeny, are not only increasing the average but also pushing the maximal life expectancy, as our bodies adapt to a new environment by investing resources into maintenance and longevity, which had not been previously possible.[97]

Prevention or delaying of aging seems to be more problematic. Still a possible scenario may be that human life will be extended to about 120 years and that man will live for 90 years healthy and active as 50-year-old today.[98] A most radical scenario has envisaged the necessity to rely on the continuous repair of damage caused by basic metabolic processes and environmental factors. This might result in permanent maintenance of physiological functions and prevention of aging, enabling people to live for thousands of years.[99]

CONCLUSION

A number of high-quality scientific debates on GE, HE, and transhumanism are available to a wider audience but so far, no public opinion on this issue has been heard.[100] This, in turn, gives ambitious groups and individuals the chance to pursue their own visions of the future and the society will be split between those pushing enhancements without limitations and those who will choose a sustainable approach to technology-aided evolution. It also seems that the public will have a tremendous interest in the technologies for the extension of the biological life, mostly because of the fear of death, fear of aging, and the desire to maintain a healthy life. However, it appears that the desire for a longer life depends on the health status and quality of life, which again raises the question of the social context and rethinking of the society. Steps noticeable in this area, are not often related to science but are instead exploited for marketing, sales, or beauty treatments and interventions that claim to overcome the effect of aging and prolong life.

While significant scientific advancements in the area of GE and HE are expected in the near future, a reasonable approach and caution in the new knowledge and technologies usage and implementation may be advised. In particular, safety issues, short- or long-term consequences of the human germline GE, an re-evaluated understanding of the concept of humanity and a person on the individual level with all facets should be explored and studied in more details prior to GE and HE consideration in medical applications. Legal, ethical, and societal issues need to be scrupulously discussed and evaluated in light of novel evidence and information to avoid critical dangers in this delicate, yet exciting era of human existence.

ACKNOWLEDGMENTS

We acknowledge the Croatian Science Foundation project "5709–Perspectives of maintaining the social state: toward the transformation of social security systems for individuals in personalized medicine", University of Rijeka research grant 13.11.1.1.11, and the project "Research Infrastructure for Campus-based Laboratories at University of Rijeka", co-financed by European Regional Development Fund (ERDF).

REFERENCES

1. Moore E. The future of our species. EMBO Rep. 2008;9:S1-S3.
2. Esvelt KM, Wang HH. Genome-scale engineering for systems and synthetic biology. Mol Syst Biol. 2013;9(1):641.
3. Wang H, Sun W. CRISPR-mediated targeting of HER2 inhibits cell proliferation through a dominant negative mutation. Cancer Lett. 2017;385:137-43.
4. Moresco EMY, Li X, Beutler B. Going forward with genetics. Recent technological advances and forward genetics in mice. Am J Pathol. 2013;182:1462-73.
5. Method of the Year 2011. Nat Methods. 2012;9(1):1.
6. Stoddard BL. Homing endonuclease structure and function. Q Rev Biophys. 2005;38(1):49-95.
7. Kim H, Kim JS. A guide to genome engineering with programmable nucleases. Nat Rev Genet. 2014;15(5):321-34.
8. Silva G, Poirot L, Galetto R, et al. Meganucleases and other tools for targeted genome engineering: Perspectives and challenges for gene therapy. Curr Gene Ther. 2011;11(1):11-27.
9. Holt N, Wang J, Kim K, et al. Human hematopoietic stem/progenitor cells modified by zinc-finger nucleases targeted to CCR5 control HIV-1 in vivo. Nat Biotechnol. 2010;28(8):839-47.
10. Gaj T, Gersbach CA, Barbas CF. ZFN, TALEN, and CRISPR/Cas-based methods for genome engineering. Trends Biotechnol. 2013;31(7):397-405.

11. Reik A, Zhou Y, Hamlet A, et al. Zinc finger nucleases targeting the glucocorticoid receptor allow IL-13 zetakine transgenic CTLs to kill glioblastoma cells in vivo in the presence of immunosuppressing glucocorticoids. Mol Ther. 2008;16: S13-S14.
12. Ousterout DG, Gersbach CA. The development of TALE nucleases for biotechnology. Methods Mol Biol. 2016;1338: 27-42.
13. Ding Q, Lee YK, Schaefer EA, et al. A TALEN genome-editing system for generating human stem cell-based disease models. Cell Stem Cell. 2013;12(2):238-51.
14. Pollack A. A cell therapy untested in humans saves a baby with cancer. The New York Times. 2015.
15. Qasim W, Zhan H, Samarasinghe S, et al. Molecular remission of infant B-ALL after infusion of universal TALEN gene-edited CAR T cells. Sci Transl Med. 2017;9(374).
16. Delhove JMKM, Qasim W. Genome-edited T cell therapies. Curr Stem Cell Rep. 2017;3(2):124-36.
17. Biffi A. Clinical translation of TALENS: Treating SCID-X1 by gene editing in iPSCs. Cell Stem Cell. 2015;16(4):348-9.
18. Dupuy A, Valton J, Leduc S, et al. Targeted gene therapy of Xeroderma Pigmentosum cells using meganuclease and TALEN™. PLoS One. 2013;8(11):e78678.
19. Makarova KS, Koonin EV. Annotation and classification of CRISPR-Cas systems. Methods Mol Biol. 2015;1311:47-75.
20. Doudna JA, Charpentier E. Genome editing. The new frontier of genome engineering with CRISPR-Cas9. Science. 2014;346(6213):1258096.
21. Shim G, Kim D, Park GT, et al. Therapeutic gene editing: delivery and regulatory perspectives. Acta Pharmacol Sin. 2017;38(6):738-53.
22. Soriano V. Hot news: Gene therapy with CRISPR/Cas9 coming to age for HIV cure. AIDS Rev. 2017;19(3):167-72.
23. Baliou S, Maria Adamaki M, Kyriakopoulos AM, et al. CRISPR therapeutic tools for complex genetic disorders and cancer. Int J Oncol. 2018;53(2):443-68.
24. Kwon D. (2017).CRISPR to debut in clinical trials. The first industry-sponsored CRISPR therapy is slated to be tested in humans in 2018. The Scientists. [online] Available from https://www.the-scientist.com/the-nutshell/crispr-to-debut-in-clinical-trials-30508 [Accessed December 2018].
25. Kosicki M, Tomberg K, Bradley A. Repair of double-strand breaks induced by CRISPR–Cas9 leads to large deletions and complex rearrangements. Nat Biotechnol. 2018;36:765-71.
26. Gallagher RR, Li Z, Lewis AO, et al. Rapid editing and evolution of bacterial genomes using libraries of synthetic DNA. Nat Protocols. 2014;9(10):2301-16.
27. Bober JR, Beisel CL, Nair NU. Synthetic biology approaches to engineer probiotics and members of the human microbiota for biomedical applications. Ann Rev Biomed Eng. 2018;20:277-300.
28. Kafkafi N, Golani I, Jaljuli I, et al. Addressing reproducibility in single-laboratory phenotyping experiments. Nat Methods. 2017;14(5):462-4.
29. Sittig LJ, Carbonetto P, Engel KA, et al. Genetic background limits generalizability of genotype-phenotype relationships. Neuron. 2016;91(6):1253-9.
30. Birling M-C, Herault Y, Pavlovic G. Modeling human disease in rodents by CRISPR/Cas9 genome editing. Mamm Genome. 2017;28(7):291-301.
31. Wefers B, Bashir S, Rossius J, et al. Gene editing in mouse zygotes using the CRISPR/Cas9 system. Methods. 2017;121-122:55-67.
32. Nunes Dos Santos RM, Carneiro D'Albuquerque LA, Reyes LM, et al. CRISPR/Cas and recombinase-based human-to-pig orthotopic gene exchange for xenotransplantation. J Surg Res. 2018;229:28-40.
33. Niu D, Wei H-J, Lin L, et al. Inactivation of porcine endogenous retrovirus in pigs using CRISPR-Cas9. Science. 2017;357(6357):1303-7.
34. Pew Research Center. U.S. public opinion on the future use of gene editing, published: 26 December 2016, retrieved on 14the December 2018.
35. de Lecuona I, Casado M, Marfany G, et al. Gene editing in humans: Towards a global and inclusive debate for responsible research. Yale J Biol Med. 2017;90(4):673-81.
36. Ma H, Marti-Gutierrez N, Park SW, et al. Correction of a pathogenic gene mutation in human embryos. Nature. 2017;548(7668):413-9.
37. Nuffield Council on Bioethics. Genome editing: an ethical review. [online] Available from http://nuffieldbioethics.org/wp-content/uploads/Genome-editing-an-ethical-review.pdf [Accessed December 2018].
38. Jackson RJ, Ramsay AJ, Christensen CD, et al. Expression of mouse interleukin-4 by a recombinant ectromelia virus suppresses cytolytic lymphocyte responses and overcomes genetic resistance to mousepox. J Virol. 2001;75:1205-10.
39. Selgelid MJ, Lorna Weir. The mousepox experience. An interview with Ronald Jackson and Ian Ramshaw on dual-use research. EMBO Rep. 2010;11(1):18-24.
40. Warmflash D. (2016). Genome editing: Is it a national security threat? [online] Available from https://geneticliteracyproject.org/2016/09/06/genome-editing-national-security-threat/ [December 2018].
41. Sample I. Experts warn home 'gene editing' kits pose risk to society. The Guardian. 2016, retrieved on 10th December 2018.
42. Regalado A. MIT Technology Review. (2015). Engineering the perfect baby. [online] Available from https://www.technologyreview.com/s/535661/engineering-the-perfect-baby/ [Accessed December 2018].
43. Hughes J. (2004). Human enhancement on the agenda. Institute of Ethics and Emerging Technologies. Retrieved on 14th December 2018.
44. Enhancement Technologies Group (1998). Writings by group participants.
45. Warwick K. Ubiquity symposium: The technological singularity: human enhancement—the way ahead. Ubiquity. 2014;2014:1-8.
46. More M, Vita-More N (Eds). The Transhumanist Reader: Classical and Contemporary Essays on the Science, Technology, and Philosophy of the Human Future, 1st Edition. John Wiley & Sons, Inc; 2013.

47. Mooney P. (2002). Beyond Cloning: Making Well People "Better". [online] Available from http://www.worldwatch.org/system/files/EP154A.pdf [Accessed December 2018].
48. Institute on Biotechnology and the Human Future. (2007). Human enhancement. [online] Available from https://web.archive.org/web/20070209224106/http://www.thehumanfuture.org/themes/human_enhancement/background.html [Accessed December 2018].
49. Allhoff F, Lin P, Steinberg J. Ethics of human enhancement: An executive summary. Science and Engineering Ethics. Springer Netherlands. 2011;17(2):201-12.
50. Bostrom N. Ethical Issues in Advanced Artificial Intelligence. [online] Available from https://nickbostrom.com/ethics/ai.html [Accessed December 2018].
51. Farah MJ. Emerging ethical issues in neuroscience. Nat Neuroscience. 2002;5(11):1123-9.
52. Greely H, Sahakian B, Harris J, et al. Towards responsible use of cognitive-enhancing drugs by the health. Nature. 2008;456:702-5.
53. Thayer KA. Mapping human enhancement rhetoric. In: Thompson SJ (Ed). Global Issues and Ethical Considerations in Human Enhancement Technologies. 2014; IGI Global. pp. 30-53.
54. Lanni C, Lenzken SC, Pascale A, et al. Cognition enhancers between treating and doping the mind. Pharmacol Res. 2008;57:196-213.
55. E. Landau (2012). So you're a cyborg – now what?. CNN. Retrieved on 14th December 2018.
56. Moss M, Cook J, Wesnes K, et al. Aromas of rosemary and lavender essential oils differentially affect cognition and mood in healthy adults. Int J Neurosci. 2003;113(1):15-38.
57. Kevin Warwick. 2014. Human Enhancement-The way ahead: The technological singularity (Ubiquity symposium). Ubiquity 2014, Article 3, 8 pages. DOI=http://dx.doi.org/10.1145/2667642
58. Hughes J. Citizen Cyborg: Why Democratic Societies Must Respond to the Redesigned Human of the Future. US: Westview Press; 2004.
59. Aguiar S, Borowski T. Neuropharmacological review of the nootropic herb bacopa monnieri. Rejuvenation Res. 2013;16(4):313-26.
60. Hart R, Norman RJ. The longer-term health outcomes for children born as a result of IVF treatment: Part I–General health outcomes. Hum Reprod Update. 2013;19(3):232-43.
61. S. Knapton. (2016) The Telegraph UK, Test tube babies could die sooner, accessed on 8th October 2018.
62. Zeng Y, Li J, Li G, et al. Correction of the Marfan syndrome pathogenic FBN1 mutation by base editing in human cells and heterozygous embryos. Mol Ther. 2018;26:1-7.
63. Knorr Cetina K. The rise of a culture of life. EMBO Rep. 2005;6:76-80.
64. Degenaar P, The Guardian UK, See the world in a new light, 2011, accessed on 9th October 2018.
65. http://transhumanist-party.org/, accessed on 9th October, 2018.
66. Commissioned report by the European Parliament implementing Framework Contract IP/A/STOA/FWC/2005-28, Technology Assessment on Converging Technologies", October 2006, retrieved on 9th October 2018.
67. Vita-More N. Transhumanist arts statement, retrieved from https://www.digitalmanifesto.net/manifestos/35/ on 1st December 2018.
68. Bostrom N. Why I want to be a posthuman when I grow up. [online] Available from https://nickbostrom.com/posthuman.pdf [Accessed December 2018].
69. Hughes J. (2005). Report on the 2005 interests and beliefs survey of the members of the World Transhumanist Association. [online] Available from https://web.archive.org/web/20060524181809/http://transhumanism.org/resources/survey2005.pdf [Accessed December 2018].
70. Bostrom N, Dafoe A, Flynn C, Policy Desiderata for Superintelligent AI: A Vector Field Approach. (2018) version 4.3 (first version: 2016). [online] Available from https://nickbostrom.com/papers/aipolicy.pdf [Accessed December 2018].
71. Humanity+. "What is Transhumanism?". November 2013, retrieved from http://hplusmagazine.com/2013/11/22/what-is-transhumanism/ on 2nd October 2018.
72. Bostrom N. A history of transhumanist thought. J Evolution Technology. 2005;14(1).
73. Hughes J. 2002. Democratic Transhumanism 2.0. [online]. Available from [Accessed December 2018].
74. Naam R. More Than Human: Embracing the Promise of Biological Enhancement. New York: Broadway Books; 2005.
75. Sandberg A. Morphological freedom–Why we not just want it, but need it. In: More M, Vita-More N (Eds). The transhumanist reader: Classical and contemporary essays on the science, technology, and philosophy of the human future. US: Wiley; 2013. pp. 56-64.
76. Hughes J. Citizen Cyborg: Why Democratic Societies Must Respond To The Redesigned Human Of The Future. Cambridge MA, Westview Press; 2004.
77. More M. (1990). Transhumanism: a futurist philosophy. [online] Available from https://web.archive.org/web/20051029125153/http://www.maxmore.com/transhum.htm [Accessed December 2018].
78. Extropy institute, http://www.extropy.org/, acccessed on 2nd November 2018.
79. Stambler I. The Longevity Party - Who Needs it? Who Wants it? IEET. [online] Available from https://ieet.org/index.php/IEET2/more/stambler20120823 [Accessed December 2018].
80. Pontin J, 2017, Silicon Valley's Immortalists Will Help Us All Stay Healthy, accessed on 9th October 2018.
81. Lucke JC, Hall W. Who wants to live forever? EMBO Rep. 2005;6(2):98-102.
82. Hughes J. The politics of transhumanism, Version 2.0 (March 2002), Retrieved December 14, 2018.
83. Lucas MS. Baby steps to superintelligence: Neuroprosthetics and children. J Evol Technol. 2012;22(1):132-45.
84. Dvorsky G. (2008). Postgenderism: Beyond the Gender Binary (IEET White Paper 03). [online] Available from https://ieet.org/index.php/IEET2/more/dvorsky20080320/ [Accessed December 2018].

85. Kurzweil R. 2005. The singularity is near: when humans transcend biology. Penguin Books Ltd, London, England, ISBN 0-670-03384.
86. Bostrom N, Cirkovic MM. Millennial tendencies in responses to apocalyptic threats. Global Catastrophic Risks. Eds. Nick Bostrom, Milan M (Eds). Cirkovic, Oxford University Press; 2008. pp. 72-89.
87. Trothen TJ, Mercer C. Religion and human enhancement: Death, values, and morality, Springer; 2017.
88. Bostrom N. A history of transhumanist thought. J Evol Technol. 2005; 14 (1).
89. Fuller S. The Sociological Review. (2017). Transhumanism and the Dialectics of Progressivism. [online] Available from https://www.thesociologicalreview.com/blog/transhumanism-and-the-dialectics-of-progressivism-response-to-whitaker.html [Accessed December 2018].
90. Stock G. Redesigning Humans: Choosing our Genes, Changing our Future. US: Mariner Books; 2002.
91. World Medical Association Declaration Of Helsinki. Recommendations guiding physicians in biomedical research involving human subjects. 1994. JAMA. 1997; 277(11):925-6.
92. Newman SA. Averting the clone age: prospects and perils of human developmental manipulation. J Contemp Health Law & Policy. 2003;19:431.
93. Rees M. Our Final Hour: A Scientist's Warning: How Terror, Error, and Environmental Disaster Threaten Humankind's Future In This Century—On Earth and Beyond. New York: Basic Books; 2003.
94. Arnall AH. Future technologies, today's choices: nanotechnology, artificial intelligence and robotics. 2003.
95. Vaupel JW, Carey JR, Cristensen K, et al. Biodemographic trajectories of longevity. Science. 1998;280:855-60.
96. Carnes BA, Olshansky SJ, Grahn D. Biological evidence for limits to the duration of life. Biogerontology. 2003;4:31-45.
97. Westendorp RG. Are we becoming less disposable? EMBO Rep. 2004;5:2-6.
98. Miller RA. Extending life: scientific prospects and political obstacles. Milbank Quart. 2002;80:155-74.
99. Post SG (Ed). Encyclopedia of Bioethics. New York, NY, USA: Macmillan; 2004.
100. Hall SS. Merchants of Immortality: Chasing the Dream of Human Life Extension. New York, NY, USA: Houghton Mifflin; 2003.

Index

Page numbers followed by *f* refer to figure and *t* refer to table.

A

Abdominal wall 59*f*
    defects 52, 57, 58*f*
Abortion 41
    risk of premature 121
Academia 30
Achondrogenesis 52
Acquired immunodeficiency syndrome 79
Acrania 52
Acrosome reaction 75
Adenomyosis 100, 100*f*
Adherence junction 3
Agnathia 54
Allele dropout 116, 117
Alobar holoprosencephaly 54*f*
Alpha-fetoprotein 124
Alzheimer's disease 136
American College of Obstetricians and Gynecologists 86
American Society for Reproductive Medicine 86
Amniocentesis 89
Amniochorionic membrane 16
Amniotic band syndrome, severe 52
Amniotic fluid 89
Anencephaly 52
Anovulation 101
Anthropology, developmental 30
Artificial intelligence, development of 138
Assisted reproductive
    techniques 93, 97, 121
    technology 19, 75
Astroglia 2
Atria 107
    compare, large 107
Atrial septum primum 108
    complete 108
Atrial spine 107
Atrioventricular canal 107
Atrioventricular endocardial cushions 108
Atrioventricular foramen 105
Atrioventricular junction 109
Auricle, malformations of 55
Autism 35
Autosomal trisomy 24

B

Bichorionic biamniotic triplets 123*f*
Big bang theory 30
Bioethical aspects 35
Biomedical technologies, current advancements of 12
Bio-optimists 131
Biopsy techniques 116
Bladder
    enlargement of 60
    exstrophy 57
Blastocyst 44*f*, 75
    inner cell mass of 15
    removal 93*f*
    stage 77
        embryos 77
Blastomere 33
    biopsy 77
Body mass index 101
Body plan, formation of 16
Body stalk anomaly 52, 57, 59
Bowel 58
Brain
    changing appearance of 24*f*
    develops 65
    factories of 9
    structure 51
    vascularity, premature 22*f*
    ventricle, single 54*f*
    vesicles, primary 65
Butterfly sign 39*f*

C

Caenorhabditis elegans 16
Cajal-retzius cells 1, 6, 7
Cardiac activity, absent 124*f*
Cardiac defects, severe 52
Cardiac tube 106
Cardiac wall, three layered 108
Cardiogenic region 106
Carnegie stage 20*t*, 106-110, 113
Catholic Church's teachings 41
Cell
    number 77
    theory 32
    zygote, single 12
Central nervous system, fetal 65
Cerebellar plate 5*f*, 6*f*
Cerebellum 51
Cerebral
    cortex 3
    hemispheres 22
Cerebro-ocular-muscular syndrome 53
Chimera 40
Chorioepithelioma 41
Chorionic fluid, less 124*f*
Chorionic villus sampling 89, 90, 126
    indications of 90
    laboratory analysis of 92
    risks of 91
    training and audit of 92
Choroid plexus 9, 39*f*
Chromosomal defect 55
Chromosomal molecular analysis 92
Chromosomal risks 90
Chromosome 13, 125
    screening platforms, comprehensive 116
Cleavage-stage scoring systems 77
Cleft lip 54
Cleft palate 54
Cognitive psychology, developmental 30
Color Doppler 56, 97
Communication skills 134
Cordocentesis 89
Coronary arteries 115
Coronary circulation 115
Corpus luteum 44, 44*f*
Corpus mamillare 5*f*
Cortical plate 2
    formation of 8
Cortical reaction 75
Cranial bones, ossification of 52
Crown-rump length 53, 124
    measurements 1

Cyclopia 54
Cystic fibrosis 93, 136
Cystic hygroma 56
Cysts, true 52

D

Dandy-Walker malformation 54
Darwinism, reception of 29
Decidualization phase 97
Democratic transhumanism 138
Deoxyribonucleic acid 92
    analysis 90
Dialogue model 29
Diencephalon 9, 22, 51
Dimeric inhibin 124
Down syndrome 15, 124

E

Early pregnancy 52*f*
    loss 96
Ears, low set 52, 55
Ear-shoulder distance, reduced 55*f*
Ectopia cordis 57
Egg activation 75
Electron microscopy 5
Embryo 12, 22*f*, 23*f*, 35, 66*f*, 67*f*, 84, 84, 109*f*, 112*f*
    and yolk sac 21*f*
    behavior of 65
    cleavage-stage 77
    coexistence of 40
    crown-rump length of 108
    culture medium, composition of 76
    escapes 14
    ethical concept of 82, 85
    implantation 96
    legal status of 38
    length of 106, 110
    moral status of 82
    neurological development of 65
    normal sonographic development of 51
    single cell biopsy from 93*f*
    to initiate pregnancy, transferring 85
    to placenta-fetoplacental circulation 45
    transfer 98, 121
    visualization, normal 19
Embryology, modern 19
Embryonal pleural effusion 24
Embryonal stage
    abnormalities 22
    system 19
Embryonal vascularity 22*f*
Embryonic brain 22
Embryonic cardiac development 105
Embryonic development, staging of 1
Embryonic disk 40
Embryonic invasive diagnostic procedures 89
Embryonic lower limb 68*f*
Embryonic malformations 52
Embryonic movements 45
Embryonic period 9, 51, 53, 89
    to adolescence 2*f*
Embryonic stage 114*f*
Embryonic stem cells 14
Embryonic upper limb 68*f*
Encephalocele 52, 53, 54*f*
Endocardial cushion fusion 110
Endocardial tube, paired 106
Endometrial cavity, central portion of 101*f*
Endometrial polyp 99*f*
Endometrial receptivity array 102
Endometrial volume, quantification of 97
Endometritis, chronic 96
Endometrium 96
    chronic inflammation of 100
    functional layers of 96*f*
    myometrium border, loss of 100*f*
Enzymes 131
Epiblast 16
Epigenetics, influence of 34
Epiphysis 5*f*
Episcopic fluorescence imaging 105
Epithalamus 22
Ethics concept of person 84
Ethylenediaminetetraacetic acid 76
Euploid embryos 78
European Society of Human Reproduction and Embryology 86
Eventration 57, 58
Exencephaly 52
Extraembryonic membranes 15
Extropianism 138

F

Facial clefts 52
Facial malformations 54
Fertilization 12, 33, 40, 75
    events of 75
    steps 75
Fertilized oocyte to zygote 44*f*
Fetal abnormalities, early 51
Fetal activity 47*f*
Fetal anatomy 51
Fetal heads 55*f*
Fetal heart 57*f*, 58*f*
Fetal hydrops 56
Fetal malformations 52
Fetal period 52
Fetus 37*f*, 45*f*-47*f*
    first trimester 55*f*, 58*f*
    side view of 56*f*
    surface demonstration of 59*f*
    with gastroschisis 58*f*
    with hygroma colli 56*f*
    with omphalocele 58*f*
Fluorescence in situ hybridization 116, 117
Follicle maturation 101
Foramen ovale 113, 115
Forebrain 3, 23*f*, 65
Four chambered heart 114*f*
Franceschetti syndrome 55

G

Ganglionic eminence 7*f*, 9
Gastroschisis 57
Gene
    defects, sampling for single 92
    disorders, single 78
Genetic hybridization, array comparative 92, 116
Genetic uniqueness 41
Genetic-obstetric counseling 89
Genetics, influence of 34
Genome 34
Genomic editing 131
    designing baby with 135
Genomic hybridization 116
    array comparative 117
Genotype 34
Germline gene 80
Gestational age 19, 105
Gestational sac, development of 20, 21*f*
Gestational twin sac, empty 127*f*, 128*f*

H

HDlive mode 51
HDlive technology 20
HDlive ultrasound 20
Heart defects 56
Heartbeat interruption 123*f*
Hematopoiesis 16
Hematopoietic stem cells 132
Hindbrain 23*f*, 65
Hippocampus 9
Holoprosencephaly 52, 53
Homologous recombination 131
Hormonal changes and implantation 101
Human being 31
Human blastocysts 15

Human chorionic gonadotropin 34, 90, 97
  beta 55, 124
Human development
  begins 33
  visualization of early 43
Human embryo 1, 3f, 4f, 14, 136
  powers of 12
Human embryogenesis, facts of 32
Human embryology 19
Human embryonic cortex 8
Human enhancement 131, 134
  technologies 134
Human genome 34
  editing 79
  project 30, 34
Human life 31
  beginning of 28, 32f, 39
Human person at fertilization 39, 40
Human superficial fetal cortex 5f
Human telencephalon 9f
Hybrid cell, single 33
Hydatidiform mole 41
Hydrops 52, 56
Hygromas 56
Hyperechogenic bowel 59
  in fetus 59f
Hypoblast 16
Hypothalamus 22
Hysterosonography 98

I

Immortalism 138
Implantation 97, 100
  assessment of abnormal 96
  assessment of normal 96
In vitro embryo 85, 86
  research with 86
In vitro fertilization 75, 84, 89, 98, 135
  pregnancies 121
In vivo embryo 86
Inflammatory disease and implantation 98
Inner cell mass 75
Interventricular foramen 107-109
  closed 110
Interventricular septum, complete 110, 113
Intracavitary fibroid 98f
Intracavitary pathology 97
Intracranial translucency 56
Intracytoplasmatic injection 89
Intracytoplasmic sperm injection 121
Intradecidual gestational sac, small 44f
Intraembryonic circulation 45

Intrauterine
  development 1
  embryonal death 26f
  fetal death, early 24f, 26f
  interventions 131
  vascularity 21f
Invasive diagnostic sampling procedures 89
Invasive prenatal diagnosis 126
Ions, molecules of 13
Isthmus rombencephali 5f

J

Joubert syndrome 53

K

Kartagener syndrome 52
Karyotype analysis 90
Kidney 17
Kousseff syndrome 55
Kurjak Antenatal Neurodevelopmental Test 47f

L

Lamina affixa 9
Lamina terminalis 3f
Libertarian transhumanism 138
Life Protection Act 35
Life
  culture of 137
  phenomenon of 30
Limb
  anomalies 60
    surface demonstration of 60f
  defects 52
Liver 58
Living indefinitely long 139
Looping cardiac tube 106
Lower limb 71f, 73f
  movements 70f, 71f
Luschka and magendie, foramina of 54
Luteal phase, late 97
Luteinizing hormone 15
Lymphatic malformation 56

M

Magnetic resonance microscopy 19
Mandible anomalies 55
Maternal blood sampling 90
Maternal serum markers 124
Mean sac diameter 51

Meckel's diverticulum 52
Meckel-Gruber syndrome 53
Medulla oblongata 51
Megacystis 52
Meganucleases 132
Memory enhancement 134
Mendelian diseases 92
Menstrual phase 96
  endometrium 96f
Mesencephalon 3f, 51, 65
Mesenchyme 5f
Metabolism, errors of 90
Metencephalon 51
Microarray platforms 118
Microglia 2
Micrognathia 55
Midbrain 22f, 23f, 65
Mid-secretory phase 97
Mitochondria 80
Mitochondria manipulation 80
Mitochondrial genetic disorders 80
Mitochondrial genome 34
Molecular scissors 131
Monogenic disorders 78
Monogenic syndrome 54
Monozygotic twin phenomenon 40
Moral status, ethical concept of 84
Morphologic changes 106-110, 113
Morula 75
  aggregation 13
Multidimensional thinking 134
Multiple pregnancy 122
Muscular interventricular septum, complete 110
Mutism 35
Mycoplasma 100
Myelencephalon 5f, 51
Myometrial cysts 100f
Myometrium 100f

N

Nager syndrome 55
Nasal bone, absent 52
Natural philosophers 28
Neocortical cerebral wall, lamination in 4f
Neocortical development 2f
Neural crest cells 106
Neural tube defect, diagnosis of 56
Neuroepithelial stem cells 3, 4
Neuroepithelium 5f
Neurogenetic events, timing and sequence of 2f

Neuronal communication 6
Next generation sequencing 116-118
Noninvasive prenatal screening 90, 125
Nonoverlapping magisteria principle 29
Nuchal translucency 124
    enlarged 55, 55f
    measurement 55
Nuclear genome 34
Nucleotide polymorphism, single 116, 117, 125

O

Obstetric ethics, professional 82
Obstetric management, counseling about 87
Obstetrics and gynecology, professional ethics in 82
Oligodendroglia 2
Omphalocele 57, 58
Omphalomesenteric duct cysts 52
One cell embryo 33
Oocyte 33
Optic vesicle 3f
Organogenesis 16
Ostium primum 107
    closed 109, 110
Otocephaly 54
Ovum activation 33

P

Pallium 4
Parvovirus infection 56
Pelvic inflammatory disease 98
Perifollicular vascularization 43
Philosophy, developmental 30
Pierre-Robin syndrome, typical sign in 55
Placenta 44, 59f
Placental tissues 89
Plasma protein, pregnancy associated 55, 90, 124
Pleural effusion, bilateral 26f
Polycystic ovary syndrome 101
Polydactyly 52, 53
Polymerase chain reaction 77, 116, 117, 131
    amplification analysis 92
    quantitative 117
        fluorescent 92
    use of 116
Postconceptional weeks 1
Postconceptual week 3
    embryo, sixth 5f
Postgenderism 138
Postovulation weeks 1
Pre-embryo 75
    assessment 77
    cryopreservation 76
    culture conditions 75
    development in vitro 75
    genetic testing of 77
    medical aspect 75
    moral
        aspects 75
        status of 79
Preimplantation genetic
    diagnosis 77, 89, 92, 116, 117t
    screening 77, 93, 116
    testing 77, 78
Preimplantation testing 77
Preimplanted pre-embryo, legal status of 78
Prenatal diagnosis 131
Prenatal invasive techniques 89
Prezygote 40
Primitive atria 106
Primitive cardiac tube, single 106
Primitive endocardial cushion 107
Primitive ventricles 106
Primordial plexiform layer 1
Pronuclear scoring systems 77
Pronuclear transfer 80
Prosencephalon 22, 51, 65
Prune belly syndrome 60, 60f
Pseudocysts 52
Pseudodecidualization phase 97
Pseudostratified epithelium 3
Psychology, developmental 30

R

Radial artery blood flow 97f
Religious teachings, different 41
Renal abnormalities 53
Reproductive medicine 84
Retrognathia 52
Rhombencephalon 6f, 22, 51, 53, 65
Rigid biopsy forceps 91

S

Saline infusion sonography 98, 99f
    three-dimensional 98f
Secretory phase, early 96
Semilunar valves 110
Senses 134
Septum primum 107
Sickle cell anemia 136
Singularitarianism 138
Sinus venosus 109f
Smith-Lemli-Opitz syndrome 55
Sonoembryology 19
    three-dimensional 19
Sonographic study, two-dimensional 65
Sperm
    capacitation 75
    oocyte binding 75
    zona pellucida binding 75
Spermatozoa 31f, 32
Spina bifida 52, 56
    small 57f
Spinal amiotrophy 93
Spinal canal, lower 57f
Spinal cord 3f
Spindle transfer 80
Spontaneous abortion 98
Spontaneous vermicular movements 65
Stoicism 35
Stomach 58
Strand breaks, double 131
Subpallium 4
    thick basal portion of 7f
Subthalamus 22
Subventricular zone 1, 4
Sugars, molecules of 13
Sulcus monroi 9
Sulcus telodiencephalic 5f
Surviving twin 123
Syngamy 33

T

Tay-Sachs disease 93, 136
Technogaianism 138
Telencephalic vesicle 3f, 4f, 5, 5f, 6f, 9f
Telencephalon 3f, 7f
Temperature index 105
Termination of pregnancy 89, 93
    counseling about 87
Thalamus 22
Thalassemia 93
Third ultrasound in first trimester 52
Thoracopagus 60f
Three-parent babies 80
Tortuous configuration 3
Traditional karyotype 92
Transabdominal chorionic villus sampling 90f, 91f
    technique 90
Transcervical chorionic villus sampling technique 91
Transhumans, rights of 137t
Transvaginal imaging, two-dimensional 39f
Transvaginal sonography, two-dimensional 38f
Transvaginal ultrasound kidneys 59
Treacher-Collins syndrome 55
Trichorionic triamniotic triplets 122f
Tricuspid regurgitation 55

Trophectoderm tissue biopsy 116
Trophoblastic cells 93f
Truncal cushion 107
Truncus arteriosus 109
    separation of 109
    single undivided 107
Tubular heart 105f
Turner syndrome 56
Twin
    conjoined 52, 60, 60f
    pregnancy 121f, 126f
        monoamniotic 60
        monochorionic 60

U

Ultrasound
    in first trimester, three-dimensional 51
    of septate uterus, three-dimensional 98f
    scans, early 126f
    three-dimensional 19, 51, 96
    transvaginal three-dimensional 65
    two-dimensional 61, 96
Umbilical artery
    single 52, 59, 60, 61f
    two 45
Umbilical cord 22f, 39f, 61f
    cyst 52
        prevalence of 52
    middle of 53f

Umbilical cysts 52
Umbilical hernia 58
Umbilical vessels 59
Unconjugated estriol 124
Unfertilized oocyte 44f
Uniformly echogenic endometrium 97f
Upper limb 71f, 73f
    left 69f
    movements 70f, 71f
Upper lip, clefts of 54
Upper palate, clefts of 54
Ureaplasma urealyticum 100
Urinary tract anomalies 59
Uterine cavity 97
    defects 97
    upper half of 98f
Uterine circulation 97f
Uterine fundus, convex shape of 98f
Uterine receptivity, assessment of 101

V

Valve movements 110
Vanishing twin 25f
    syndrome 121, 124, 126, 127
        effects of 123
        influence of 124-126
Vasculogenesis 16
Vena cava valve 108
Ventricular cells 4
Vertebra, primary ossification of 56
Villous chromosomal examination 25f

Vitelline circulation 45
Vitrification method 76

W

Walker-Warburg syndrome 53
Warnock committee 78
Water, molecules of 13
Window of implantation 96
Wrist 71f

X

Xeroderma pigmentosum 132

Y

Yolk sac 20, 22, 24, 37f, 66f, 67f, 69f-73f
    abnormality 52
    echogenic shrunk 26f
    large 24f, 25f
    to embryo 45

Z

Zagreb neuroembryological collection 3f
Zinc
    finger nucleases 132
    sparks 75
Zona pellucida 33
    penetration of 75
Zona reaction 75
Zygote 33